Textbook of Hospital Pharmacy

Textbook of Hospital Pharmacy

EDITED BY

M. C. ALLWOOD PhD MPS

Principal Pharmacist, Research and Development
Addenbrooke's Hospital, Cambridge

J. T. FELL PhD MPS

Lecturer, Department of Pharmacy
University of Manchester

Blackwell Scientific Publications
OXFORD LONDON EDINBURGH MELBOURNE

© 1980 Blackwell Scientific Publications
Editorial offices:
Osney Mead, Oxford OX2 0EL
8 John Street, London WC1N 2ES
9 Forrest Road, Edinburgh EH1 2QH
214 Berkeley Street, Carlton, Victoria 3053, Australia

First published 1980

British Library Cataloguing in Publication Data

Textbook of hospital pharmacy.
  1. Hospital pharmacies—Great Britain
  I. Allwood, M C   II. Fell, J T
  362.1'1   RA975.5.P5

  ISBN 0-632-00631-5

Distributed in U.S.A. by
Blackwell Mosby Book Distributors
11830 Westline Industrial Drive
St Louis, Missouri 63141,
in Canada by
Blackwell Mosby Book Distributors
86 Northline Road, Toronto
Ontario, M4B 3E5,
and in Australia by
Blackwell Scientific Book Distributors
214 Berkeley Street, Carlton
Victoria 3053

Set in Monophoto Baskerville
Printed and bound in Great Britain by
Butler & Tanner Ltd, Frome and London

Contents

SECTION III. Patient services

SECTION IV. Provision of information

Contributors

J. W. Barnett
Area Pharmaceutical Officer, Hereford and Worcester Area Health Authority, Worcester.

C. W. Barrett
Area Pharmaceutical Officer, City and East London Area Health Authority, London.

Irene Coupar
Principal Pharmacist (Quality Control), Royal Infirmary, Glasgow.

N. Driver
Principal Pharmacist (Quality Control), Withington Hospital, Manchester.

J. Fereday
Area Pharmaceutical Officer, Brent and Harrow Area Health Authority, London.

Celia Feetam
Staff Pharmacist, Rubery Hill Hospital, Birmingham.

A. L. Glenn
Senior Lecturer, Department of Pharmacy, University of Manchester.

Joan C. Greenleaf
Regional Pharmaceutical Officer, North East Thames Regional Health Authority, London.

R. Hambleton
Lecturer, Department of Pharmacy, University of Manchester.

C. Hetherington
Area Pharmaceutical Officer, Leeds Area Health Authority.

J. B. Kay
Formerly Principal Professional and Technology Officer, Department of Health and Social Security, 14 Russell Square, London; presently Technical Director, Contactasol Ltd, Ruxley Towers, Claygate, Esher, Surrey.

W. A. Little
Principal Pharmacist, The Liverpool Clinic, Liverpool.

J. A. Myers
Chief Administrative Pharmaceutical Officer, Lothian Health Board, Edinburgh.

P. J. Noyce
District Pharmaceutical Officer, Harrow Health District, Northwick Park Hospital, Middlesex.

M. L. Rogers
Principal Pharmacist, Drug Information Services, The London Hospital, London.

A. J. Ross
Area Pharmaceutical Officer, Bolton, Bury and Rochdale Area Health Authority, Bolton.

I. H. Stockley
Lecturer, Department of Pharmacy, University of Nottingham.

E. Van der Kleijn
Apotheek en Klinische Farmacie, Sint Radboudziekenhuis, Nijmegen, Netherlands.

Preface

Role of the Hospital Pharmacist (*Report of the Working Party on the Hospital Pharmaceutical Service*, Chairman Sir Noel Hall; DHSS 1970):

'The pharmacist can no longer be regarded only as a dispenser of medicines. He has an important consultative and management role. He should be responsible for the planning of pharmaceutical services and the establishment and maintenance of safe systems of work within his department, and the collection of data on drug use. He has also to co-operate with medical and nursing staff in securing the most effective, safe and economical use of drugs.'

The Noel Hall Report recommended that hospital pharmacists should play a more positive role in the hospital team. We have set forth with this possibility in mind, and with considerable trepidation, to produce a book which attempts to describe pharmacy within the context of the modern British hospital environment. It is essentially concerned with the amalgamation of management and science which is a distinctive requirement of hospital pharmacy. Within any system of hospital pharmacy certain guidelines can be set down. Although the book uses the British hospital system to draw on for examples, much of the work described is universally applicable. The book should be of particular interest to postgraduate students and recently qualified pharmacists, but we hope that it contains information and discussions useful to the experienced hospital pharmacist in Britain and elsewhere.

The topic is divided into sections although we do not pretend that the subdivisions are exclusive. We commence with the various facets of organisation and management in hospital pharmacy within the National Health Service. This is followed by more detailed discussions of the production of medicines. The third part of the book is devoted to the clinical aspects of modern pharmacy, and finally, chapters describing the provision of drug information services.

A relatively large number of authors were invited to contribute in order to obtain as broad a spectrum of expertise and opinion as possible. All of the authors, when approached, agreed that there was a clear need for the book and have consequently tackled the project with enthusiasm and commitment. We are indebted to all of them for their efforts to complete the assignment.

Because hospital pharmacy is in a state of transition, the eventual outcome of which is uncertain, some novel concepts of the role and activities of the pharmacist in the NHS are discussed. We feel that it would be short-sighted to shun some of the ideals expressed, although they may appear impractical. In a multiauthor book such as this, some duplication is inevitable and there are instances in which the grouping of material for editorial convenience may seem unrealistic. Nevertheless we hope that, as editors, we have linked the contributions into a reasonably coherent text to produce a valuable description of British hospital pharmacy in the late 1970s. In bringing the book to fruition we trust that it will prove to be a worthwhile contribution to professional pharmacy.

M. C. Allwood
J. T. Fell

Acknowledgements

The following figures are taken from the literature and are reproduced by permission of the copyright owners:
Fig. 12.1 from Van der Kleijn *et al* (1977) In *Plasma digitalis concentration and digitalis therapy*, ed. T. Godfriend; Editions Arsia, Brussels. Fig. 12.3a from Van der Kleijn *et al* (1977) *Acta Pharmacologica et Toxicologica* **41,** suppl. 1, 168. Fig. 12.3b from Van der Kleijn *et al* (1975) *Pharmaceutische Weekblad* **110,** 1222. Fig. 12.5a as Fig. 12.3b. Fig. 12.5b as Fig. 12.1. Fig. 12.5c from Schobben *et al* (1975) *European Journal of Clinical Pharmacology* **8,** 97. Fig. 12.9 from Reuning *et al* (1973) *Journal of Clinical Pharmacology* **13,** 127. Figs. 12.10 & 12.12 from Jonkman (1977) PhD Thesis, University of Groningen. Fig. 12.13 from Van der Pohl *et al* (1975) *Journal of Pharmacokinetics and Biopharmaceutics* **3,** 99. Fig. 12.14 from Vree *et al* (1975) *Pharmaceutische Weekblad* **110,** 1257. Fig. 12.15 from Guelen & Van der Kleijn (1978) *Rational antiepileptic drug therapy*; Elsevier, Amsterdam. Fig. 12.16 from Van Ginnekan *et al* (1974) *Journal of Pharmacokinetics and Biopharmaceutics* **2,** 395. Fig. 12.17 from de Zeeuw *et al* (1978) *8th Meeting of the European Poison Control Centres, Utrecht.* Fig. 12.19 from Blom & Guelen (1976) *Proceedings of the 3rd International Workshop on the Determination of Antiepileptic Drugs*, ed. C. Gardner-Thorpe; Pitman, Oxford. Fig. 12.21 from Knop & Edmunds (1976) *Abstracts, Symposia and Communications of the 17th Dutch Federation Meeting, Amsterdam.* Fig. 12.22 from Hulshof *et al* (1977) *Pharmaceutische Weekblad* **112,** 326. Fig. 12.23 from Pitlick & Levy 1976) *Journal of Pharmaceutical Sciences* **65,** 462. Fig. 12.24 from Van der Kleijn (1974) *Clinical Pharmacokinetics, A Symposium*, ed. G. Levy; American Pharmaceutical Association.

I
Provision of services

1

The Region

J. C. GREENLEAF

Hospital pharmacy today includes provision of a pharmaceutical service to clinics and other community services. The reorganisation of the National Health Service in 1974 aimed at integration of the hospital service with general practice and the community health services provided by local authorities. Integration is far from complete and provision of medical and pharmaceutical services to the community by general practitioners is administered separately on a contractual basis. Hospitals form a major part of the managed service, but the trend in health care is away from hospital treatment and towards domiciliary care and prevention. The effects of this are complex but may be summed up as fewer hospitals but more intensive diagnosis and treatment within them. Increasingly the hospital pharmacist must look outside the confines of his pharmacy and of the hospital, and take domiciliary care into account.

At the present time, the management arrangements of the health service are under review and the Royal Commission on the National Health service has examined the working of the entire Service (DHSS 1979). Management structures may come and go but the management needs of the pharmaceutical service will not change substantially. Pharmacy management needs to be able to produce an efficient, cost effective service, adapting readily to change, and able to keep pace with rapid developments in therapy. It would be unwise, however, to consider hospital pharmacy management without trying to understand the management of the Health Service as a whole. Pharmacy plans must be related to need, and if they are to succeed, they must be presented in the right way, at the right place and at the right time.

THE HOSPITAL PHARMACEUTICAL SERVICE

The objective of the hospital pharmaceutical service is to provide safe effective medication for all patients attending hospitals and clinics. Pharmacy managers must work together to achieve this objective within available resources. They must strive to make the pharmaceutical service safe, efficient, economic, equitable and progressive. This is no mean task as pharmacy has to compete for resources with many other needs in the Health Service. Pharmacy managers must be realistic in their demands but will need to be prepared to fight to

3

make sure that pharmacy gets a fair 'slice of the cake' when resources are allocated. The duties of the pharmaceutical service include purchase, storage, processing, control and supply of medicines and associated products for use in wards and departments; dispensing prescriptions for inpatients and outpatients; and providing an advisory service on medicines. The pharmacy service has a responsibility for advising on suitable, safe and secure storage of medicines wherever they are kept in hospitals and clinics, that is in wards and departments as well as in the pharmacies. Medicine as a science is changing very rapidly; it is essential that the pharmacy service should keep pace. Pharmacy managers need to continually review their methods and streamline operations if they are to be able to meet that challenge.

NHS ADMINISTRATION AND ORGANISATION

The National Health Service Reorganisation Act was passed in 1973 with the object of unifying the Health Service. Management arrangements for the reorganised service which had been foreshadowed in the 'grey book' (DHSS 1972a) were published by the Department in a series of Health Reorganisation Circulars; pharmacy was dealt with in HRC (73) 28. There are three levels of management: District, Area and Region, while general practitioners remain independent contractors.

The District

The District is the basic unit of provision of the service but is not in itself a statutory authority. The District is a unit within which it can reasonably be expected that all the main types of health care should be provided for the population. It usually represents a population of about 250 000–300 000 persons, and the catchment area of a District General Hospital. There is no District Authority, all District staff being employed by the Area Authority and the District Management Team is responsible directly to that Authority.

The Area

The Area Health Authority (AHA) is a statutory authority, made up of members appointed by various bodies including the Regional Health Authority and the local authority. Day-to-day management is carried out by an Area Team of Officers (ATO). The Area's function is to plan and manage the service. The Area is the level at which the Health Service is matched to local authorities. This was thought important for integration as many local authority functions, such as housing, social services and homes for the elderly, have a direct effect on health care. In single district areas the functions of the District and Area are merged. There is a single team of officers which is known as the Area Management Team.

The Region

The Region is the strategic planning level of authority. The Regional Health Authority (RHA) is composed of members appointed by the Secretary of State, universities, and other bodies. Day-to-day management is carried out by a Regional Team of Officers. The Regional Authority's prime function is strategic planning, but it is concerned also with allocation of resources. The Department of Health and Social Security (DHSS) allocates resources for the Health Service to Regions, issues broad guidelines for health care (DHSS 1977) and indicates a few items which should be given priority, for example care of the elderly and the mentally handicapped. The Regional Health Authority has to work out guidelines for use within the Region, decide on priorities and allocate funds between Areas. In doing this, the Regional Officers have to consider many factors such as changes in the age of the population, population movements, for example from city centre to new towns, and changes in emphasis in health care, for example from hospital care to care in the home. The Regional Authority must estimate need and calculate the number of hospitals, health centres and clinics which will be needed over the next decade and where they should be sited. Pharmacists at Regional level are expected to estimate the associated need for pharmacy services and see that plans are shaped accordingly.

The planning system

The Region does not make these decisions in isolation from the people operating the service. The Health Service Planning System (HSC (IS) 126) is a two-tier system operating simultaneously at strategic and operational levels. Strategic plans, covering the NHS for 10–12 years ahead are produced by Regions and Areas. These are reviewed and updated annually, in the light of operational plans or any changes in strategic guidelines and are revised overall every fourth year. Annual operational plans examine in detail action proposed for the next 3 years ahead. These annual plans are produced at District, Area and Regional levels against the background of the strategic plan. Plans will be firm for year 1, provisional for year 2 and in outline for year 3. Strategic and annual plans are subject to wide consultation at Region, Area and District, as are the broad ideas underlying the plans. Once the system reaches a steady state, nothing in the annual plans for year 1 should come as a surprise to those involved in planning. They will have had an opportunity to influence the

evolution of strategy and yet further opportunities for influence as an outline plan for year 3 proceeds successively through year 2 to a firm plan for
year 1.

The Health Service Planning System therefore is based on plans formulated at grassroots level. Plans put forward by hospital departmental heads are
considered by the District Management Team along with local proposals for
new hospitals, etc. Plans which are accepted are passed in priority order to
the Area. The Area Team of Officers considers competing priorities put forward by the Districts within the Area and makes recommendations to the Area
Authority. The Area's plans in order of priority are passed to Region where
a similar process is carried out. The Region considers plans from all the Areas,
measures them against Regional and National guidelines, estimated need and
competing priorities. It then decides on the major capital building programme
and the allocation of resources to Areas for running the service. In considering
Area plans, the RHA has to take account of some special problems. Although
the general philosophy is that every health district should have a full range
of medical care, there are some specialities which it is not justified to duplicate
in this way. The RHA has responsibility for ensuring that such specialist services are provided adequately in the Region, but not overprovided. Teaching
hospitals present another problem. It is essential that a proper range of facilities
is provided for teaching undergraduate and postgraduate medical and dental
students. 'Centres of excellence' and associated research facilities are essential
if medical science is to progress. Unfortunately, there is a danger that these
may demand an unfair proportion of scarce resources and result in continuing
neglect of other essential but more mundane areas of health care such as care
of the elderly and the mentally handicapped. It is an important function of
the Regional Authority, in consultation with the universities, to see that a
proper balance is kept within the Region. Similarly, with the pharmaceutical
services, it is necessary to keep a balance between the specialised needs of teaching hospitals and those of other types of hospital in which, in pharmacy, as
in many other disciplines, there has been a tradition of neglect.

Allocation of resources

Each year funds are allocated by the DHSS to Regions. Although a rough
estimate of the sum is known in advance, the actual amount is subject to budget
changes according to the state of the National economy, and political factors
influencing public spending. This makes planning difficult and sudden
changes of direction inevitable from time to time. The amount allocated to
each Region is based on what was spent in previous years, and on agreed developments. A redistribution factor recommended by the Resource Allocation
Working Party (RAWP) (DHSS 1976) is applied to correct inequalities in
health care and to try to equalise over a decade the amount spent on health

per head of population in various parts of the country. A similar redistribution is taking place within Regions.

Capital and revenue

Funds are allocated as capital and revenue. The precise definition of these is complex and redefined by the DHSS from time to time. In general, capital may be thought of as large sums of money used once and for all for building or for purchasing equipment. Revenue is the running costs of the Health Service and includes replacement of minor equipment, maintenance and upgrading of buildings, and staff costs. For instance in 1977, single items of building costing over £10 000 or equipment costing over £5000 were defined as capital, while items under these sums and staffing costs were defined as revenue. Revenue is further subdivided into non-recurring (once-only items such as upgrading or purchase of equipment) and recurring (salaries, rentals, service contracts etc.). Capital and revenue allocations to Areas are made annually after negotiation between Area and Regional Officers. Major building works are agreed and capital allocated accordingly. An additional 'discretionary' capital allocation is made to each Area to cover small schemes, and revenue allocations also are made. Some small interchange between capital and revenue is allowable, the exact proportion being recommended by the DHSS each year. Some Regional Authorities hold reserves, but others allocate all available money to areas at the beginning of the year. During the year, accounts are published regularly to show how actual spending is matching up with estimates and allocations. Under- and overspending is monitored by the RHA and at all other levels. The service is now working within strict cash limits so overspending has to be corrected by economies in the Area or District concerned, or by transferring funds from one Area or District to another. A small overspending may be carried forward to the next year, but may result in further difficulties, so is strongly discouraged. It is accepted that in periods of national economic difficulty, developments should be self-financing (i.e. additional money should be spent only if it can be demonstrated that it would save money in future).

There is more likelihood of underspending of capital than revenue allocations. The capital programme is given a time scale for expenditure, but there are frequently difficulties during building such as unforeseen structural problems or industrial action which cause work and hence payments to fall behind schedule ('slippage'). About halfway through the year, the Region and Areas take a realistic look at progress of all schemes and revised estimates are published. At this stage, additional short-term schemes may be added to the building programme and extra money released to Areas for immediate use for small upgradings and purchase of equipment.

Guidelined allocations

Regions vary in the amount of control they exert over spending by Areas. In some cases, capital and revenue allocations may be 'guidelined' to Areas for specific purposes, for example pharmacy, while other Regional Authorities believe that Areas should be given full discretion to decide their own priorities within very broad Regional guidelines. The amount of influence Regional Pharmaceutical Officers can exert on pharmacy funding in Areas will vary accordingly.

Capital building programme

Building is a major concern of Regional Authorities. Architects, engineers, quantity surveyors and support staff are employed. Schemes submitted by Areas are checked for feasibility within estimated costs. Many schemes are delegated to Areas for implementation, while some larger schemes may be carried through to a detailed design stage by Regional staff. Construction work may be carried out by Health Authority employed staff or put out to contract. The contractor may be responsible just for construction, or the contract may include some detailed design work. It is important that pharmacy managers should understand the building and contracting operation, as misunderstandings and friction often result. For example, after a certain stage, alterations may not be possible without invalidating the contract. It is essential that specifications are detailed, unambiguous and correct before the contract is made. Many design teams have little experience of pharmacy building, so the pharmacy manager must take the initiative and make sure that the specifications include all the points which are important. A description of the planning and building process is given in the DHSS Health Building Procedure Notes 1–6. Under the general title 'Capricode' (Capital Projects Code) these include information on procedures for planning and processing individual building projects, planning policies, functional content, development control plans, schedules of accommodation and cost control.

MEDICINES ACT

The Regional Health Authority has a special responsibility in relation to the Medicines Act. The Secretary of State, when deciding not to rest on Crown privilege but to apply the Medicines Act to Health Authorities, made the Regional Health Authority the 'licensing authority'. The RHA is responsible for ensuring that Medicines Act standards are applied throughout the Region. Reports of inspections are sent to the RHA through the Regional Administrator and the RHA is required to ensure that satisfactory quality control arrangements are in operation, and to designate a person responsible for quality control in the Region. The RHA also has a responsibility for ensuring that the pharmacy building projects included in the capital building programme conform to Medicines Inspectorate standards.

PHARMACY WITHIN THE NHS

The pharmaceutical arrangements in the reorganised Health Service were set out in HRC (73) 28. These arrangements were a compromise, fitting the pharmacy Area service recommended by the Noel Hall working party (DHSS 1970) into the structure of the reorganised NHS. The basic concepts for the service are that hospital pharmacy should be organised on a scale large enough to make proper use of staff and equipment, and to provide a career structure for hospital pharmacists and technicians.

There has been some disagreement about the place of the District in pharmacy organisation, or perhaps more correctly, the place of pharmacy in the District. It seems clear that in most cases, the District cannot support a hospital pharmacy service which meets the criteria of the Noel Hall report and that, consequently, pharmacy should be an Area-managed service. It must be remembered, however, that the District is the basic unit of health care, in which the District General Hospital plays an important part. Each District in an Area needs an adequate pharmaceutical service, and District Management Teams and other District staff need to be quite clear to whom they should turn for pharmaceutical advice. In considering the way pharmacy fits into the overall structure of the NHS, it must be remembered that Regions and Areas differ not only in geographical and demographic features, but also in philosophy and management styles. Some Regions devolve a great deal of responsibility to Areas, while others believe in holding the reins rather more tightly; similarly with Areas and Districts.

Regional pharmaceutical organisation

The amount of direct pharmaceutical management at Regional level will depend, to a large extent, on the policy of devolution in the Region. The pharmaceutical organisation at Region is headed by the Regional Pharmaceutical Officer (RPhO). The RPhO is directly responsible to the Regional Health Authority and has direct access to its Chairman, although for most day-to-day purposes, he will work through the Regional Team of Officers. An outline job description is included in HRC(73)28. The RPhO is responsible for advising the RHA on all matters concerning pharmacy, represents the RHA in discussion of pharmacy matters with the DHSS, manages any pharmacy services which are not delegated to Areas, and monitors and coordinates all pharmacy services in the Region. The Regional Pharmaceutical Officer's relationship with the Area Pharmaceutical Officers is a monitoring and coordinating one, and is similar to that of the relationship of the Region itself with Areas. The RPhO is responsible for producing strategic plans for pharmacy services and for advising on priorities. He is responsible for coordinating Area plans for pharmacy to produce a coherent Regional service which makes optimal use of resources. He is responsible for ensuring that legal requirements and agreed minimum safety standards are maintained in all parts of the Region, and he has special responsibilities of this type in relation to the Medicines Act. He is responsible for coordinating postgraduate education and training of pharmacy staff in the Region and for seeing that acceptable standards are maintained.

It should be remembered that, except in the case of those services which are directly regionally managed, Regional Officers produce service to patients only by working through the Areas. The RPhO's relationship with APhOs is crucial to the success of the pharmaceutical service in the Region. He will need to work very closely with the APhOs, holding meetings, visiting Areas and trying to get to know as thoroughly as possible the particular circumstances in each Area.

Regional Pharmaceutical Committee

The Regional Health Authority and the Regional Pharmaceutical Officer are advised on professional matters by the Regional Pharmaceutical Committee. This is a statutory committee set up as part of the Health Service advisory machinery (HRC (74) 9). It is made up of hospital and general practice pharmacist representatives from each Area together with a representative from a school of pharmacy. The Regional Hospital Pharmaceutical Committee is made up of the hospital pharmacist members of the main Regional Pharmaceutical Committee. The RPhO will receive the papers and attend all meetings of the Regional Pharmaceutical Committee and Regional Hospital Pharmaceutical Committee. He will convey the Committees' recommendations to the RHA, the Regional Team of Officers and to the Area Pharmaceutical Officers although the Committees have right of direct access to the Regional Health Authority and its Chairman. The Regional Pharmaceutical Officer should work closely with the Chairman of the Pharmaceutical Committee and try to ensure that all policy documents of the Regional Authority which may affect pharmacy are referred to the Committees for comment. The Regional Health Authority is required to supply administrative support for advisory committees. It may be a member of the RPhO's administrative staff who will service the Pharmaceutical Committees, but the work of the Committees should be kept independent of the RPhO and it should be clear to the Committee members that the RPhO does not influence unduly the actions of the Committee or the minutes.

Objectives and priorities

One of the major management tasks of the RPhO is to set realistic objectives and priorities for the pharmaceutical service. These must take heed of the National and Regional priorities and will need to be continually reviewed. In pharmacy, as in other disciplines, the acute services are the most immediately professionally rewarding. The RPhO has a responsibility to see that other services such as those to geriatric and handicapped patients get sufficient attention. The RPhO must sort out competing priorities and try to avoid unnecessary duplication. He will advise the Regional Team of Officers on plans for pharmacy services submitted by the Areas. If he has had sufficient discussion with the Area Pharmaceutical Officers during preparation of the plans, there should be little conflict at this stage. If an Area has given insufficient priority for a scheme to get into the programme, and the RPhO is convinced it is essential to the maintenance of a satisfactory level of service, he can ask the Regional Team of Officers to refer it back for reconsideration. He should realise of course that unless he does this in a responsible way, it will be counterproductive. If the RPhO declares every pharmacy improvement top priority, the Team will soon learn to take little notice of him. This is equally true at other levels of the service.

Pharmacy planning

Pharmacy plans come up from Districts and Areas to the Region. The RPhO needs to know about the plans before they reach the RHA because the timing for the various stages of the planning cycle are short. The planning system is a cyclical operation with an annual review when new plans are added. Pharmacy planning must be treated in the same way. Plans should be prepared as the need arises, given a priority rating and put forward with supporting evidence at the appropriate time in the year. Plans and priorities should be reviewed annually to see if they are still appropriate.

Planning advice available

There are various guidelines for building and equipping new hospitals and departments. The RPhO and APhOs need to be fully conversant with all those which may affect pharmacy. Those include *Hospital Building Note No. 29* (DHSS 1973), *Health Equipment Note No. 29* (DHSS 1975), Capricode, Hospital Technical Memoranda, guidance on the Medicines Act (HSC (IS) 128), radiation safety (DHSS 1972b), health and safety at work (DHSS 1974), and fire precautions (HTM 16). There is a good deal of planning help available at Regional and Area level, although there is sometimes a lack of experience of planning pharmacies. Area Pharmaceutical Officers will be wise to involve the Works Officers closely in planning. At Regional level, in particular, there is a wide range of technical expertise available. Regional Authorities, having a heavy involvement in building programmes, have a large specialist staff. It is important to make sure that the expertise is used to the advantage of the pharmacy service rather than against it. For example, a plan which has been poorly prepared from an engineering point of view at hospital level, may be excluded from the programme for this reason when it reaches Area or Region. The observant APhO and RPhO working together can often forestall that sort of problem by enlisting the help of the Area and/or Regional engineer or other technical officers at an early stage. The Scientific and Technical Branch of the DHSS may be able to offer guidance on a wide range of engineering and equipment problems. The Pharmaceutical Division of the DHSS may also give help on a number of problems as the pharmacists in that division have broad knowledge of current activities in Health Service pharmacy. There are other sources of expertise available in the Regions which can be of help in pharmacy planning. All Regions have statistics divisions which can supply and evaluate data which will affect the pharmacy service (i.e. likely future changes in bed numbers, type, occupancy etc.). Some Regions also have Management Services divisions with Work Study and Operational Research sections which can advise on layout, scheduling, forecasting, etc.

Regionally managed services

Certain pharmacy services such as production, quality control, drug information and education and training in some Regions may be managed at Regional level. In other Regions, such services may be managed by an Area on behalf of the Region, on an agency basis. In either case, the RPhO will be responsible for ensuring that the service is run efficiently. Reports of output, workload and costs should be produced and monitored regularly, and regular meetings held with the specialist managers and users of the service. There are a number of different ways of managing and funding Regional services. The service may be run on a charge-to-user basis or as a 'free' service. This decision must be taken in consultation with other Regional Officers and will be in accordance with general Regional policy. A 'free' service saves accounting work at all levels, but care must be taken to guard against unnecessary demands being made on the service by users. Proper financial provision for replacement of equipment and staffing will need to be made. That will depend on accurate records of demand being kept and forecasting of future trends being carried out. A charge-to-user service is in many ways easier to run. A method of costing should be developed in consultation with the treasurers. Charges to consumers should be sufficient to allow reserves to be built up to cover equipment replacement and periodic modernisation of facilities.

Drug contracts

Although in general drugs are purchased at Area or hospital level, there may be price advantages to be gained by Regional contracting for some items.

There are certain basic standard procedures for competitive purchase in the Public Service which must be observed, but the details of the contracting operation will vary from Region to Region. The Regional Pharmaceutical Officer will work closely with the Regional Supplies Officer in the preparation of contracts. The main stages of the procedure will be decision on the range of items to be included in the contract, estimation of demand, invitation to tender, collation of offers to supply, adjudication, and notification to suppliers and consumers of results. In some Regions, the administration of contracting arrangements is carried out by the Supplies Officer, in others by the RPhO's staff. The important thing is that the RPhO must be responsible in ensuring that there is adequate pharmaceutical involvement at the adjudication stage, both from the point of view of control of quality of the item and acceptability to the purchasing pharmacists in the Areas. Arrangements must be set up for obtaining and testing samples from would-be suppliers before contracts are awarded, and for testing materials received from the successful contractors during the course of the contract year. National collaboration between Regional Quality Controllers can avoid an unnecessary duplication of effort in this respect. In the case of contracts for dressings, pharmaceutical containers and sundries, there also should be pharmaceutical involvement in the quality of items purchased, whether or not the items are purchased and supplied by the pharmaceutical service.

Education and training

The Regional Pharmaceutical Officer has responsibility for coordinating all postgraduate education and training for pharmacy staff in the Region, usually having specialist pharmacists to help with this task, and also working closely with schools of pharmacy and the Regional Education and Training Officer. It is envisaged that Regional Education Committees will be established in all Regions to plan and control postqualification education of all pharmacists working in the Health Service (education and training is discussed in detail in Chapter 4).

Research

Funding for research in the Health Service is available from a number of sources. The DHSS will fund some major projects and this type of funding may be available for scientific and operational studies. Funds are allocated also to Regions under the arrangements for locally organised research (HSC (IS) 148). Pharmacy research projects will be considered for funds in competition with other disciplines by the Regional Research Committee. Funding for operational research projects sometimes may be obtained indirectly by running these projects jointly with one of the Region's specialised divisions (e.g. computer services or operational research science), or with a school of pharmacy.

AREA PHARMACY ORGANISATION

Although at present under review, pharmacy is likely to continue as an Area managed service, and Area Pharmaceutical Officers are likely to continue having responsibility for managing the hospital pharmaceutical service and coordinating that service with the services provided by general practice pharmacists who are independent contractors whose conditions of service, along with those of general medical, dental and optical practitioners, are regulated by Family Practitioner Committees. The Area Pharmaceutical Officer is responsible to the Area Health Authority and has direct access to that Authority and its Chairman, although for many day-to-day purposes he will work through the Area Team of Officers. The APhO is advised professionally by the Area Pharmaceutical Committee (APC) which is made up of equal numbers of general practice and hospital pharmacists from the Area. The APC is a statutory committee as is the Area Chemists Contractors Committee (Local Pharmaceutical Committee).

REFERENCES

DEPARTMENT OF HEALTH AND SOCIAL SECURITY (1970) *Report of the Working Party on the Hospital Pharmaceutical Service*. The Noel Hall Report. HMSO, London.

DEPARTMENT OF HEALTH AND SOCIAL SECURITY (1972a) *Management Arrangements for the Reorganised National Health Service*. HMSO, London.

DEPARTMENT OF HEALTH AND SOCIAL SECURITY (1972b) *Code of Practice for the Protection of Persons against Ionizing Radiations Arising from Medical and Dental Use*. HMSO, London.

DEPARTMENT OF HEALTH AND SOCIAL SECURITY (1973) *Hospital Building Note 29 (Pharmaceutical Dept)*. HMSO, London.

DEPARTMENT OF HEALTH AND SOCIAL SECURITY (1974) *Health and Safety at Work Act: advice to employees*. HMSO, London.

DEPARTMENT OF HEALTH AND SOCIAL SECURITY (1975) *Health Equipment Note 29 (Pharmaceutical Dept)*. HMSO, London.

DEPARTMENT OF HEALTH AND SOCIAL SECURITY (1976) *Sharing Resources for Health in England. The report of the resource allocation working party*. HMSO, London.

DEPARTMENT OF HEALTH AND SOCIAL SECURITY (1977a) *The Way Forward. Priorities in the Health and Social Services*. HMSO, London.

DEPARTMENT OF HEALTH AND SOCIAL SECURITY (1977b) *Guide to Good Pharmaceutical Manufacturing Practice*. HMSO, London.

DEPARTMENT OF HEALTH AND SOCIAL SECURITY (1979) *Report of the Royal Commission on the National Health Service*. HMSO, London.

Official circulars and memoranda issued by DHSS

Health Building Procedure Notes 1–6 (1969–76) *Capricode (Capital Projects Code)*.

Health Service Reorganisation Circulars: HRC (72) 1–9; HRC (73) 1–40; HRC (74) 1–38.

HRC (73) 28: *Organisation of the pharmaceutical services.*
HRC (74) 9: *Local advisory committees.*
Health Service Circulars (interim series)
HSC (IS) 126: *The NHS planning system.*
HSC (IS) 128: *Application of the Medicines Act to health authorities.*
HSC (IS) 148: *NHS locally organised research scheme.*
Hospital Technical Memorandum
HTM 16: *Fire precautions.*

2

The Area

A. J. ROSS

The Noel Hall Report (DHSS 1970) indicated the causes of many problems experienced in hospital pharmacy. One of the main difficulties arose from the small scale on which the service was organised which resulted in:

1. Duplication of effort, inflexibility in the deployment of resources and the lack of adequate supporting staff.

2. The small department being particularly vulnerable to staffing shortages, leading to the curtailment of the services provided both at ward level and in dispensing to outpatients.

3. Restricted opportunities for the younger pharmacists to extend and develop their skills.

To sum up, hospital pharmacy had entered a vicious circle where lack of job satisfaction and poor remuneration had led to poor recruitment, thus increasing the load of more and more routine work falling on the remaining staff.

Since the introduction of the National Health Service in 1948, pharmacy had developed independently in all but the smallest hospitals. Prior to the reorganisation in April 1974 hospitals were organised in groups under the control of a Hospital Management Committee. In some cases a group pharmaceutical service had been set up, but even then little progress was made towards the integration of the pharmaceutical work because the group pharmacist was not given the authority to introduce changes and improve the efficiency of the systems in use.

Noel Hall recommendations

The report recommended that to overcome the difficulties the operational unit for providing the pharmaceutical service to hospitals should be based on a geographic area and so provide a very much larger organisation. The organisation of the Area Service is designed to fulfil the following criteria:

The basic unit of organisation must:

1. Provide an area of work large enough to ensure that pharmacists, technicians and other supporting staff can be fully used on the work appropriate to their training and skills, and that resources are not wasted by the duplication of services.

2. Be of such a size that the scope and responsibility of the work justify the employment of a top-class pharmacist and manager in the post of pharmacist-in-charge, enable staff to be deployed at levels appropriate to the length and quality of their experience, and make it possible for those pharmacists now working single-handed or in isolated independent departments to become members of a pharmaceutical team.

3. Offer a wide range of pharmaceutical work, which provides diversity of experience to younger pharmacists to fit them for further responsibility, and at the same time allow for some specialisation by more senior staff.

4. Have sufficient flexibility in its staffing to enable the pharmacist-in-charge to move staff between pharmacies and sections to provide cover during staff leave, sickness or periods of particular strain, and to release them for the substantial measure of further training that will be required in the future.

The size of an Area is in many cases defined by geographical considerations such as road communications and the need for the boundaries to be coterminous with the administrative Districts and Areas. There is, however, a minimum size below which the requisite number of pharmacists and supporting staff cannot be employed on duties which are appropriate to their skills. It has been recommended that the minimum number of pharmacists in an Area should be eight. Many Areas are considerably bigger than the quoted minimum. The increased size produces improvements in efficiency because of the employment of a higher proportion of supporting staff and the introduction of mechanisation for some of the routine work.

A larger Area organisation may mean increased flexibility in staffing but this cannot be obtained if staff are inconvenienced by the distances they have to travel. The limiting factor for the size of an Area is probably the time and cost of transport over the distances between the hospitals. However, it may well be feasible to obtain the benefits of production on a larger scale by setting up multiarea or regional manufacturing facilities where considerable cost savings can be demonstrated.

Integration of the National Health Service

The reorganisation of the Health Service came into operation in April 1974. This involved the integration of the three previously separate branches of health care:

1. General practitioner services.
2. Local authority health services.
3. Hospital services.

Hospital pharmacy therefore had to undergo two separate upheavals more or less concurrently: the 'Noel Hall' reorganisation which was entirely pharmaceutical and the NHS reorganisation insofar as it impinged on the running of the hospital pharmaceutical service. Two effects of the NHS reorganisation became immediately apparent:

1.   The change and extension of the duties and responsibilities of those Area and Principal Pharmacists who were appointed Area and District Pharmaceutical Officers.

2.   The extension of the hospital pharmaceutical service to take in the supply and control of medicaments to the former local authority clinics and health centres.

There will undoubtedly be further changes in the functions of the hospital pharmacy in relationship with general practice pharmacy. Improved contact between the two branches of the profession can benefit both and thus also benefit the patient, for example in the maintenance and supply of rarely used materials or those which are in short supply. The meetings of the Area Pharmaceutical Advisory Committee provide a platform for the exploration of mutual problems. Joint projects include the provision of drug information to all pharmacists from a regional specialist unit.

Time will be needed before the barriers between the sections of the profession can disappear. While the differences between the terms of employment of the two are so great, difficulties will naturally arise in arranging free interchange. Nevertheless, experimental projects are already under consideration (Pritchard 1972) in which the exchange of pharmacists between hospital and general practice pharmacy is being carried out. Recommendations have been made that the general practitioner pharmacist might take part in the ward service to peripheral hospitals (DHSS 1974).

MANAGEMENT OF AN AREA HOSPITAL PHARMACEUTICAL SERVICE

Functions of the Area Pharmacist

The Area Pharmacist is the manager of the Area Hospital Pharmaceutical Service and is responsible for all the pharmaceutical activities within the Area and is concerned with the overall planning, effectiveness and efficiency of the service. As a manager the Area Pharmacist should not be involved in the day-to-date activities of the pharmacies but should be in a position to stand back from the problems and look at the overall picture. The job description for the post covers the following responsibilities:

1.   To manage the pharmaceutical service within the Area.

2.   To advise the constituent authorities on the development of the pharmaceutical service in the Area.

3. To advise on pharmaceutical matters within the Area.

4. To establish future staffing requirements in the Area and advise on the appointment of staff.

5. To ensure that safe systems are used within the departments.

6. To give advice on the safe and effective use of medicines.

7. To represent the pharmaceutical service at meetings of all committees at which matters affecting pharmacy may be discussed.

The day-to-day work of the Area Pharmacist can be divided into several different spheres. Firstly, as part of the planning function, it is essential that any proposals for alterations or extensions to the service provided by the Area Authority are considered in relation to their effect on the pharmaceutical service. This entails scanning all the minutes and reports of meetings of the Health Care Planning Teams, the Area and District Team of Officers, medical committees and many others. If a subject is to be discussed at a coming meeting and has pharmaceutical implications, it will be necessary to obtain copies of earlier reports and to attend the meeting. In addition the Area Pharmacist must be aware of any shortcomings in the pharmaceutical service, formulate plans for their elimination, and discuss the proposals with everyone concerned.

The second range of duties involves the overall management of the service. The running of the departments is left to the Principal and Staff Pharmacists but the Area Pharmacist must ensure that the work carried out is undertaken in a proper manner. Safe systems of work are laid down for all procedures and these must be adhered to. Any activities which are carried out on an area basis must be coordinated and an eye has to be kept on the running of the system. Staff training may involve the transfer of personnel between departments to obtain experience in specialised techniques and the organisation of the transfers has to be undertaken.

The third and by far the greatest demand on the Area Pharmacist's time is the need to visit every department in the Area frequently to discuss problems as they arise and to maintain contact with the staff at all levels. In addition it is necessary to know the senior medical, nursing and administrative staff in each of the hospitals and try to form personal relationships with each of them. Without a direct knowledge of the people concerned it is very difficult to obtain any useful discussion of problems or proposals.

Lastly, every Area Pharmacist in each Region is involved in the discussions which take place at regional level on policy and there may be a considerable amount of work involved in assembling information for these meetings.

Organisation of the service

The term 'management' can be defined as the direction and control of an organisation to obtain optimum results. The manager has to specify the aims and objectives of the organisation and then set out a programme or method by which the aims may be achieved. Efficiency can be measured by the effectiveness of use of the resources available. The resources in pharmacy are the buildings and equipment in the pharmacy and, most important of all, the manpower available. All organisations can be represented by a very simple diagrammatic scheme (Fig. 2.1).

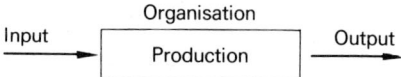

Fig. 2.1   Schematic representation of an organisation unit.

Within the organisation, the work can be subdivided into the direct production and 'service' activities which feed the production. Each 'service section' can of course be similarly subdivided into 'production' and 'service' components (Fig. 2.2).

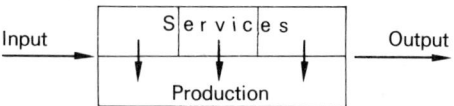

Fig. 2.2   Schematic representation of the subdivision of an organisation into 'production' and 'service' activities.

In the pharmacy the input represents drugs and preparations and the output treatments. The 'service' activities are such sections as manufacture, sterile products, quality control, stores etc.

Integration and centralisation

Reorganisation of the hospital pharmaceutical service has been directed towards the accruing benefits of increased scale. Four major objectives have already been stated (see p. 16) but a further advantage can be obtained. With increased size, economies can be made by the introduction of factory-like organisation in some sections (Ross 1973).

The different functions within the field of hospital pharmacy have to be approached in different ways. Some activities, such as dispensing for outpatients, must be carried out at the hospital at which the clinic is held. Others (e.g. manufacturing) can be undertaken at a remote point and the products transported to the 'user pharmacy'. With concentration of manufacturing at one centre the sizes of batches can be increased, mechanisation introduced and significant savings in manpower achieved. This particularly applies to the production of sterile fluids and to the repacking of solid and liquid oral dose forms. There are two possible ways of achieving increases in production batch size, by integration and by centralisation:

Integration. The concentration of a particular process at one unit, this unit depending on other units for supplies of other types of products.

Centralisation. All facilities and staff are concentrated at a central point so that a very large unit is achieved.

The advantages to be gained from centralisation have been widely accepted, but very often what was, in fact, being referred to was the integration of several units to try to obtain the same advantages without the capital cost of building and equipping a new large central unit capable of handling the total workload.

Medicines Act

The application of the Medicines Act (1968) to the production of pharmaceuticals in hospitals has induced a fundamental reappraisal of hospital manufacture. The philosophy of 'make do and mend' and develop slowly could no longer be accepted. The standards of hygiene and design of the facilities to be used which were demanded by the Medicines Inspectorate were in many cases considerably more stringent than could be met in the existing pharmacies. Manufacturing sections were closed down and in many units restrictions placed on the range of products which could be prepared. The effects of many years of underinvestment in pharmacy had suddenly been brought to light. This action by the DHSS prevented the development of dual standards between hospital and industry for the preparation of medicines. The effect was for hospital production to be centralised in those units which were satisfactory, and plans had to be drawn up for the replacement or improvement of others which exhibited shortcomings. As the replanning of the manufacturing facilities had to be undertaken during the period of national stringency, the economics of providing manufacturing units at every District General Hospital or even in every Noel Hall Area was questioned. It became obvious that it made good sense to centralise the manufacture of certain types of products on a Subregional and even Regional basis. Though it may be desirable for every Area or large District General Hospital to have some manufacturing capability for 'specials' (items which are only used in bulk locally) it can be foreseen that no Area Authority will ever again be entirely independent in this field.

The need to provide a considerable capital investment in the manufacturing function resulted in a review of the range and types of products which had traditionally been prepared within the hospital department. Each product has to be challenged not only on the economics of manufacture versus purchase, but also on the necessity for its use at all. Every one in the range of 'variations on a theme' type of formulation has to be critically examined to cut out unnecessary duplications. In addition, with the introduction of automatic and semiautomatic machines, the flexibility with which different pack sizes and types can be produced is much reduced. An extensive exercise is necessary to try to find the common denominator in pack size and type so that as many as possible different demands can be met with a single presentation.

As centralisation proceeds some advantages may be gained:

1.   Economy of manpower.
2.   Quantity discounts.
3.   Reduced duplication of stock.
4.   Flexibility in the reissue of stock.
5.   Flexibility in staffing.

However, with a centralised unit a breakdown in production could be disastrous as there are no alternative sources of supply. A high degree of specialisation of the staff involved will develop which in itself may cause problems.

The introduction of automatic or semiautomatic machinery is expensive and can only be justified if maximum use is made of its capabilities. A properly equipped large unit may well be able to serve two or three Area Pharmaceutical Services with all their needs in a certain range of products. Progress towards centralised manufacture will promote the development of sophisticated stock control systems both at the central unit and in the pharmacies which depend on the central unit for their supplies. 'Out of stock' situations cannot be tolerated and the manufacturing section will no longer be able to produce materials on request. Hospital manufacturing units will in future tend to complement the service provided by the industry and not compete as they have in the past.

Manufacturing and costing

Before manufacture is undertaken, it is essential to ensure that adequate costing is carried out. Products will fall into one of several categories:

1.   Items which are more expensive to manufacture than to purchase from trade sources and so must be purchased. As the raised standards mentioned above are applied, it will be found that the number of items falling into this class will increase.
2.   Items which are cheaper to prepare in the department thereby giving a financial incentive for manufacturing.
3.   Items which cannot be purchased and therefore must be made within the hospital.

Hospital pharmacists have been accused of not calculating the true cost of manufacturing when comparing hospital preparations with those of industry. The costs of manufacture will include many factors. The following list shows those which will need to be included in any calculations: ingredients; labour; heating and lighting; power (steam and electrical); quality control, (finished product plus ingredients); transport; containers and labels; stock holding; ordering/storekeeping; maintenance of equipment; in-process control; depreciation of equipment.

In addition it may be necessary to include rent and rates even though these do not strictly apply in Crown property. If new building is involved then again an apportionment for this will have to be included. Only when the true full cost of all the aspects of manufacture have been identified is it possible to compare the economics of hospital manufacture against the cost of purchasing from trade sources.

Comparison of workload

Many factors affect the level of work in the individual pharmacy, by far the most important being the prescribing activity of the medical staff. Others include the extent to which manufacturing is carried out, the methods used within the department, the services offered to the other professions in the hospital and the extent to which these services are used. In addition there may be a considerable amount of work involved in the provision of supplies for the community services. Comparisons may be invidious but it is essential for the manager of the service to have some index of the workload of the department so that decisions on the allocation of resources can be made in a fair manner. A technique is needed which will enable the activity and workload of a department to be measured. At present the only indicators available are the total expenditure on drugs and the number and type of beds served. The total number of items issued can be recorded and this will indicate the workload in the dispensing and ward supply sections. There must, of course, be a definition of an 'item' which can be best described as: 'the smallest unit which can be issued properly labelled to the patient or nurse' (e.g. a bottle of tablets, a box of ampoules). The totals so collected will give some crude indication of the work carried out and will show any trends in the demands made upon the department.

To enable a direct comparison of the workload between two departments some allowance must be made for the complexity of the work being carried out. The basic unit of work, as defined above, is the container filled and handed out ready for use. The situation where there is the minimum possible work involved is the labelling of a ready packed item. If any manipulation is involved, be it merely the counting of the tablets or the preparation of a complex ointment, a 'complexity loading factor' would have to be applied to enable the work to be related to other types of items issued. Records of items issued in the various complexity groups would have to be kept and the appropriate loading factor applied to obtain a 'workload figure' for the department. In addition the totals of all items produced or handled in the 'service' sections would need to be compiled and again a loading factor applied to allow for the differences in the work involved. The total workload figure for each department is useful in a variety of ways. For example, comparisons between workload per person in different departments will give some indication of the different efficiencies between the departments (or some complexity loading factor which has not been correctly estimated).

Parameters of efficiency

Two parameters which give a useful indication of the effectiveness and efficiency with which the department is being run are the ratios:

1. Number of items prepacked to total items issued. Prepacking is a much more efficient system than piecemeal filling of containers and the ratio (expressed as a percentage) should be as high as possible. If, however, there is a move in the future to purchase a much higher proportion of medicines in a ready-for-use pack this ratio may have to be reassessed or the prepacked definition extended to include the purchased packs.

2. Number of orders placed on suppliers to total items issued. The cost of placing an order on a supplier is considerable and the number should be kept to the minimum compatible with the maintenance of adequate but not excessive stock levels. If the ratio (again as a percentage) rises, lack of adequate stock control is indicated.

Management structure

The Area Pharmacist's first task is to develop the management structure of the organisation. This involves the construction of a chart showing the formal lines of responsibility delegation between the senior managers and the middle managers of the various sections of the pharmacy. Responsibility may be for a specific technical activity (e.g. sterile products or quality control) or for the service to a geographic section of the Area. In the development of a viable structure within the organisation, it is necessary first to identify all of the activities undertaken. Once the list is complete the activities must be grouped together to form the sections of responsibility, whilst accepting that certain constraints operate (for example, that one person cannot be responsible for both production and quality control). With the groupings selected to form the sections, the next step is to ascertain the grade of staff needed to take control of each section. A decision has then to be made as to whom the section (middle) manager reports. Again constraints will appear with the need for specialised knowledge or geographic distance from the senior manager. A simple orthodox type of management structure chart is shown in Fig. 2.3. As can be seen Principal Pharmacists, each of whom are responsible for the pharmaceutical services of a large District General Hospital, are responsible to the Area Pharmacist. Beneath them are Staff Pharmacists who act as section managers and report to the Principal Pharmacists. In certain isolated circumstances a Staff Pharmacist may report directly to the Area Pharmacist if, for example, the Staff Pharmacist carries the responsibility for a specialised function in two or more District General Hospitals.

There are disadvantages to the construction and operation of the type of management structure which is outlined above. Firstly, staff are allocated to a particular section and specialisation rapidly builds up. Though specialists

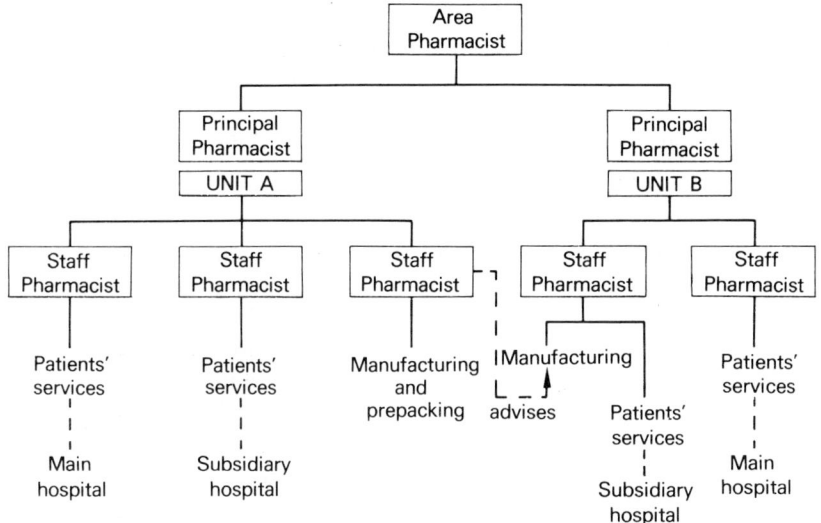

Fig. 2.3　A simplified management structure; solid line, line of responsibility; dotted line, advice.

are necessary and probably inevitable in a large and complex organisation, a staff composed almost entirely of highly specialised personnel can lead to difficulties when any member is absent on leave or through sickness. In addition overspecialisation can lead to problems when the specialist applies for promotion. A pharmacist who has specialised in this manner may find it difficult to gain promotion back into general activities. The second disadvantage is the formation of compartments beyond which communication is difficult. For instance, in Fig. 2.3 the specialist staff pharmacist in unit A in charge of manufacturing is supposed to advise on the manufacturing carried out in unit B. However, is the advice to be given directly to the technical staff or must communications be via the Principal Pharmacist?

Communications

Pharmaceutical

The second task for the Area Pharmacist is the setting up of channels of communication both between himself and and his staff and among the staff themselves. There are three possible communication pathways within the Area Pharmaceutical Organisation:

1.   Vertical. Between the Area Pharmacist and the remainder of the pharmaceutical staff. It is, of course, important that communications work both ways and that the lower grades of staff have the opportunity of communicating upwards as well as hearing what is happening at the top. Even more important, it is essential that the communication channel is not used just to promulgate 'edicts from on high'.

2.   Horizontal. Between similar grades of staff in different units.

3.   Extraterritorial. Discussions with other area organisations.

To achieve these three lines a complex system of meetings is needed. For vertical communications, the Area Pharmacist meets with the Principal Pharmacists (or heads of departments). In turn the Principals hold departmental or group meetings and the staff are made aware of the discussions at Area meetings and feedback of comments is made to future Area meetings.

Horizontal communication links are much more difficult to achieve. Various schemes have been attempted. Interchange of staff for short periods for training will produce some contact. Similar meetings between all staff in the Area may be useful. However, no matter how much effort the manager may put into developing this, there will always be the possibility of a 'them and us' situation developing. There are two methods which may be useful in overcoming distrust. Complete integration and interchange between the various units can be instituted though this may not be feasible due to geographic separation. Alternatively the manager has to accept the situation and try to make use of the antagonism by introducing an element of friendly rivalry. The third element of communication between Area organisations will tend to be more sporadic. However, contacts made between members of staff are rarely valueless and opportunities should be given for people to visit other departments. A more formal and regular contact will be maintained between Area Pharmacists by meetings at Regional level. Breakdowns in communication within the pharmaceutical service usually show in one of two ways. Either someone complains that they 'did not know/were not told', or action is taken on an agreed policy but in the wrong manner. It is particularly difficult to ensure that schemes which are under discussion are not started prematurely before all the groundwork has been completed. The Area Pharmacist must try to chat informally with all the members of the staff to try to find if information is being misconstrued or if anxiety is developing about any proposals under discussion.

There are special problems involved where the Noel Hall Area Service includes more than one administrative district or area. In such a case it is necessary to form an interdistrict or interarea administrative working party to achieve a coordinated approach to developments, particularly where one of the authorities is being asked to provide a service for the others and the setting up and running costs have to be met by the user authorities.

Interdisciplinary

Pharmacy as a profession does not act in isolation. The service provided is used by the nursing and medical profession and is designed to benefit the patient. A hospital is a very complex organisation and the communication pathways needed to obtain effective working are extremely complicated. It is necessary to ensure that proposals and requests which affect a number of disciplines are brought to the attention of everyone concerned.

Three levels of discussion can be identified:

1. Policy determination. Proposals for changes in policy must be discussed with the senior members of all the professions, e.g. medical, nursing, administration, treasurers.
2. Application of policy. Agreed policy must be fully discussed and explained to the members of the hospital staff who are affected.
3. Day-to-day problems. Discussions will be needed between the members of the professions concerned, preferably at equivalent seniority and 'face to face' wherever possible rather than over the telephone.

Communication on treatment

Four parties are involved in the treatment of each patient (Fig. 2.4) and breakdown of communication between them occurs far too frequently. This can

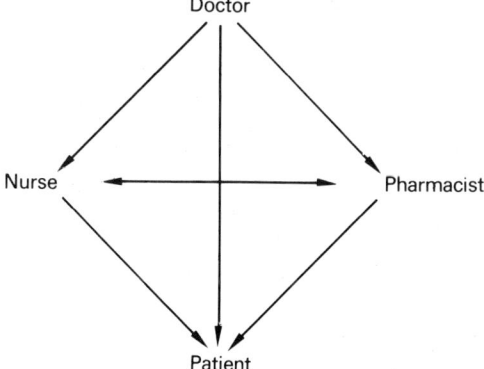

Fig. 2.4 Communications on treatment and the four people involved.

lead to considerable difficulties for the patient. For instance, wrongly requisitioned material by the nurse can be due to a misunderstanding of the doctor–nurse message. The label on a discharge medication does not always correspond to what the nurse has told the patient. The possibilities of error are infinite. To overcome some of these problems, complex systems of requisitions, prescription forms and dose record sheets have been developed. These are described in later chapters.

Objectives and setting targets

Clearly, the main objectives for the pharmaceutical service include:

1.   Integration and centralisation of manufacturing activities with the provision of units in which good conditions can be attained, and the introduction of full quality control for all the products manufactured, including 'in process' checks.

2.   Small-scale facilities will be needed in each Area, if not at every district general hospital, for the manufacture of sterile and non-sterile preparations, the repackaging of solid oral dose forms, mixtures and lotions to supplement the centralised manufacturing units.

3.   Ward pharmacy service for all beds and extension of visits to those clinics previously administered by the local authorities.

4.   Supply service to all wards and departments daily or more frequently with a topping-up system for commonly used stock items and individual patient dispensing for others.

5.   Provision of extended hours service to cater for requirements on the wards outside the normal 'nine-till-five' period.

6.   Intravenous additive service available on an extended hours or 24 hours-a-day basis as needed.

7.   Information service to answer queries and to routinely supply background information on the products in use.

8.   Provision of good training schemes for preregistration pharmacists and student technicians.

9.   Development of facilities for undertaking investigations, of stability and formulation problems and for carrying out research on pharmaceutical topics.

It is extremely difficult to measure the progress towards given objectives, particularly when improvements in the quality, as apart from the quantity, of a service is being aimed at. The manager has to set out the details of the objective and then a series of steps which will lead towards the goal. It is essential that the manager is able to obtain the commitment of everyone concerned to the proposals presented. In each step one or more aspects must be chosen which can be measured and these measurements used to determine the progress which is being made. If the introduction of ward visits as part of the ward pharmacy service is the objective, then a count of the visits made indicates some progress. However, if the objective is to improve the standard of contact between the visiting pharmacist and the junior medical staff, it is necessary perhaps to log the frequency with which useful discussions took place or the number of times advice was sought by the doctors. Whatever the objective, it is essential that feedback is obtained on progress (or the lack of it). In many cases it is necessary to set target deadlines for the completion of the preparatory stages or the starting point will never be reached. Where new techniques have been introduced it is also necessary to lay down monitoring procedures to ensure that the technique is maintained. All too often experience will show that the methods used have slipped back to the old way because of some small hitch developing with the new technique.

Staff and staffing

Many different grades of staff are employed within the pharmaceutical service. Pharmacists from preregistration student to area pharmacist, together with technicians, senior technicians and students plus pharmacy assistants, make up the technical staff. In addition there are the storekeepers and storemen, clerks and secretaries, cleaners, drivers and porters, all of whom have an important role to play in the organisation. To make most effective use of the staff available it is necessary to ensure that each person is employed on tasks for which they are adequately trained. It is also essential to make sure that they are not spending time on jobs which could be carried out by lower grade staff. To be able to grade a vacancy accurately it is necessary to analyse in detail the tasks to be carried out. In an existing situation many anomalies will come to light and these may require the reallocation of the tasks or a change in the grade of the post.

Job descriptions

When a job analysis has been carried out a job description should be compiled. Job descriptions should outline the duties and responsibilities of the post and also give some indication of the relative importance of the various facets of the work. It is important to state clearly to whom the person is responsible and over whom the person has control. In addition, it is as well to include a general outline of the conditions of service.

Definitions of the grades

The grades of pharmacists and the definitions attached to them in the context of hospital pharmacy are as follows:

Regional Pharmaceutical Officer

The pharmacist responsible to the Regional Health Authority for the functions given in the Noel Hall report (see Chapter 1).

Area Pharmacist/Area Pharmaceutical Officer

The pharmacist responsible for the pharmaceutical services of an Area Pharmaceutical Service.

Principal Pharmacist/District Pharmaceutical Officer

A pharmacist responsible to the Area Pharmacist for the pharmaceutical services of a large District General Hospital which is not the headquarters of the Area Pharmaceutical Service, and/or Deputy to the Area Pharmacist in a large Area, or undertaking special responsibilities, possibly including those that extend beyond the boundaries of one Area.

Staff Pharmacist

A pharmacist responsible for the pharmaceutical services either of a medium-sized hospital or of a number of smaller hospitals, or of a major section of work of the Area Pharmaceutical Service or of a large hospital pharmacy department or engaged in specialist work at a sufficiently high level.

Pharmacist, Basic Grade

A pharmacist undertaking basic duties normally requiring some element of direction by a senior colleague.

Preregistration graduate student

A postgraduate, preregistration student undergoing training.

Senior technicians

A senior technician (Whitley Councils 'B'; DHSS 1972a) should be looked upon as the section leader for a particular function within the department. They must be given the responsibility to run the activities of their section within the guidelines which have been set down. The guidelines will be contained in the procedure manual for the sections, but only the pharmacist-in-charge of the section will have the authority to allow deviation from the set procedures.

Technicians

The place of the technician in the future will be at the dispensary bench, where, under supervision, they will carry out the bulk of the dispensing. Technicians should not be employed as labour in the manufacturing and prepacking sections as the routine filling of bottles does not require the degree of training which has been provided for them.

Student technicians

The student will be expected to gain experience in all sections of the pharmacy, dispensing under tuition in the dispensary and working alongside the semi-skilled assistants at routine jobs.

Pharmacy assistant

This is probably the most undervalued grade in hospital pharmacy at present. A great deal of routine work at present carried out by more highly trained staff could easily be undertaken by this grade of staff. In addition the entrants are often middle-aged women who form a stable and hard-working team within the department.

Storekeeper, clerk

Highly trained technical staff and pharmacists should not be expected to carry out routine clerical duties. Given properly laid down procedures the complete operation of ordering, stock control, invoice clearance and costing can be left to the storekeepers and clerks with minimal oversight from a pharmacist.

Cost of staffing

It is often necessary to estimate the cost of alternative staffing structures. Money allocated for staff can be calculated on the basis of the mean of the salary scale plus additional expenditure involved in the payment of national insurance, superannuation etc. These expenses must not be overlooked in the totalling of the cost of any appointment.

This method is based on the supposition that, overall, as members of staff move up the salary scale they are promoted and are replaced by more junior people; this does not, however, necessarily apply to senior posts where movement of staff is much less frequent.

Training and promotion

Preregistration pharmacists

A great deal of thought and effort has been expended on setting up training schemes for preregistration pharmacists. At hospital level the new appointee is first given an orientation session on the activities of the department by the principal pharmacist. Then, having been given time to find out what actually goes on in the department, the graduate should be taken round the hospital to learn its geography and also to visit departments, for example: administration; treasurer; pathology; CSSD, wards; X-ray; supplies; theatre; casualty; CCU.

If arrangements can be made for a short period to be spent actually working in some of these other departments (such as pathology, X-ray, treasurers, records) considerable benefits can be reaped in understanding how the pharmaceutical service fits into the hospital organisation. The new entrant should first work in each section of the pharmacy so that the handling of all the equipment can be mastered. Then, later in the year's training, the preregistration pharmacist should work alongside the manager of each section and be allowed to take some administrative responsibility, at least towards the end of this period. To obtain the fullest range of experience the preregistration pharmacist would be expected to spend some time in each of the departments in the Area and, in fact, should, if necessary, be sent to hospitals outside the Area to gain experience in specialised techniques. Time must also be allocated to enable the graduate to see and read medical and other literature. Formal tuition on specific topics should be organised on a regional basis and should be linked with the opportunity to visit pharmacies in other Areas. Involvement in a project of either a research or review nature will undoubtedly benefit the preregistration pharmacist, and, provided that the subject is carefully chosen, will enable him to relate some of the theoretical information which he has at his command to his work.

Pharmacists

Once the preregistration pharmacist has completed the required 12 months' training and has registered, the duties undertaken should be arranged to enable a wide range of tasks to be undertaken. It would be expected that the pharmacist would work in more than one department either by transfer within the Area or by applying for posts in others. Courses for newly qualified pharmacists on technical subjects are arranged on a regional basis and the pharmacist should take full advantage of these opportunities. Similarly, it is desirable that the individual undertakes a considerable volume of reading and possibly also takes part in a research project. Attendance at a first-line management course would also be very beneficial. After 2–3 years the pharmacist would have gained a considerable depth of experience and knowledge over a wide range of activities and would be ready for promotion.

Staff Pharmacists

The Staff Pharmacist grade posts are normally advertised on a specialist basis, though in fact the responsibilities are rarely limited to a specific section. To ensure that adequate all-round experience is gained some scheme should be operated within an Area which allows the Staff Pharmacists to change round. However, a regular move round on a 'so-many-months' basis may be counterproductive as the pharmacist does not necessarily identify with the job and its responsibilties. At some stage in the training of pharmacists attendance at a multidisciplinary management course is essential. A Staff Pharmacist before promotion to principal grade ought to have attended courses up to middle management level.

One great danger in career planning is the possibility of overspecialisation where a Staff Pharmacist with experience in a particular section obtains a post as a specialist principal pharmacist at a regional unit. This would lead to a 'dead end' as it is essential for Principal Pharmacists to have a great deal of experience in the administration of hospital pharmacies to be eligible for appointment as Area and Regional Pharmaceutical Officers. There may well be a need for a promotional structure in the specialised functions up to Area Pharmacist level.

It can be argued that the specialisation at Staff grade level ought to be matched by a similar specialisation at Principal Pharmacist level. Each Principal Pharmacist in an Area could be asked to maintain a special interest in one of the technical branches as well as carrying the responsibility for the running of the service to the particular hospital. In this way breaks in continuity of the management of a section from the promotion or transfer of the Staff Pharmacist can be overcome. However, the existence of the Principal with special responsibility will decrease the effectiveness of the management role of the Staff Pharmacists and may be undesirable on this account.

Budgets

Functional budgets

Departmental or functional budgets are a recent introduction in hospital pharmacy. Basically the system operates by allocating the senior functional manager (the Area Pharmacist) a global sum of money within which he has to operate the service to the best advantage. Funding under this scheme has the advantage that the manager has the opportunity to divert money from staffing to equipment or the reverse to make optimum use of the facilities available. However, the manager has the responsibility of ensuring that the budget figure is not exceeded. This improved flexibility allows for adjustments in the balance of the various grades of staff employed, in relation to developments. For instance, it enables the numbers of pharmacy assistants to be increased at the expense of other grades of staff, and to enable the introduction of factory type production without employing trained technicians on laborious and tedious tasks. (Under the previous system money was allocated for specific purposes and to use funds which were earmarked for staffing to purchase equipment was administratively difficult.)

The expenditure on drugs should be included in the medical budget. The pharmacist is charged with the task of 'ensuring the effective use of drugs'. Towards this end Ward Pharmacists will advise prescribers on the treatment for individual patients and the Principal Pharmacist will be involved in the discussions on prescribing policies within the hospital. Effective prescribing may well be more expensive than the inefficient use of drugs, but if the patients can be discharged more quickly there will be a considerable overall saving to the hospital. Savings in the expenditure on drugs can be achieved by contracting arrangements carried out within each region by pharmacists and supplies officers working together. The pharmaceutical budget will therefore cover the internal organisation of the service (e.g. equipment, staffing and information services).

Medical budget

A direct interest is taken in the cost of providing health care in the hospital service. Figures must be produced so that the cost of treatment per patient or for each specialist can be calculated. At some stage investigations into the cost effectiveness of alternative treatments are necessary. Various schemes are now in use although on a small scale. Computer systems are being used in which each issue to every ward and department is coded and charged. Alternatively, the costs of a sample of supplies can be calculated and used as a basis for the apportionment of the total expenditure. Sampling systems can be extended to provide average costs for various types of supplies thereby reducing the amount of work involved in the collection of the data. If the average cost of an item supplied to a ward is known and the number of items supplied to each ward is recorded for workload analysis purposes a running total of expenditure for the ward can very easily be calculated. Purchases of medicines are usually analysed under categories (analgesics, anaesthetics, antibiotics etc.) to enable trends in consumption of the various categories to be recognised. The information collected, however, may be of little use as it is not sufficiently specific. The only costing of issue which is carried out universally is the charging out of supplies sent to other hospitals, as this is required by the treasurer's department to compile the annual cost statement for each hospital. This figure is obtained either by pricing all the requisitions for supplies or on a sample period basis. One alternative system which has been tried is to monitor the consumption of a small range of the more costly items used and apportioning the remainder of the expenditure on the basis of the ratios of these figures. However, a slight change in the quantities of any one of these expensive items would have a disproportionate effect on the total figure for that unit and produce wide fluctuations.

Estimates

Two forms of estimates are required in the Health Service. The first is the estimated cost of maintaining the existing services from the revenue provided for the Area Authority. Figures are produced for pharmacy for 'drugs' (more properly 'medicines') and for staffing. These estimates are prepared by the Area Treasurer's department on the basis of the previous year's figures with an allowance for inflation, the upward trend in the cost of treatment in the case of drugs and incremental rises in the case of staff. The second type of estimate is that of the cost of any proposals for the extension of the services provided for the replacement of equipment and facilities at present in use. Here the cost is allocated to 'capital expenditure' (i.e. non-recurrent) though there may well be revenue cost consequences of the scheme. If there are to be increases in the cost of running the service due to the proposals under discussion it is necessary to ensure that they are not overlooked in the early stages of the planning process. Where the service provided by other sections of the hospital is being extended, for instance by new wards or departments being built, it is essential that the effect on the pharmacy is considered. There may be a need for capital work for the pharmacy to be included as part of the main building scheme. Alternatively there may be a need to increase the staff establishment to cope with the increased workload. It is the Area Pharmacist's duty to ensure that he is aware of all developments being planned.

Major equipment has a finite life and the need for replacement must be brought to the attention of the Area Authority well before the equipment is beyond repair. It is unreasonable to expect large capital sums to be found immediately and the replacement must take its place in the Authority's capital programme.

Departments themselves need money spent upon them to keep them at maximum efficiency, especially as the service provided changes over a period of years. These requests will have to take their place in the capital programme in a similar way to replacement of equipment.

Obtaining allocation of funds for developments depends on the strength of the case submitted to the authority. Cases can only be judged on facts and it is important that the submission includes as much factual information as possible. Clearly, a case which shows in detail the advantages to the hospital, will gain much greater acceptance than a scheme which promises vague benefits. In all cases it is obvious that a great deal of detailed information is needed to support the submission and on this detail the success of the proposals will rest.

REFERENCES

DEPARTMENT OF HEALTH AND SOCIAL SECURITY (1970) *Report of the Working Party on the Hospital Pharmaceutical Service*. The Noel Hall Report. HMSO, London.

DEPARTMENT OF HEALTH AND SOCIAL SECURITY (1972a) *Whitley Councils; Pharmaceutical Profession and Technical 'B' PTB Circular 280*. DHSS, London.

DEPARTMENT OF HEALTH AND SOCIAL SECURITY (1972b) *Whitley Councils; Pharmaceutical Committee 'C' PH Circular 51*. DHSS, London.

DEPARTMENT OF HEALTH AND SOCIAL SECURITY (1974) *Community Hospitals; their role and development in the National Health Service*. HMSO, London.

PRITCHARD A. D. (1972) *Pharmaceutical Journal* **209**, 292.

ROSS A. J. (1973) *Pharmaceutical Journal* **210**, 582.

3

The Department

J. FEREDAY & C. HETHERINGTON

The Pharmaceutical Area, comprising approximately 4000–6000 beds, provides the basis for planning the pharmaceutical service. While some services will only be required at one site in an Area, others, particularly patient services, should be available in all hospitals where a pharmacy department is viable. This chapter describes the basic organisation and management of such a department. (The reorganisation of pharmaceutical services has naturally been based on the facilities which were previously available. Although ideally several functions, particularly manufacturing and prepackaging, can be more effectively organised on an Area scale, the nature of existing facilities has limited the extent to which services can be rationalised in the initial stages.)

DEPARTMENTAL DESIGN

Size

Hospital Building Note 29 (DHSS 1973) gives recommended areas for rooms within pharmacy departments based on the number of acute beds served. These, however, must be considered in the light of special local requirements and the information provided should be used only as a guide. In the overall planning of a department an addition of 30% must be made for internal circulation space, and internal walls and partitions. Mechanical ventilation and engineering plant are normally accommodated in separate plant rooms which may be situated within the department.

Location

The position of the pharmacy in relation to other parts of the hospital is important. For the convenience of outpatients the pharmacy should be close to the outpatient and accident and emergency departments. There must be good access to the goods-receiving area for the largest delivery vehicles anticipated and sufficient room for turning. For ease of distribution of supplies to the wards, and access for hospital staff, it is also desirable that the pharmacy should be situated close to the ward areas. To satisfy all these requirements some degree of compromise may be necessary.

Large manufacturing units may be established with independent collection, storage and delivery arrangements. There is no need for such units to be close to a main hospital pharmacy department, and they may be situated distant from patient treatment areas.

Internal relationships

If possible the pharmacy department should be situated entirely on one floor. The movement of staff and particularly goods between floors can be very time wasting. However, accommodation on the floor where the dispensary is best positioned is often at a great premium, and manufacturing and storage areas may best be accommodated on separate floors. The practice of providing a separate dispensary for outpatient dispensing is undesirable as this necessitates duplication of stocks, and reduces flexibility in the use of staff.

It is important to consider the flow of materials and products through the department, from receipt to issue. A well-organised flow can increase the efficient running of the department by making the best use of available space and reducing unnecessary work.

Development planning

All substantial alterations to departments must be carefully planned. From the initial outlines, detailed plans are prepared and the building and engineering requirements determined by the appropriate officers. At this stage there must be consultation within the organization to ensure that the implications of change are fully understood, for example increased cleaning services, security, access etc. Furthermore it is necessary to confirm that the requirements of Building Regulations, Fire Regulations, and if relevant, the Medicines Act, are met.

The interval between preliminary planning and commissioning is considerable. After planning and local approval, the scheme must be costed and allocated a priority with other developments. Only when funds are available can the scheme be implemented. For substantial schemes the minimum time elapsing between preliminary planning and completion is unlikely to be less than 2 years, and may be considerably longer if there is strong competition for funds. During this period it is necessary to ensure that plans are updated to meet any changes in requirement, for example in working conditions, equipment requirements or workload.

Accommodation

Stores

Reception

In all main pharmacy departments it is desirable to have a clearly defined area for storage. The external entrance for goods may be shared with other departments, but it is essential that part of the loading area is reserved solely for collection and delivery of pharmaceutical supplies. The storekeeper's office, situated within the pharmacy, should allow observation of the loading area in the interests of security. Goods should enter the store through a separate receiving area, where supples are unpacked and checked before storage. Discarded packing materials, a potential fire hazard, must be stored tidily and cleared from the area as frequently as possible.

Drugs store

The wide variety of packs held in the store, from small vials to sacks and drums, requires the use of different methods of storage to obtain optimum use from the store. The majority of goods are best stored on adjustable steel racking arranged in bays. Heavy containers and bulky items such as sterile solutions are suitable for pallet storage and transport. Mobile racking may be used when space is severly limited, but it is better suited for slow-moving items. It is important that goods are stored in a clearly defined order. Subdivision into major groups such as tablets, injections, liquids, solids, with alphabetical arrangement within each section, is a simple, acceptable system. It is essential that any item may be easily located in the store by all staff, and more complex arrangements, such as grouping of goods by manufacturer to simplify ordering, may require staff to seek further information before locating any item. It is essential that stock is used in rotation, and it is helpful if all containers are stamped with the date of receipt before storage. Wherever possible new stock should be placed behind existing stocks so that the oldest stock can be taken from the front. It is important that potentially hazardous substances, for example acids and solvents, should be stored in a safe place to avoid breakage and spillage. They should never be stored above eye level, or on mobile racking.

In addition to the main drug store, there is a requirement for other specialised stores.

Returnable container store. This provides storage for empty drums and other containers which are returnable to the supplier and is conveniently situated adjacent to the loading bay.

Flammable store. A store for inflammable materials should be constructed as a separate building isolated from the main building. If the store is shared with other users, the stock of pharmaceutical materials should be clearly separated from any other contents.

Cold store. In large departments the stock of thermolabile materials may warrant the construction of a walk-in cold store within the main store. This consists of a specially constructed room with a refrigeration unit. The door must be capable of being opened from both sides.

Security store. Special security arrangements are required for controlled drugs and other drugs liable to misuse. A special store located within the main store is acceptable, preferably avoiding the use of an outside wall. Arrangements for security should comply with the current recommendations of the D.H.S.S.

Container store. This is required for the wide range of containers (bottles, jars, tubes etc.) and closures used for large-scale packing and individual dispensing. Since the degree of security required is relatively low, this store may, if necessary, be separate from the main drug store.

Dressings store. In recent years there has been a tendency for the routine supply of dressings to be taken over by supplies departments. Thus it is unlikely that there will be requirement for a special store within most pharmacy departments. Small quantities may be kept for outpatient dispensing purposes.

Cylinder store. Although piped supplies of gases are becoming more widely used, there is still a considerable requirement for cylinder storage. This must provide suitable storage for horizontal and vertical storage as appropriate, and there must be adequate arrangements for the separate storage of full and empty cylinders. The store must be accessible outside normal working hours, and, although it should be adjacent to the main goods entrance, need not be adjacent to the main pharmacy store.

Raw materials store. Raw materials should be placed in quarantine when received, pending approval by the Quality Controller. A separate area should be maintained for this purpose, but may conveniently be provided within the main drug store. When approved for use, all containers should be appropriately marked.

Storage for manufactured goods

Manufactured and prepacked items should not be stored in manufacturing areas, and appropriate storage should be provided, either within the main store or separately. A clearly defined area must be allocated to manufactured goods in quarantine, pending approval by the Quality Controller, so that there is no possibility of confusion between approved batches and those under test (see Chapter 5).

Patient services section

Dispensary

A single dispensary should be provided for the dispensing of prescriptions for inpatients and outpatients as previously discussed. There are wide differences in views on the best layout for a dispensary, and a great deal can be learned by examining as many different existing arrangements as possible. Individual working stations, sliding storage units, and division of work between areas for special purposes, for example tablet dispensing, liquid dispensing, and extemporaneous ointment preparation, may prove useful according to local requirements and accommodation. Generally a square room is preferable to a long, narrow area as unnecessary movement is reduced, and attention must be paid to the geographical arrangement of working areas, particularly island benches.

The issue of ward and departmental stock drugs may be performed in the dispensary, but if the workload is heavy a separate area may be preferred. Great savings in time are made if all such items are prepacked, and stored in sequence corresponding to the sequence of a preprinted requisition form. Provision must be made for the storage of empty and full transit containers, sorting and disposal of empty bottles and a logical sequence of operations within the section. The use of sloping shelved storage units, loaded from the back may help to reduce the required storage space and ensure use of stocks in the correct chronological sequence. Shelving or racking should be provided for transit containers as indiscriminate stacking may constitute a hazard, particularly where there is a high level of staff movement.

Messengers' waiting area

This should be situated adjacent to the dispensary, and be separated from the outpatient waiting area.

Outpatient waiting area

This area must be adjacent to the dispensary and should be comfortably furnished. A wide service counter is preferable to a number of small hatches which are not conducive to satisfactory consultation between patients and staff. However, an open counter should be designed to provide some privacy for individual patients when receiving their medicines. If prescription payments are to be made in the waiting area, suitable accomodation must be provided for a clerk.

Emergency drug store

Medical staff will require access to a range of drugs outside normal working hours if a 24-hour service is not provided. In order to maintain security in the pharmacy it is preferable to provide a separate cupboard or room outside the department, stocked with a suitable range of drugs (see Chapter 10).

ORGANISATION

The key to a successful pharmacy department is a well-defined organisation, with policies understood and practised by each member of the staff. It is important for all staff to know what duties they are expected to perform and to whom they are directly accountable for their work. The knowledge of one's role in the organisation should promote efficient working, increase job interest and satisfaction, and should eliminate the 'grey areas' of uncertainty which can hinder the efficient working of the department. In all but the smallest departments there should be a clear division of work into sections. The distribution of duties will vary according to the nature and volume of work. It may be desirable, for example, to separate responsibility for inpatient and outpatient services, or alternatively to combine these under the general heading of 'Patient Services' and subdivide the duties into dispensary management, ward visiting services and bulk distribution. There is no universally preferred scheme of organisation as the wide variation in demand, resources and local personal preference are all justifiable influential factors.

It is important that there should exist clearly understood working procedures which should be comprehensive and in written form. The initial production of formal procedures can be an onerous task, particularly if there are insufficient agreed policies in existence to form a basic policy manual. However, the formation and recording of procedures alone justify the exercise. The benefits of written procedures include:

1. The provision of guidance to new staff.
2. Ensured continuity in the application of policy.
3. Improved efficiency.
4. Reduction in the possibility of error.

It is important that any written manual is kept up to date, and this in itself can provide an ideal method of informing staff of changes in procedural policy. In addition to a departmental policy it is also necessary to produce, in conjunction with other disciplines, formal policies concerning the ordering, storage and use of drugs, and relationships with other departments, for example maintenance, domestic, transport and finance.

PROVISION OF OUT-OF-HOURS SERVICES

In those hospitals where pharmacists have become clinically involved it very soon becomes apparent that the service they provide from the pharmacy is one which must be geared to meet the needs of 'their' patients and not one to which the hospital must be restricted. The Ward Pharmacy Service which extends to a stage where the needs of individual patients are of prime concern soon involves the pharmacy in work which previously the doctor or the nurse on the ward would have been left to manage in the best way they could. The pharmacist in such a service is able to identify work and procedures which, in the interests of the patient, would be better performed by staff specially trained, using proper facilities found in the pharmacy department and not on the wards in the hospital. Every clinical pharmacist could cite examples; suffice to quote only two which illustrate the point.

1. A patient is having difficulty in swallowing large delayed-release potassium chloride tablets. The nurse asks the pharmacist, because he is available, to provide a suspension (which in his absence she would have attempted to prepare herself by crushing the tablets). The pharmacist would identify the problem and suggest a more suitable dosage form, such as a flavoured solution for oral administration.

2. A paediatric surgeon initiates a parenteral feeding regimen which he wants to continue for at least 2 weeks, for a 2-week-old baby suffering from intestinal obstruction, who has undergone extensive surgery. Treatment involves a variety of solutions with additives all required in small doses to be given intravenously. The pharmacist's involvement in preparing unit dose presentations reduces the possibility of error which may result when conventional intravenous fluid containers are used and additives made in the ward.

Both these examples show the way in which the treatment for the patient can be made safer if the special expertise of the pharmaceutical services in a hospital can be called upon by doctors and nurses when required.

In the absence of 24-hour service, so often the other members of the health care team will 'make do' themselves, as it means dragging someone in to do a special job, rather than turning to the pharmacy and having their expertise available as part of the team treating the patient. Psychologically there is a deterrent to asking someone to come in and do a job if by alternative means one can 'make do', even recognising that it may not be the ideal.

The case for out-of-hours services

Work undertaken outside normal hours is an extension of those duties routinely carried out during the day. The distribution of workload in hospitals is such that the majority of work arises during the day, but it must be remembered that acute admissions account for a large proportion of hospital work and these are fairly evenly spread throughout the 24 hours of a day. Those that arrive outside normal daytime hours require the same attention as those arriving during office hours. In some ways the need is greater outside normal hours as these cases are treated by junior medical staff who would value the support which a pharmacist could provide.

Dispensing

In busy general hospitals the Accident and Emergency Department is seeing patients at all hours of the day and night (many of these require drug treatment)—one can argue that the Casualty Officer can give a patient a supply of medication, which has been prepackaged and labelled, from an emergency cupboard; on the other hand, when is pharmacy and the pharmacist necessary and when just a luxury that can be done without? It is very difficult to understand how the pharmacist can argue that certain procedures require his expertise from 9.00 a.m. to 5.30 p.m. Monday to Friday and 9.00 a.m. to 1.00 p.m. on Saturday while at all other times a doctor or nurse is capable of performing them. It is as well to remember that the pharmacy hours in the majority of hospitals are only some 25% of the total 168 hours in a week.

Intravenous additives

Addition of drugs to intravenous fluids is a procedure which has received a great deal of attention in recent years (see Chapter 10). An intravenous additive service has many direct benefits to the pharmacist and the other members of the team. When involved in presenting intravenous fluids with additives the pharmacist is soon brought into the discussion of therapy and, especially in paediatrics, the preparation of solutions not commercially available. This contact can so easily be the basis for the pharmacist's wider acceptance into the discussion of treatment by the therapeutic team.

Drug information

The provision of drug information has become an important aspect of modern hospital pharmacy practice and recognised as such in the Noel Hall report. Like intravenous additives, this service must be continually available to be most effective. As with additive programmes the provision of drug information soon commits the pharmacist to a greater concern for the individual patient and leads to clinical pharmacy. Information services along with the other aspects of pharmacy service represent reason enough for a pharmacist to be available at all times, certainly in the very large hospitals of each Area or District within the reorganised National Health Service.

Work load

Table 3.1 shows the work undertaken in the pharmacy of the General Infirmary at Leeds outside normal working hours (8.45 a.m. to 6.00 p.m. 7 days per week) for a 12-month period.

Table 3.1 Work undertaken in Leeds General
Infirmary outside normal working hours in a
12-month period

Task	No.
Outpatient prescriptions	3276
Inpatient prescriptions	9950
Calls to Poisons Information Bureau	2163
Intravenous additives	3824
	19213
Calls for service after midnight	1498 (7.8%)

Although the number of items of service provided vary considerably from one night to another over a period of a year these figures are fairly constant and certainly do not indicate any increasing demand or abuse of the service. Calls for service after midnight are approximately 8% of the total and are mainly calls to the Poisons Information Bureau or for unstable intravenous additives.

Advantages of a 24-hour service

1.   The pharmacy service is recognised by other members of the *team* as 'caring' about their patients and also their colleagues; accepting its share of responsibility for ensuring that standards of care are maintained irrespective of what time of day or night they are provided.
2.   The pharmacy can be consistent in its advice (e.g. intravenous additives *always* performed in the pharmacy).
3.   Available to operate services which otherwise it would have to decline (e.g. Poisons Information Bureau).
4.   Greater security on the premises when someone is working compared with the 'lock up' department.
5.   Pharmacy staff relieved from on call duties at home, which can become a burden for staff in large hospitals.
6.   Opportunity for the service to develop into 'clinical pharmacy' where the needs of individual patients become very important.
7.   Provides an opportunity for the young pharmacist to gain extensive experience and insight into the operation of a hospital and its various systems, by being 'around' in the 'quiet' hours.

Difficulties

These are considerable because the majority of pharmacists have been conditioned during their training to expect a job involving at worst shop hours of 9.00 a.m. to 6.30 p.m. 6 days a week, probably with a half-day holiday each week. The major problem is therefore convincing pharmacists that hospital practice requires this kind of commitment and that it will be to their eventual advantage to have gained such experience. Abuse of the service for trivial requests is cited by some as a possible danger but to a large extent this depends upon the control which the pharmacy has on its total workload. It is possible to operate systems of pharmaceutical supplies distribution which are pharmacy controlled and in such situations the possiblity of requests for trivial supply needs are eliminated or at least reduced to a minimum. Security must always be considered, particularly as the value of drugs on the black market increases. Care must be taken to ensure that staff working alone at quiet hours are adequately protected against possible incidents; open hatchways and the use of waiting rooms inside the pharmacy should be discontinued for service at night.

Staffing

Out-of-hours service can be provided by a rota of staff, either specifically responsible for the service or by a group of day staff who are available on rotation resident in the hospital. The hours to be staffed are large, approximately 6.00 p.m. to 9.00 a.m. for 7 days or 105 hours each week. However, in Leeds, a group of three pharmacists each working 39 hours a week can provide a service, with cover for holidays, for this 1200-bed teaching group of hospitals. This should apply to all similar groups providing that the geographical structure is suitable.

Communications

In a department providing a 24-hour pharmacy service although one individual may be responsible for the patient services pharmacy in a management sense, a number of pharmacists will be involved in a rota of duties both daytime during the 7 days of the week and at night. It is therefore essential that a procedure is devised to ensure that there is a proper handover between one period of duty and another. In Leeds it is found satisfactory to have half an hour overlap between the day staff and night staff both in the morning and in the evening. This provides the opportunity for the pharmacists involved to communicate any necessary information. As staff will often be working alone and required to cover a whole range of services it is necessary to ensure that a file of resource material is available on unusual items. A newsletter recording such information as the taking into stock of new products, resiting of materials in a store, announcement of a new clinical trial, amendments to operating procedures and other matters of importance can be published regularly. As some pharmacists may for long periods work nights only it is essential to arrange departmental meetings on a regular monthly basis, when all staff can attend and discuss the operation and development of the service. Such meetings can serve an educational purpose by including a topic for presentation and discussion.

The future

As clinical pharmacy is introduced into hospitals the need for such services will become more evident and in time much easier to justify for, as the pharmacist becomes more involved with direct patient care, the need for him to be around will become more readily accepted. In these situations it will be necessary to extend the pharmacy service hours.

With the reorganisation of the National Health Service and the integration of services it may be in the future that the hospital pharmaceutical services could be the centre from which the general public obtain its emergency pharmacy service. It is no longer economical for general practice pharmacists to provide such a service, but the general public should have the benefit of a pharmacist's expertise in providing medications at all times.

FURTHER READING

DEPARTMENT OF HEALTH AND SOCIAL SECURITY (1970) *Guide to Good Practices in Hospital Administration.* Management Services (NHS) Report 1. HMSO, London.

DEPARTMENT OF HEALTH AND SOCIAL SECURITY (1971) *The Organisation and Work of Hospital Pharmaceutical Departments.* Management Services (NHS) Report 3. HMSO, London.

DEPARTMENT OF HEALTH AND SOCIAL SECURITY (1973) *Hospital Building Note 29 (Pharmaceutical Dept).* HMSO, London.

DEPARTMENT OF HEALTH AND SOCIAL SECURITY (1975) *Health Equipment Note 29 (Pharmaceutical Dept).* HMSO, London.

HASSAN W. E. (1973) *Hospital Pharmacy.* Lea & Febiger, Philadelphia.

4
Education and training

P. R. NOYCE

Traditionally, in the United Kingdom, Schools of Pharmacy have been the main organising bodies for education and training in pharmacy. The Pharmaceutical Society of Great Britain (PSGB) relinquished its examining responsibility in 1970 and subsequently has not been intimately involved in the education and training of pharmacists. It does, however, formally monitor and approve undergraduate courses through its system of quinquennial inspections of colleges and universities and is establishing a forum for the continuing education of all pharmacists through the Regional Postgraduate Education Committees. The professional society is also the registration body and as such potentially has considerable influence over the nature of the preregistration period. Currently it merely requires that a graduate should obtain experience in various aspects of pharmacy practice, in this case, in hospital. If pharmacy departments can provide the required range of experience, then they are deemed suitable for preregistration purposes. The Department of Health and Social Security (DHSS) is unlikely to provide general advice or guidelines on the education and training of hospital pharmaceutical staff. Nonetheless, postgraduate education and training of pharmacists could successfully be organised on a national basis as undertaken in Sweden by Apoteksbolaget, the National Corporation of Swedish Pharmacies (Brånstad 1977).

PHARMACY BACCALAUREATE IN PERSPECTIVE

The design of undergraduate courses is the province of pharmacy teachers rather than pharmacy practitioners, but the following points are intended as a perspective:

1. Hospital pharmacists within their professional activities are expected to undertake duties for which they have received no formal training, for example, developing microbiological quality control programmes, providing evaluated information on medicines and drugs, or establishing prepacking units. Their lack of relevant knowledge and skills also hinders them from developing other appropriate functions, (e.g. provision of therapeutic advice in specialist clinical areas such as renal units and paediatrics, or patient counselling).

47

2.   The undergraduate course is essentially didactic and this is followed abruptly by an experiential phase of training during the preregistration year. Learning in these two situations is in stark contrast, for on the one hand it is rigidly structured and assessed, whilst on the other there is minimal organisation of learning and no assessment. In the current process of pharmacy education and training, the student has to accommodate these differences alone, for neither the practising pharmacist nor the academic tutor is familiar with both learning situations. Not suprisingly, the student frequently becomes disorientated and disillusioned.

Medical undergraduates gradually move from the classroom atmosphere of their preclinical years to the ward experience of their 'house' appointments. In nurse training, periods of didactic and experiential training alternate. Thus in both professions, the academic and professional contents are integral parts of the students' basic education and training. A similar integration is achieved in the pharmacy sandwich course organised by Bradford University, in which the preregistration year is incorporated into the undergraduate course to give two 6-month periods of vocational experience in the second and fourth years respectively.

3.   There is continuing debate about the desired contents of the undergraduate course (Baker 1976; Turner 1977) with the Schools of Pharmacy tending to favour a course in pharmaceutical sciences, whilst the profession needs the pharmacy baccalaureate to be a foundation for vocational training. There is confusion about what this divergence of opinion means in reality, for some pharmacy teachers are concerned that the desired changes in the course would be so incisive as to denigrate the academic status of the course, whilst others sincerely believe that the same syllabus can meet both aims. The change in orientation and emphasis required by the profession would mean restructuring parts of the course, particularly the third year, and the introduction of new material, but much of the course substance would remain substantially unchanged.

4. It is unrealistic to expect the undergraduate course to provide other than basic pharmaceutical knowledge and skills. A bachelor degree should be viewed as an educational foundation rather than an education endpoint in itself. Programmes of postgraduate education and training are necessary for hospital pharmacists to meet their professional commitments competently. These could either be university based as with current MSc courses, or professionally based, as are those of the medical colleges of practice.

Staff in training grades (student pharmacy technicians and preregistration pharmacists) should undergo a scheme of structured in-service training which integrates with the academic component of their studies. For such in-service programmes to be complete, work experience needs to be supplemented with off-the-job seminars, study days and courses. Indeed, some see the preregistration year as a 'fourth' year of basic education and training in which vocational material could be taught. The practicalities of the situation dictate otherwise; for except in one or two Regions that have succeeded in creating posts for student pharmacy technicians and preregistration pharmacists which are supernumerary to establishment, staff employed in training grades have a full service commitment. In most circumstances, training posts have been created from within the staff establishment agreed as necessary to meet the service commitment of a particular department and no administrative recognition is given to a department's training commitments. Thus training interests may be compromised by service demands and this is particularly so in teaching hospitals where preregistration pharmacists form a significant component of the staff complement.

Although in the interests of training, it would be sensible to create supernumerary training posts, this would undoubtedly lead to a drastic reduction in the number of trainees employed. Indeed, solely on the basis of manpower requirements, the current number of training posts within the hospital pharmaceutical service cannot be justified.

CAREER AND DEVELOPMENT

A complete metamorphosis occurs in the nature of work on moving up the promotional ladder from Preregistration Pharmacist to Regional Pharmaceutical Officer. This means that if one attains the grade of Pharmaceutical Officer the job performed is totally different from that when one joined the service as a Preregistration Pharmacist, in terms of nature of work, work cycle and environment. It also means that the education and training received for one's original job becomes less applicable and more relevant knowledge and skill have to be acquired. Fig. 4.1 demonstrates the faculties required of pharmacists at different levels within the service.

Whenever there is a change in the nature of a job, learning must occur for the incumbent to perform his new job competently. The greater the change, the more learning needed and undoubtedly the greatest change occurs in the preregistration year in gaining knowledge and skills of a professional/technical nature. In moving from Pharmacist to Principal Pharmacist grade, there is a gradual consolidation of one's professional/technical knowledge and skills, compounded by experience. Concomitantly, there is a need to develop and strengthen one's management abilities, for at Principal level, management constitutes a significant part of one's work. At Pharmaceutical Officer level one becomes, in the main, detached from 'bench' activities and becomes absorbed in duties of an administrative and managerial nature. This is reflected, in the diagram, by the gradient of the interface between technical and managerial components in moving from Principal Pharmacist to Area Pharmaceutical Officer.

The time between registration and retirement is generally not less than

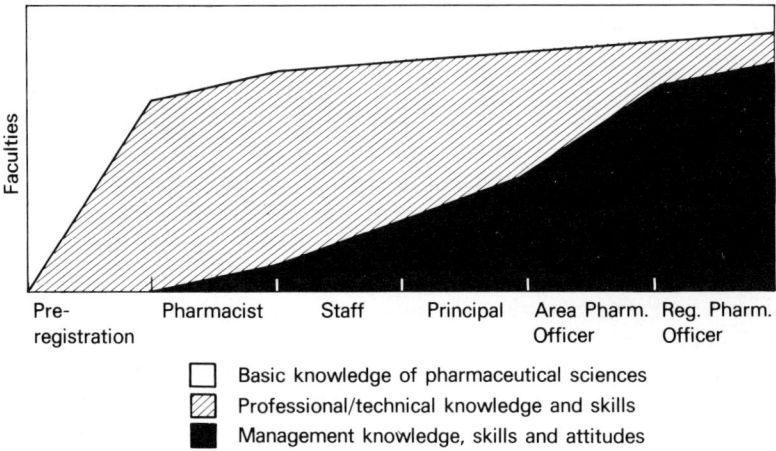

Fig. 4.1   Knowledge and skills (faculties) required of pharmacists at different levels within the Health Service.

30 years and within this period considerable changes will occur in the therapeutic management of patients, professional practices, and available drugs, equipment and techniques. We work in a continually dynamic environment in which aims and priorities constantly change. Thus there is a need to maintain a programme of continuing education simply to remain abreast of the current scene.

CONCEPTS OF EDUCATION AND TRAINING

Learning is a complex process which varies with the individual, his innate skills and stage of development, the nature and substance of what is to be learned and the reason for learning. In hospital pharmacy, interest in learning is limited to that which is necessary for pharmaceutical staff to perform their duties competently. The formal devices of education and training are used to assist the process. Education is concerned with the development of fundamental understanding through the learning of principles, concepts and facts. Training is a conditioning process through which skills are learned. Practice or experience reinforces training.

Concepts related to 'learning' may be more comprehensively explored through the model of learning to drive a car. The first stage in learning to drive a car is an *educational* one, since there is a need to know that the accelerator or throttle increases the speed of the vehicle and the brake slows or stops the car. More difficult concepts that must be grasped are an understanding of the clutch mechanism and the principle of gears. When these principles are mastered, the pupil understands the fundamentals of driving but is not in any demonstrable way nearer to being able to drive the car than before the learning process began. A caricature of these situations is expressed in quips about graduates such as 'knows all the theory, but hasn't a clue about what to do in practice'. In a similar vein, a sound understanding of various management theories does not necessarily confirm good management nor does an appreciation of systems such as the planning cycle or functional budgeting, alone, ensure that one can plan or budget effectively. Knowledge without the skill to apply it is worthless in terms of performance!

Education, however, is fundamental in nature and returning to our driving pupil, once he understands the principles of throttle, brake, clutch and gears, he will then appreciate the basic operation of all other machines which incorporate these features, without further learning.

The next stage in learning to drive a car is a *training* process in which the pupil must learn to recognise and acquire the skills necessary to control the vehicle (e.g. steering, speed control, clutch control and changing gear). Although the driving instructor provides guidance, these skills can only be acquired through actually attempting the various operations. Skills cannot be learned simply by having processes explained or demonstrated, but necessitate *experience* of appropriate situations.

'*Practice* makes perfect' is probably an exaggeration in reality, either due to lack of commitment, or inability to refine skills sufficiently. Practice, however, is an important factor in developing any skills, even though some people are more gifted than others. The contribution that practice makes is readily recognised when learning to speak a foreign language or play a musical instrument. Indeed, whilst learning to drive, the bulk of one's lessons is occupied in practising new techniques. Conversely, if one fails to use or practice an acquired skill, then one loses the 'knack' or becomes 'rusty'.

Once the basic skills of driving have been acquired, the pupil is introduced to more complex manœuvres which incorporate these skills (e.g. reversing around corners). When these composite skills are mastered, the success of the learning process in attaining its aims is assessed by means of a Driving Test in which the candidate's *competence* is judged against criteria considered to be in keeping with an acceptable level of efficiency and safety.

Only after a considerable amount of driving experience subsequent to formal learning does one feel *confident* to drive and the processes involved become second nature. After reaching this stage, one's performance can still be adversely affected by unfamiliar situations, such as driving abroad or in different vehicles. Similarly, the operational effectiveness of experienced managers can be affected by changes in organisation and systems.

The process of teaching a person to drive a car is fairly simple in training terms compared with, for example, training a pharmaceutical officer to manage an area pharmaceutical service. Thus a rigidly structured approach known as instructor training can be used, which involves the instructor in explaining principles, demonstrating techniques, providing guidance and encouragement to pupils whilst developing skills, and setting criteria for, and providing feedback on, performance. Obviously for developing more intricate skills, particularly behavioural skills, more complex, flexible and subtle training methods are necessary. In general, the appropriate method of training is largely determined by the nature of the skills required, although much training in hospital pharmacy occurs by default, in 'sitting by Nellie' situations. The main disadvantage from the aspect of the student's ultimate performance is that he adopts the standards and practices of 'Nellie' whether these represent a satisfactory level of performance or not.

The value of formal training programmes may be called into question when many people are seen to operate effectively without training, merely by harnessing their natural skills and learning through the experience of 'trial and error'. In this situation, one's competence is a product of one's cognitive powers and the faculty to develop appropriate skills. If training is considered as a process of supervised exposure to concentrated experience, then, whatever one's propensities, training enhances learning efficiency.

At this stage, the following generalisations can be made about learning and its processes:

1.   Learning is a complex process; style and speed vary individually and with circumstance.
2.   Education is a process for developing knowledge whilst training is a vehicle for developing skills.
3.   Skills can only be acquired through appropriate experience and adequate practice.
4.   Training techniques vary with the skills to be learned.
5.   Training is not an essential prerequisite of effective performance, but is an efficient aid to development.

EDUCATIONAL AND TRAINING PROGRAMMES

Fig. 4.2 illustrates the stages involved in organising effective learning programmes.

Most educational/training schemes or events for pharmaceutical staff do not follow this rational process and are only active at the second and fourth stages of design and implementation. If stage one is omitted, then inappropriate or unnecessary learning can result, so compromising the contribution which education and training can make to performance. Terminal evaluation of courses is not uncommon, but the merit of this as an assessment of effect on performance is doubtful. Validation is generally non-existent. Although there is little justification in running schemes or events that are not of proven worth, the devising of practical parameters for measuring the value of much education and training is no easy task. Pharmacy, however, could take leads

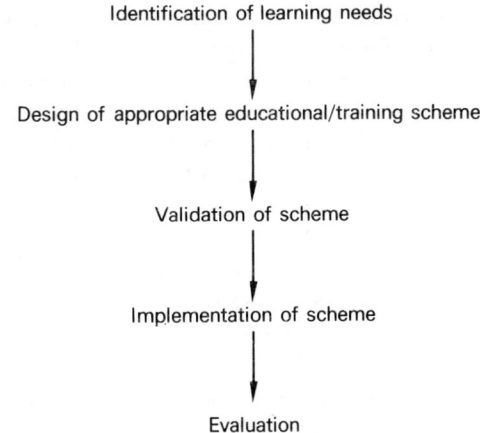

Identification of learning needs

Design of appropriate educational/training scheme

Validation of scheme

Implementation of scheme

Evaluation

Fig. 4.2 Stages in organising effective learning programmes.

from the work of Freeman and Byrne (1976) on assessment of vocational training.

Education and training of hospital pharmaceutical staff may be broadly subdivided into in-service training and continuing education. Under in-service training, induction training, professional training and management education and training are considered in turn.

In-service training

The term in-service training covers all job-related education and training whether this be undertaken on or off the job. For pharmaceutical staff the two major areas of in-service training comprise professional training and management training. Formal courses of education leading to academic awards are not usually included under the title of in-service training, even though they may be undertaken during worktime and sponsored by the employing Health Authority. However, the complete education and training programme for student pharmacy technicians will be considered in this section, for convenience.

The crux of in-service training is unquestionably the on-the-job component, which involves learning about work at work. A good on-the-job training scheme requires the provision of a wide range of relevant experience, high standards of work and diligent coaching. Many will argue over the semantics of 'on-the-job training' versus 'experience'. The basis of on-the-job training is structured experience. An on-the-job training programme should provide the trainee with the widest relevant experience possible and his programme of work and progress should be closely supervised. If the trainee is considered simply as another 'pair of hands', his range of experience will probably be limited and the potential for learning consequently suffers. Service demands easily and effectively smother training interests unless prevented, and experience, as a vehicle for learning, can range from very valuable to practically worthless, if left uncontrolled. Like other teaching/training processes, on-the-job training should have definite aims and be organised in such a way that these are achieved. At present the quality of in-service training in hospital pharmacy is quite variable, although rotational schemes of work are mandatory for preregistration pharmacists, common for student pharmacy technicians, and are being increasingly adopted for pharmacists. Perhaps the development of training 'packages' for in-service schemes would be helpful. These should specify aims, provide guidelines and standards for organising schemes and incorporate some training aids, such as a series of overhead slides to demonstrate a process.

Induction training

Induction schemes should be devised for all staff, but are particularly important for unskilled workers. Although pharmacy assistants are expected to perform only straightforward tasks, they do need to be familiar with the work situation in order for them to work efficiently and safely. Indeed, because of their general unfamiliarity with pharmacy, they require more comprehensive induction programmes than most other pharmaceutical staff. A list of aims for the induction of pharmacy assistants is proposed and lesser variants will be applicable to other grades of staff. Induction programmes for pharmacy assistants should:

1. Explain the various functions of hospital pharmacy and how these are executed in a particular department.
2. Explain their duties, responsibilities and restrictions, the duties of those with whom they work and how they relate to other personnel.
3. Identify the 'boss'.
4. Make them aware of the practices in that department with respect to checking, ordering, meeting requests from wards etc.
5. Provide basic information on the materials to be handled including a simple legal classification of medicines in order that they appreciate the different processes involved in handling various preparations.
6. Provide instruction in the various processes in which they will be involved (e.g. replenishing ward boxes, prepacking and cleaning of equipment).
7. Familiarise them with procedures for safe working, including the safe handling of materials and operation of machinery.

If duties are changed, practices or processes altered, or new machinery installed, then reorientation training needs to be provided.

Professional training

Student pharmacy technicians

Currently there are two recognised examining bodies for pharmacy technicians, the City and Guilds of London Institute and The Society of Apothecaries of London. The qualifications awarded are Dispensing Technician's and Pharmacy Technician's Certificates respectively. The syllabuses and modes of examination closely concur. The practical advantage of City and Guilds examination to most students is that they may sit the examination at local centres whereas the Dispensing examination for the Society of Apothecaries can be taken only at Apothecaries Hall in London. Both examining bodies require that student pharmacy technicians undergo a formal course of education and training which is supplemented by a 2-year period of practical experience under the supervision of a pharmacist. The curriculum demands a minimum of 360 hours of study which is usually accommodated by a local technical college on a day-release basis over 2 years.

The college-based syllabus is common for both student pharmacy technicians undergoing training in retail and hospital pharmacy and comprises elementary aspects of pharmaceutics, physiology and pharmacology, a working knowledge of pharmaceutical legislation, and training in the manipulative skills of dispensing. The minimum entry requirement to the 2-year course is three GCE 'O' levels although some technical colleges do provide a year's preliminary course for those who have not reached this entry requirement. Certificate candidates sit two theory papers, one covering pharmaceutical topics and the other physiology and pharmacology. A practical dispensing examination is also taken which has an oral component. Under the aegis of the West Midlands Regional Health Authority, an advanced course for pharmacy technicians is run in Birmingham, which is a further 2 years' part-time study.

Technician education and training in all fields is under rigorous review. In 1973, the Technician Education Council (TEC) was instituted with a view to establishing a common framework for the education and training for all technicians. TEC, unlike City and Guilds and the Society of Apothecaries, is not an examining, but a validating body. It does not therefore assess individual students but in order for students to be awarded a TEC qualification they must have undergone a course of study which has been approved and moderated by TEC.

Within the TEC framework, each programme of study is based upon defined educational objectives and is subdivided into a number of units of study, each with its own objectives. Each unit comprises 60–75 hours' tuition and has a designated level (I, II, III). Some units, for example physiology, are common to several courses of study. For entry to level I units, a student is required to have attained an acceptable level in agreed subjects, probably at the level of CSE grade III. For entry to a level II unit, a student must have either satisfactorily completed an appropriate unit at level I or attained an appropriate GCE 'O' level or CSE grade I subject. Entry to level III units is usually through appropriate level II units. TEC provides for four levels of qualification, but in the case of pharmacy technicians, the most elementary (certificate) level will be adequate for most purposes. A TEC certificate course has a minimum of twelve units of study, which is roughly equivalent to 900 hours of tuition, with not less than two level III units and not more than five level I units. Since most level I units appropriate to a pharmacy technician course are basic sciences, exemption from these can be gained through the possession of the appropriate GCE 'O' levels. Thus with an entry requirement of five GCE 'O' levels, a pharmacy technicians' certificate programme could be reduced to 600 hours of tuition which could be accommodated, as now, on a 2-year day-release basis. General studies occupy 90 hours of this study period, and unlike City and Guilds, is a compulsory subject within TEC programmes. Another difference is that study undertaken at work is admissible and thus practical units of study, such as dispensing techniques, could be accommodated outside college time. All units would, of course, be subject to a common assessment procedure.

A potential obstacle to the inclusion of pharmacy technicians within the TEC system is the level of the TEC certificate. This is roughly equivalent to the Ordinary National Certificate (ONC) which is significantly above the level of the present pharmacy technicians' syllabus. However, in Scotland, a pharmacy technician's course has already been accommodated within the framework of the Scottish Technical Education Council.

Programmes of work rotation through the various sections of a hospital pharmacy department are arranged for most student pharmacy technicians, although, unfortunately, the experience of some is limited to a specialist hospital or a single section. As mentioned earlier, experience is a vague term and unless structured, leaves the student's learning to chance. Both City and Guilds and Society of Apothecaries whilst providing syllabuses, do not offer guidelines for students' practical experience. At present there are no clear aims for the experiential part of a pharmacy technician's training. If pharmacy technicians do come within the scope of TEC, then practice-based training would be scrutinised if it formed a contribution to the formal curriculum.

In a recent survey undertaken by the author, most student pharmacy technicians considered that although there was someone at work whom they could ask about material that they did not understand, there was a total absence of practice-based 'tutors'. Many supervising pharmacists supported their students by checking their understanding of college lessons but none had devised on-the-job training programmes. Perhaps, again, the provision of training packages which state aims, provide guidelines and include training aids for supervising pharmacists would improve the situation. Recently, Ameer and Johnson (1977) have demonstrated the value of adopting a rational approach to the in-service training of pharmacy technicians.

Supervising pharmacists may not feel any identity with the teaching staff of the local college and an integrated programme of learning necessitates a close liaison between college and hospital. This problem has been overcome in some Regions where the Health Authority's Education Pharmacist acts as an internal tutor and also organises the college-based course. A single training manual is provided in which exercises undertaken at college alternate with those done at work. This undoubtedly helps students to relate their formal education and training to practice.

Preregistration pharmacists

In the Pharmaceutical Society's publication of 1972 providing guidance on the nature and organisation of the preregistration period, reference is made to preregistration experience' and the words 'education' and 'training' are tactfully avoided. The notes of guidance applicable to hospitals state that 'the graduate should be given a comprehensive experience of all aspects of hospital pharmacy'. They further state that 'the graduate should be fully integrated into the work of the pharmacy department and should gain experience in the provision of a full hospital pharmaceutical service, including dispensing, ward supplies, small and large-scale manufacture of sterile and non-sterile products, the ordering, storage and supply of drugs, medicinal gases and other medical supplies, professional contacts with allied professions and patients, the advisory service on the action and uses of drugs and medicines, and administration and staff control'. Other requirements are that the department should 'be of adequate size for the provision of a comprehensive service' and 'contain such equipment as to enable the provision of a comprehensive pharmaceutical service'. Although these statements give guidance on the areas of work to which a graduate should be exposed during his period of preregistration experience, they provide no indication of what the preregistration pharmacist is expected to learn during this period. If the preregistration period is without assessable learning objectives, then there is little probability, let alone guarantee, that graduates at the point of registration who have undertaken their year's experience in hospital pharmacy, will have common competencies. At present, the 'responsible pharmacist' has to rely on his subjective, if experienced, professional discretion in deciding whether a graduate at the end of his preregistration period is suitable for admission to the register of pharmaceutical chemists. No objective criteria are provided for the 'responsible pharmacist', upon which to judge whether a candidate has appropriate and sufficient knowledge and skills to practise competently as a pharmacist.

For preregistration experience to be established on a rational basis requires the setting of appropriate and definite aims and devising realistic means of assessment. The starting point in this process is the agreement of a list of competencies expected of a pharmacist at the point of registration. An appropriate mode of assessment then has to be devised and guidelines prepared on the education, training and experience necessary during the preregistration period for candidates to attain the designated competencies prior to registration. Undoubtedly, the total scheme would be a substantial albeit worthwhile, undertaking, but fortitude and guidance may be taken from a successful attempt in California (Day 1975).

The development of a preregistration period along the lines discussed would probably entail periods of off-the-job training and the routine monitoring of preregistration pharmacists. It would also require 'responsible pharmacists' to develop some expertise in in-service training. Any scheme must accommodate the various situations in which graduates undertake their preregistation experience: as a single graduate in a District General Hospital; as one of several graduates in a teaching hospital; as a participant in an Area/Regional supernumerary scheme or as a sandwich course student.

What can graduates currently expect from preregistration experience in hospital pharmacy? Unfortunately there are still preregistration graduates in situations where, if not actually considered as, they are certainly treated as, 'another pair of hands'. Whether this is due to pressure from service commitments; a sincere belief that experience, whatever the nature and level, is what the preregistration graduate most needs at this stage of his career; or whether the 'responsible pharmacist' has no clear perspective of what a student needs to learn during his preregistration period or indeed how to instruct him, is open to question. For most students there are a series of study days arranged during the year either at Area or Regional level on therapeutic subjects, aspects of hospital pharmacy practice, and management topics. There may also be visits to departments/centres of interest (e.g. pathology or blood transfusion). Some hospitals with several students, and many Areas, organise tutorials on a weekly or fortnightly basis, at which a similar range of topics are covered. The greater frequency, however, allows more subjects to be considered in greater depth. (An Area preregistration scheme has been described recently by Longshaw and Skews 1977.) Where preregistration pharmacists are supernumerary, there are greater opportunities for off-the-job education and training and in one Region approximately 25 days of formal study are provided. These comprise a 3-day induction course, a 1-week practice course, a 1-week clinical pharmacy course, three 2-day seminars on specialised aspects of hospital pharmacy practice, three 1-day visits and a 2-day education course. Some hospitals provide the opportunity during the preregistration period for graduates to familiarise themselves with the wide area of drug usage, through visits and secondments to wards, outpatient clinics and theatres.

Projects are frequently allocated to preregistration pharmacists and undoubtedly are of interest. Where they relate to real problems, they do provide a valuable opportunity for preregistration pharmacists to 'cut their teeth' on real situations. However, if projects are ritually allocated, then, from a training viewpoint, they probably do little more than reinforce the principles of scientific method inculcated at undergraduate level.

Although work experience needs to be supplemented by off-the-job education and training, the most significant feature of the preregistration period is the quality of work experience. In this there is considerable variation between different hospitals and frequently it is a sad reflection of the differences in level of service. The point may be taken from a survey in which 20% of women and over 30% of men considered that they had not undergone a 'planned programme of experience' (Johnson 1977) during their preregistration period.

Although there are no official guidelines for assessment of performance during the preregistration year, some hospitals do already routinely review a graduate's progress at regular intervals during the preregistration period, both through written appraisal and interview. Others maintain check lists to ensure that students have acquired experience in the processes and procedures deemed necessary.

Qualified staff

At the point of qualification in the case of pharmacy technicians, and registration in the case of pharmacists, staff are deemed to have acquired a level of competence necessary to practise. From this point onwards, staff are responsible for their professional actions, but need to consolidate their experience and gain professional confidence before becoming proficient in their vocation. In various skilled trades, the period of apprenticeship is traditionally followed by a spell as an improver or journeyman, before recognition as a skilled tradesman is achieved. Newly qualified staff can be considered in the improver category and indeed the working party on postgraduate education and training (Pharmaceutical Society of Great Britain 1975) recommended a 6-month 'period of acclimatisation' immediately after registration during which a pharmacist would be subject to a 'degree of supervision'. Unfortunately, the low level of remuneration that existed in hospital pharmacy until recently, led to an erosion of the basic grade. More propitious circumstances mean that sufficient time is now spent at the pharmacist grade for this to provide a meaningful period of in-service training. Some large hospitals have adopted rotational schemes of work for staff at this level, which provide periods of experience varying from 3 to 6 months, in the various branches of hospital pharmacy. The experience differs from that at preregistration level, for apart from being longer, the level of involvement is at decision making and problem solving rather than familiarising oneself with processes.

During the evolution of the newer support specialities of quality control, drug information and radiopharmaceutical preparation, little provision has been made for on-the-job training. Specialist staff are still being appointed, frequently in situations of professional isolation, with merely the acquaintance of preregistration experience in the specialty. This is due to a dearth of specialist posts at pharmacist grade which would provide the necessary opportunities for young pharmacists to develop alongside experienced specialists.

Off-the-job support for learning is variable. Courses are organised by Schools of Pharmacy on radiopharmaceuticals and aspects of quality control. The Hospital Engineering Centre at Falfield runs joint courses for pharmacists and engineers on such topics as steriliser maintenance and piped medical gases. Meanwhile, the information specialists have implemented their own off-the-job education and training programmes for staff with information responsibilities. One School of Pharmacy provides tutorial support programmes for small groups of pharmacists who are developing clinical pharmacy services in nearby hospitals. In the circumstances, much work needs to be done in designing rational in-service training programmes for qualified staff in all aspects of hospital pharmacy.

Management education and training

Management is a vast subject, much larger than pharmacy. It is also quite different in nature, for pharmacy is rooted in 'hard' sciences whereas much of the practice of management is founded on 'softer' behavioural sciences. Many people consider management to be a matter of common sense and that managers are born, not made. Some folk obviously have a natural aptitude for man management, but this does not mean, by implication, that others cannot acquire the skills of management. Perhaps the DHSS (1974) memorandum puts the situation in perspective best: 'Management is not a distinct body of knowledge that can be learnt like a discrete academic subject. Whilst drawing on a wide range of theory for its concept and techniques, the real meaning of management is not learned until it is experienced by actually managing.'

As with any area of performance, the learning of management can be subdivided into knowledge and skills components. The knowledge required is of organisational structures, systems, procedures and practices. The relevant skills are behavioural or intellectual in nature (e.g. planning, negotiating and monitoring). Pharmacists readily recognise that knowledge is useless without technical skills but generally are less aware that the same principle applies in management with respect to behavioural skills.

In the NHS, management education and training have been organised at three levels: first-line or supervisory level, second-line or middle-management level and senior management level. First- and second-line management education and training are organised at a local level, either by NHS training staff based at Region/Area/District level or, on an agency basis, by colleges of further education. Conventionally, first-line management courses are 3 weeks in duration and middle management, 2 weeks. The approach and course contents vary considerably and within the North West Thames Region alone, there are five different agents, each with their own style, providing training at supervisory and middle-management levels.

There are three general approaches to the management education and training of NHS senior managers, all using various academic institutions. The most common is the senior management development course which is designed specifically for recently appointed NHS officers. Such courses are run at King's Fund College, Manchester University, Birmingham University and Nuffield Centre, Leeds. These courses are 4–6 weeks in length and at Birmingham and Leeds are organised on a modular basis. Experienced senior managers' courses are organised at Leicester Polytechnic and Leeds for NHS managers who have been in post for longer than 3 years. These courses are shorter than development courses but modular in nature. For senior managers who are likely to benefit from the experience, the DHSS sponsors several places annually on multiprofessional courses run at the London and Manchester Business Schools and the Staff College, Henley.

First-line courses cover such topics as: organisation and control of work and allocation of duties; deployment of staff; techniques for securing and maintaining discipline; and effective utilisation of local resources. They are intended to accommodate the needs of supervisory staff. Of all the disciplines in the NHS, nursing has the largest number of managers, and therefore these courses are primarily aimed at Staff Nurses and Sisters. Many first-line courses are limited to nurses.

Second-line management courses are concerned with the education and training of middle managers. The following list provides a selection of topics covered at this level: interviewing and selection of personnel; presentation of information; group decision making and problem solving; medium-term planning, forecasting and programming of workload; and budgeting and cost control.

Middle-management courses are multidisciplinary, but generally there is a preponderance of nurses in the course membership.

In principle, this approach to the training of junior and middle managers would seem reasonable, but in practice is less than ideal for training pharmacy managers for several reasons:

1. For nurses, the General Nursing Council encourages the introduction of management principles to nurses undergoing training and, as mentioned, supervisory courses are organised for Staff Nurses and Sisters. Although management topics are included in some pharmacy undergraduate courses, for most pharmacists, their first taste of management training is at middle-management level, by which time the material is unpalatable.

2. Selection for courses is often based on status rather than the management content of the job. Pharmacy is not a labour-intensive discipline when compared with nursing, domestic services or catering and Principal Pharmacists are, in general, more appropriate candidates for middle-management courses than the Staff Pharmacists who so often attend.

3. Pharmacists can experience difficulty in the 'transfer' of material to their own work particularly if courses concentrate on unfamiliar work areas such as nursing.

4.   The superiors of many of the course participants are unfamiliar with the process of management training and little benefit has resulted from some courses because participants are unable to apply the principles or skills learnt when they return to work.

Nowadays there is a move away from the prescribed format for first-line and second-line management courses. In the new approach, there is a common multidisciplinary foundation course of 1–2 weeks' duration and this is followed by a number of modules, usually of 2–6 days' duration. Each module is devoted to a particular topic, such as interviewing and selection, employment legislation and industrial relations, budgetary control or staff development. This flexible approach allows superiors to select modules which are appropriate to the needs of individual staff, rather than their having to attend a course of which only a part is relevant.

Management education and training should incorporate the following principles according to a DHSS (1974) memorandum and as such should be:

1.   Comprehensive. This commends that the education and training needs of managers in particular disciplines should be specifically accommodated, in addition to those needs common to all NHS managers. The schemes devised for these two situations should obviously be complementary.

2.   Integrated with work. Managers cannot be solely trained through the isolated experience of a management course: the process begins and continues away from the classroom at the workplace.

3.   Progressive. Management training programmes should be viewed as episodes in a continuing development process.

4.   Collaborative. The process of management training should not be limited to trainee and trainer but involve the trainee's 'boss', others who affect the trainee's role and the parent organisation.

5.   Related to organisation needs. Management education and training should be designed to improve the trainee's performance in handling real situations within his job.

6.   Related to individual needs. Management education and training, in both substance and method, should be organised to meet individual needs. Rigidly structured courses do not meet this criterion.

7.   Monitored and evaluated. Programmes need to be assessed against real aims which are related to performance at work.

These principles emphasise that management education and training should

    a. Meet individual needs in specific situations.
    b. Be closely integrated with work experience.
    c. Involve not only the trainee but all those that have an organisational relationship with him.

For management education and training to be optimally effective, it must be part of a staff development programme which includes appraisal, coaching and counselling.

Sound selection, precourse preparation, participation of immediate superiors and postcourse review are essential ingredients of any successful formal programme for learning. A recent study (Toman 1977) of a sample of nurses who had undergone a management training programme revealed the following characteristics: 13% attended as a result of an appraisal interview; 13% were sent by their immediate superior; 45% were given precourse material and 28% reviewed the courses with their immediate superior. No wonder that 81% considered that the management course was an isolated experience, detached from the real life problems of managing hospital services!

With the implementation of the Noel Hall structure and, in close succession, the reorganisation of the NHS, senior pharmacists were appointed to posts which had no pharmaceutical precedent. Most of those appointed were formerly Chief Pharmacists or Group Chief Pharmacists and, as such, had been accustomed to the day-to-day management of hospital pharmacies.

In their new posts, senior pharmacists were expected to work at an administrative level, away from professional activity. They were introduced to management principles involving 'coordination' and 'monitoring'. Their horizons were extended to include the provision of pharmaceutical services in the community. Area Pharmacists and Pharmaceutical Officers became responsible for managing Area pharmaceutical services. This was a new level of organisation, which is particularly difficult to manage where there is no Area budget for pharmacy. In other words, the nature, scope and level of work of senior pharmacy managers has undergone a complete change from the pre-Noel Hall days. This metamorphosis of role was accompanied only by written guidance from DHSS (1972, 1973).

Organisational development does not occur simply through a change in the paper structure and organisation and the assignment of new titles. It happens through people beginning to 'live' the new jobs created in the organisation, by the understanding and adoption of new responsibilities, and learning to operate effectively in the new working environment by developing appropriate skills and relationships. In an organisation the size of the NHS, the transitional process takes several years.

Recently, a focus for senior management training has been established with the opening of the NHS Training and Studies Centre in Harrogate in 1976 (Smith 1977). A Pharmaceutical Services Workshop for Regional and Area Pharmaceutical Officers was convened there in autumn 1976 with the express intention of exploring the roles of pharmaceutical officers in depth. This Workshop developed into a 6-month role development scheme during which participants, on returning to work, developed particular aspects of their job which, as a result of their role reviews, they considered they were not performing appropriately and/or effectively. The scheme terminated in a second module in which participants reviewed, from a learning viewpoint, individual's experiences encountered in role development, explored concepts critical to their effective functioning, such as strategic planning, and agreed in general terms, the training needs of senior pharmacy managers.

From this Workshop, a national training scheme for senior pharmacy managers (Area Pharmaceutical Officers and Area Pharmacists) was evolved. This scheme, based at Harrogate, extended over a 10-month period. The first module of the scheme which was 4 days long, was devoted to the identification of individual training needs and securing commitment to a role development programme for the duration of the scheme. The design and contents of successive modules, of which there was provision for five during the 10-month training period, was decided solely on the basis of identified needs. The modules punctuated a role development programme allowing review of what was learned during the periods of intervening work experience.

This training scheme for senior pharmacy managers has been developed and organised by a team jointly comprising training staff from the Harrogate Centre and pharmacists. Thus the management training needs of pharmacy managers have been considered and accommodated specifically. Hopefully the outcome of this scheme will not only be more able senior pharmacy managers but also, within Regions, the development of rational training programmes for pharmacy middle and junior managers through the initiative and involvement of pharmaceutical officers. This does not, by implication, suggest that all management training for pharmacists should be undertaken on a single professional basis, for both uni- and multidisciplinary courses have their place. Nonetheless, it is up to pharmacy as a discipline to take the initiative with regard to management education and training within the profession.

Continuing education

The undergraduate course should only be expected to provide an educational foundation for pharmacists. To become proficient in any aspect of hospital pharmacy requires the acquisition of further knowledge. The level and nature of the knowledge to be acquired will largely determine whether appropriate and sufficient learning can be undertaken informally at work or if a formal education programme is necessary. Several universities (e.g. Aston in Birmingham, Bradford, Manchester and Strathclyde in Glasgow) have responded to the advanced education needs of hospital pharmacists by organising appropriate MSc courses, usually in close liaison with their local Health Authorities. Specialist hospital pharmacists have found that postgraduate degrees and diplomas in such subjects as chemical analysis and information science satisfy their education needs.

Having established competence to practise, one is faced with maintaining this competence. Nevertheless, most people once admitted to a profession, receive a licence to practise for life. Recently this has caused concern and a committee of enquiry has already reported on competence to practise within the medical profession (Committee of Enquiry into Competence to Practise 1976). In 1974, the Pharmaceutical Society elected a Working Party on Postgraduate Education and Training and this recommended that participation in continuing education programmes should be a requirement for continued registration (Pharmaceutical Society of Great Britain 1975). The Working Party considered that 'any profession, the members of which base their professional service on knowledge which is continually expanding and changing must embrace the philosophy that continuing education is an integral part of professional practice'. The Council of the Pharmaceutical Society, whilst acknowledging this principle, did not endorse the Working Party's proposal for mandatory continuing education.

Continuing education, like any learning strategy, should have specific aims. Houle (1974) proposed a number of goals for the continuing professional education of pharmacists:

1. To keep abreast of new knowledge required to perform responsibly.
2. To keep up with changes in the relevant basic discipline.
3. To prepare for changes in personal career from specialist to generalist or in moving from one speciality to another.
4. To retain the power to learn.

Continuing education programmes should accommodate the needs of particular student populations (e.g. the general professional needs of specialist hospital pharmacists or pharmacists qualified longer than 20 years). Indeed the DHSS (1975) encourages the organisation of courses specifically designed for married women contemplating a return to pharmacy.

Continuing education needs to be planned and organised on a rational basis. Hopefully the Regional Postgraduate Education Committees which bring the continuing education of all pharmacists under the same umbrella will foster this development; but will do so only if effectively coordinated. At present there is considerable disparity in the continuing education organised across the country, for this is largely dependent on local enthusiasm.

Most courses currently organised for contractor pharmacists cover therapeutic topics (Pharmaceutical Society of Great Britain 1977) and are organised by Schools of Pharmacy. Hospital pharmacists, whilst patronising these courses, also have Study Days and courses organised within the service. These hospital educational events cover a similar range of topics to those for contractor pharmacists, but sectional interests are also accommodated. Sometimes the specialist needs of hospital pharmacists are met through the resources of Schools of Pharmacy, in such areas as sterility testing and radiopharmaceuticals. As yet, no Region has a definite rolling plan for continuing education, based on specific aims, for hospital pharmacists and pharmacy technicians.

Traditionally, continuing education has been provided through the medium of the formal lecture, although educational films are sometimes used. Large group teaching is not necessarily the best approach to continuing education. It is an inflexible means of attempting to meet individual learning needs and styles, apart from the practical problems such as timing or situation, that it inherently causes. However, it does have the advantage of being a familiar mode of presentation and probably the social component encourages attendance. Small groups (the staff of a single department or specialist pharmacists in a single Area/Region) can be accommodated using slide/tape or slide/cassette presentations. The Pharmaceutical Society has prepared several topics using this format and Regional Training Departments have adopted this vehicle for topics of common interest (e.g. SI units). Video recordings have the advantage of being animated, and although video equipment is not as widely available as projection/recording equipment, its application is increasing. A course on pharmacokinetics, using videotape and a work manual, has been prepared by the University of London Audiovisual Centre. Adopting the approach of the Open University, the Inner London Education Authority has established a closed circuit television network (Sharp 1976) that has been used for continuing education programmes on therapeutic topics.

Individual self-learning in the field of continuing education is commended. Several American universities have prepared, mainly for hospital pharmacists, courses of material on cassette which are available with accompanying course manuals. The latter contain lecture outlines, figures, self-test units and glossaries of terms. Other institutions have produced correspondence courses.

Many pharmacists try hard to meet their continuing education requirements through diligent reading. Several series of articles in *The Pharmaceutical Journal* make it a potential organ for continuing education. An approach worthy of consideration is the 'add-on' journal such as *Medicine*. This publication is produced monthly and provides structured reading organised in

Table 4.1   Educational requirements of hospital pharmacy staff

Grades of staff	Learning process		
	Professional training	Management training	Continuing education
Pharmacy technicians			
Student	×		
Technician	×		×
Senior		×	×
Pharmacists			
Preregistration	×		
Pharmacist	×		×
Staff		×	×
Principal/Area		×	×
Pharmaceutical Officer		×	×

a standard format: each instalment is concerned with a single clinical area (e.g. skin diseases).

Who should be learning what?

Table 4.1 provides a résumé of the education and training which various grades of staff within hospital pharmacy require.

REFERENCES

AMEER B. & JOHNSON K. E. (1977) *American Journal of Hospital Pharmacy* **34,** 383.

BAKER J. A. (1976) *Pharmaceutical Journal* **217,** 272.

BRÅNSTAD J. O. (1977) Presented at the *International Symposium on Clinical Pharmacy,* The Hague, 1–3 September 1977.

COMMITTEE OF ENQUIRY INTO COMPETENCE TO PRACTISE (1976) *Competence to Practise.* Chairman E. A. J. Alment. CECP, London.

DAY R. L. (1975) *American Journal of Pharmaceutical Education* **39,** 569.

DEPARTMENT OF HEALTH AND SOCIAL SECURITY (1972) *Management Arrangements for the Reorganised National Health Service.* HMSO, London.

DEPARTMENT OF HEALTH AND SOCIAL SECURITY (1973) *Operation and Development of Services: Organisation of Pharmaceutical Services* (HRC (73) 28).

DEPARTMENT OF HEALTH AND SOCIAL SECURITY (1974) *Management Education and Training in the Reorganised NHS.* Personnel Management in the National Health Service, Memorandum 1 (HSC (IS) 47).

DEPARTMENT OF HEALTH AND SOCIAL SECURITY (1975) *Memorandum on Continuing Education for Pharmacists Providing Part IV Pharmaceutical Services.*

FREEMAN J. & BYRNE P. S. (1976) The assessment of postgraduate training in general practice. In *Research into Higher Education Monograph no. 20,* 2nd edn. Society for Research into Higher Education, Guildford.

HOULE C. H. (1974) From Lemberger M. A. & McCormick W. C. (1976) *American Journal of Pharmaceutical Education* **40,** 170.

JOHNSON R. C. (1977) *Journal of Clinical Pharmacy* **2,** 23.

LONGSHAW R. N. & SKEWS R. D. (1977) *Pharmaceutical Journal* **219,** 380.

PHARMACEUTICAL SOCIETY OF GREAT BRITAIN (1972) *Pre-registration Experience Requirements.* PSGB, London.

PHARMACEUTICAL SOCIETY OF GREAT BRITAIN (1975) *Pharmaceutical Journal* **214,** 546.

PHARMACEUTICAL SOCIETY OF GREAT BRITAIN (1977) *Pharmaceutical Journal* **219,** 197.

SHARP D. R. (1976) *Medical and Biological Illustration* **26,** 235.

SMITH D. (1977) *Health and Social Service Journal* **86,** F1.

TOMAN J. P. (1977) *Nursing Times* **73,** 1041.

TURNER P. (1977) *Pharmaceutical Journal* **219,** 251.

II
Production of medicines

5

Manufacture of pharmaceutical preparations

J. B. KAY

The general facilities available for the manufacture of pharmaceutical products will always influence the quality of the final product. This chapter will deal with the design of a unit required for the preparation of these products. It will also examine the practicalities of operating a production unit by examining the protocols and documentation systems required to ensure product security and efficiency of production. Continual reference will be made to systems operating under the British Health Service, but the philosophy underlying the system should be universally applicable. The *Guide to Good Pharmaceutical Manufacturing Practice* (DHSS 1977; 'Orange Guide') should be referred to since it embodies the ideals of good pharmacy practice. Obviously, the more a project is split and delegated within a hospital pharmacy, the more people of less specialised training become involved and consequently the more relevant to the hospital scene the 'Orange Guide' becomes. However, the factor of human error is common to all, and this fact gives the 'Orange Guide' a place in hospital pharmacy.

Planning

An early stage in the design procedure is to consider the basic facilities required for the products and add to these the necessary support systems, such as changing facilities and storage areas. These basic facilities will generally be the most expensive and should have a life expectancy, in both practical and technological terms, of about ten years if this period is relevant to the function of the unit. During planning, the need for versatility and possible future expansion should be borne in mind. Once the basic facilities have been reconciled to production and quality control (QC) requirements it will then be necessary to examine flow patterns and feasibility in detail for the particular site. The space available for a unit may be finite and this limits both the range and number of products manufactured. Alternatively, a range of products and required outputs may be the design criteria, in which case the space requirements will then have to be decided.

During various stages of development, consultation will be required with the 'Orange Guide', management services and technical support. It is at this stage that feasibility patterns will emerge and management services will assist in decision-making exercises. The balance between capital and current costs, amongst other factors, will be carefully considered in relationship to the life expectancy of the unit. It is important to correctly organise the ergonomics of the unit since this will influence not only the efficiency of, but also the product security within, the unit. 'Cross paths' and 'backtracking' must be avoided whenever possible, and it is important to avoid this adverse situation when designing sterile product facilities which must be clearly segregated into various categories of environmental control.

At this early stage the design and working parties should be planning, simultaneously, the protocols, procedures and documentation systems required since these will have a considerable influence on the detailed design of the facility. The first priority of any pharmaceutical manufacturing department is that the product be of the correct quality and fit for its intended use: efficiency and other considerations are secondary and can be negotiated.

The working environment

Three levels of environment are required for the various types of medicines which may be prepared within a hospital (Kay 1978). The least sophisticated of these is the socially clean area where high standards of cleanliness and hygiene are required for the preparation of items such as oral liquids, tablets, ointments and non-injectable sterile water used for the moistening of wound packs and the rinsing of gloved hands and instruments in theatre. The second category of environment is the clean room area where clean room technology is applied in order to provide not only socially clean conditions but also an atmosphere free from small particles (e.g. $>0.5\,\mu m$ size), since products such as intravenous fluids must be free from such contamination. The most demanding environmental condition is the aseptic area where clean room technology and aseptic techniques are applied in order to provide an atmosphere ostensibly free from microorganisms for the manufacture of products which are not sterilised in their final sealed containers but rely for their microbiological quality on the techniques used and the environments in which they are assembled and processed.

If each environmental category is given a different and distinct colour code as the environments progress from a street condition to a socially clean area (black), to a clean room area (white), to an aseptic area (red) (Fig. 5.1), and these colour codes, along with a written indication, are clearly marked on all entrances and exits and certain equipment (e.g. cleaning equipment) within the department, then daily supervision and formal self inspection at all levels will be made easier and all staff will accept and respond better to the importance of this segregation.

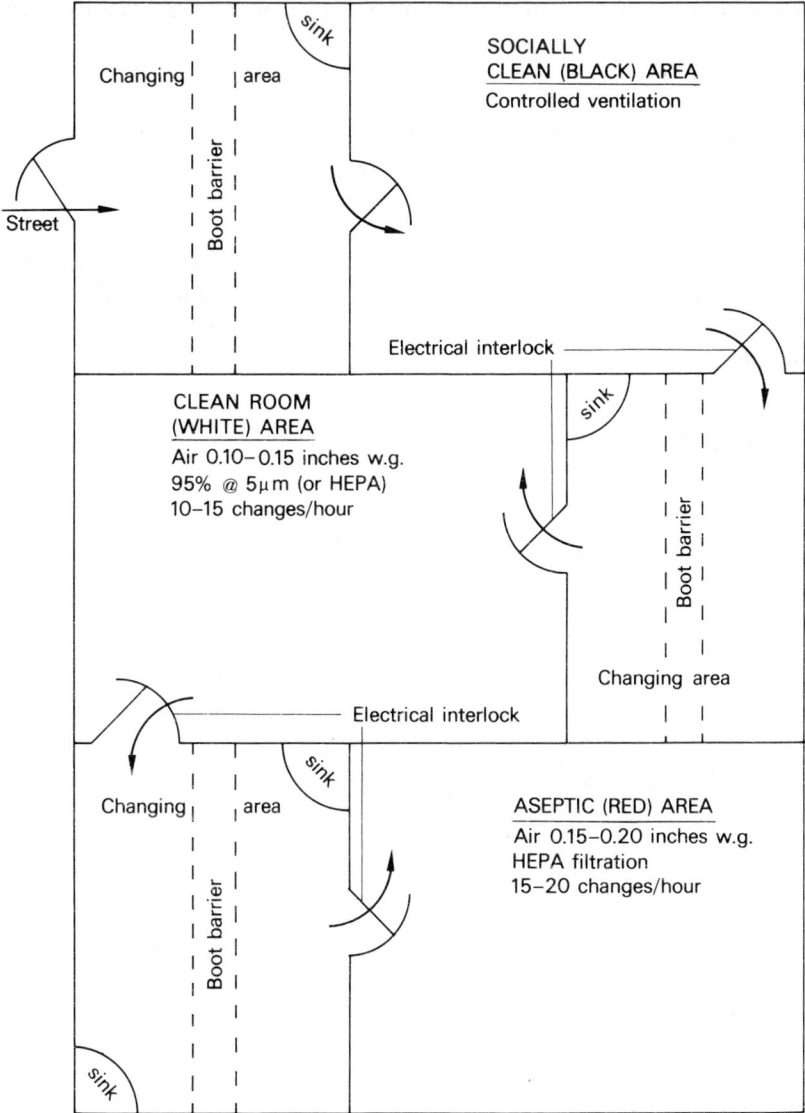

Fig. 5.1 Basic design of a manufacturing facility to indicate the stages in environmental control.

The objectives of environmental control in these areas are to reduce the particulate contamination of the working environment and to reduce and control the population of microorganisms, since their presence in parenteral products prior to terminal sterilisation must be kept to the lowest possible number. When a clean room area of this type is being designed, it is very important that the design team should fully commit themselves to the working standards which will be set and maintained by daily surveillance of the facility when in use.

MANUFACTURE OF PARENTERAL PRODUCTS TERMINALLY STERILISED IN SEALED CONTAINERS

The flow pattern set out in Fig. 5.2 indicates the usual sequence of events during the manufacture of a batch of intravenous fluids filled into glass containers. A shaded box in Fig. 5.2 indicates that a clean room area condition is required for that activity, whereas socially clean area standards are required for the remainder.

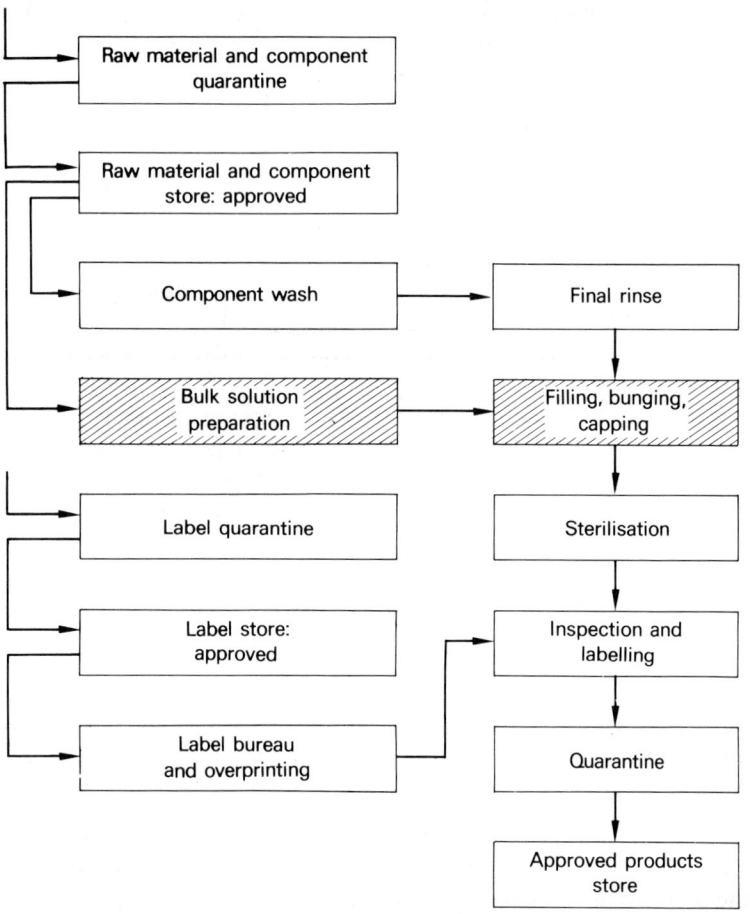

Fig. 5.2 A diagrammatic representation of the usual sequence of events for the manufacture of parenteral fluids in glass containers. Shaded boxes indicate a clean room area is required.

Since clean room area conditions are difficult and expensive to achieve and maintain, it is important not to undertake any work in such areas which does not require these high standards (e.g. inspection and labelling of bottles, weighing of powders, delabelling of bottles). The clean room area should only be used for the preparation of the intravenous solution and sealing of this solution into the container. Consequently, environmental standards and procedures will be considered firstly for clean room areas and secondly for the adjacent socially clean areas.

Reduction of particulate contamination

A clean room designed for the preparation of the bulk solution and the filling of parenteral sterile products makes use of adequately filtered and conditioned air brought into the area through (preferably) terminal filters located in the ceiling and exhausted either through return air ducts or pressure relief systems located near the floor around the periphery of the room. Action is taken to limit the contamination introduced into the air in the room by controlling the personnel, operation and materials inside the facility. Personnel are required to wear low particle-shedding type garments and all materials must be cleaned before being introduced into the area. In addition, the particular zone within the room where the filling exercise takes place should be given further protection from particulate contamination by the use of physical barriers and horizontal or vertical laminar flow units. The following points should be considered as 'guidelines' when considering the design of a clean room for the bulk manufacture and filling of intravenous products.

The room should undergo a minimum of 10–15 air changes per hour. All incoming air should be passed through filters with an efficiency of at least 95% when tested at the manufacturer's factory according to British Standard 2831 : 1971 using test dust number 2. In addition, terminal High Efficiency Particulate Air (HEPA) filters may be installed at only a modest increase in cost. The added advantages of such an upgraded system are that such terminal filters can be tested for integrity after installation and routinely thereafter to a set standard (see p. 100) and the environment can be checked to a fixed level of particulate contamination (e.g. class 10 000 Federal Standard 209B 1973 and class 2 BS 5295: 1976; see Tables 5.2 and 5.3). The room should be designed to operate at a minimum positive pressure of 0.05 inches water gauge (w.g.) and in most cases it is preferable to commission the unit at 0.15 inches w.g. and review the installation if this pressure drops below 0.10 inches w.g. Access to the room should be by air lock systems with interlocked doors arranged such that the clean room itself can never be inadvertently opened directly to the outside environment. A minimum number of access air locks should be installed. Air temperature and humidity are important factors and must be controlled carefully, since operators will be wearing constrictive clothing (see p. 95). All materials used in the construction of the clean room or brought into the clean room should be assessed in terms of liability to shed particles. Wall to floor and wall to ceiling joins should be coved and there should be a minimum of projecting ledges. Walls, floors and doors may be covered with a smooth resistant plastic sheeting to obviate cracks or joins where particles could accumulate. Exposed woodwork should be avoided. A clear differentiation should be made between a socially clean condition (black), a clean room condition (white) and an aseptic condition (red). Any items or personnel entering an area subjected to higher standards of cleanliness to that being left should undergo a formal documented procedure to reduce the possibility of contamination being brought about by this route. An air lock should be subdivided, preferably by a physical barrier at floor level, to indicate where one environmental condition 'ends' and another 'begins'. This is a tangible representation to the process worker where one discipline ends and another begins. The safe manufacture of sterile products is fundamentally a question of disciplines being upheld by people of varying abilities; the more tangible and demonstrable a discipline is, the easier it is for process workers to follow the rules, and for more senior staff to undertake supervision (and sometimes vice versa!). A physical barrier such as a boot barrier has the added advantage that people are less likely to walk unthinkingly across the boundary. Boot barriers represent a useful means whereby personnel can sit and swivel from one class of area to another; pigeon holes installed in each side of the barrier then provide useful footwear storage areas, but they must be designed with ease of cleaning in mind. The use of 'tacky' mats at strategic points within the manufacturing area helps to reduce the quantity of free particulate contamination brought in underfoot. By simple observation one may gain some idea as to the amount of contamination crossing into this zone, and such surveillance may help in the maintenance of good discipline.

Since 85% of the particulate contamination generated in a clean room may originate from the personnel using it, it is obvious that the number of people in the facility compared to its size, the extent of movements undertaken by these people and their mode of apparel, will have a major influence on the quality of the environment. In most applications of clean room technology as applied to the manufacture of intravenous fluids, a normal yardstick is 60 square feet per person for a facility with a headroom of between 10 and 12 feet. The processing should be designed to take place with a minimum of movement of personnel and materials. Consequently, it is advisable to arrange for the bulk solution manufacture to take place away from the filling zone, and to erect a physical barrier from floor to ceiling between the two interconnected zones. The (normally) horizontal or vertical laminar flow unit within the filling zone will be constantly 'cleaning' the air by its recirculating action. However, like all tools, clean rooms and laminar flow units are not a guarantee of quality in themselves. Operator techniques, skill, intelligence and dedication are vital if product quality is not to be compromised.

When deciding on the design of a laminar flow unit some factors relevant to this section should be borne in mind. Large particles such as skin debris will fall almost vertically through laminar flow air (Austin 1970). Consequently, laminar flow systems should not be relied upon to protect open containers over which the operator may have to reach (to adjust a machine, fill a hopper etc.); a physical barrier should be installed to protect such exposed situations (Diamond 1972). Ideally, the unit should be built into the wall of the filling area such that there is no protrusion of the outer top surface. Since it is inadvisable to move some free-standing laminar flow units without a subsequent check being made to reaffirm filter integrity, the unit should be positioned and installed in such a way that cleanliness of all surfaces exposed to the area can be monitored and checked.

Reduction of population of vegetative microorganisms

The bulk manufacture and filling complex of an intravenous fluid production unit must be designed, used and monitored in such a way as to ensure a low level of microbial contamination. One of the most practical ways of achieving this objective is to ensure that all items of equipment can be washed with hot aqueous detergent, soaked for 10 minutes in water at 80°C and then allowed to dry quickly and remain dry until required. In general, if an item or surface is difficult to clean, then it is difficult to disinfect. The use of chemical disinfectant solutions in the production area should be unnecessary, since it merely introduces into the unit a further margin for error. If disinfection with hot water is not possible, then the surface should be moistened with 75% v/v aqueous ethyl or isopropyl alcohol and left to dry. Cleaning equipment can itself be a major source of infection and written procedures must be described for the cleaning and disinfection or, preferably, sterilisation of mops and other items (Maurer 1974). 'U-bend' traps require special consideration (see p. 91), and overflow systems should be avoided, since they are very difficult to clean and disinfect.

Cleaning and clothing systems

Adequate cleaning facilities and suitable clothing is vital if a clean room area is not to be contaminated to unacceptable levels by the personnel entering such zones. The principles and techniques required for these systems have much in common with those required for aseptic areas, and are covered in a later part of this chapter (see p. 93).

Preparation of the bulk solution

The object is to provide facilities within a clean room area for the preparation, in the main, of aqueous solutions suitable for use as intravenous products. In most units it will be necessary to provide for the preparation of *one* batch (i.e. one homogeneous mix) at a time. However, if it is envisaged that more than one batch will be undergoing preparation at any one time, then strict measures will have to be taken to ensure that a cross contamination or mix-up will not occur. This will involve the erection of physical barriers between the various products. If this cubicle system is required within a clean room area, then the effects on the air circulation system must be accounted for by suitable siting of intake and extract services; furthermore, the injectable grade water (IGW) source should be common and within easy access of all the cubicles.

If chemicals used in the preparation of bulk solutions are to be stored permanently in the clean room, then they should be delivered to the area in containers that are compatible with clean room principles and which have been approved individually by QC. An alternative is to establish a central dispensary for all chemicals required in the pharmacy for the preparation of pharmaceutical products and for the exact quantity of each material to be delivered to the bulk manufacture zone in a suitable container as required.

All services should be installed so as to create a minimum of disruption within the clean room when maintenance or routine servicing is required.

If IGW is collected daily, then a minimum number of collection tanks should be installed (ideally one). IGW should not be allowed to stand at room temperature for periods in excess of 4–6 hours as discussed later. The tank should be equipped with a well-fitting lid and a simple drain control tap. The same principles should be applied to mixing vessels as are applied to the cleaning and disinfection of the IGW collection tanks. Mixing vessels will obviously vary in size and construction with the batch size being produced. Sufficient headroom should be provided to allow for inspection if large tanks are to be employed. Washing facilities must be provided for scoops and other general equipment. Stirrers and heaters will either be installed as a part of the mixing vessel structure or be portable pieces of equipment, and should be designed for easy cleaning and inspection. A stirrer can cause problems by oil leakage from the bearings or gear-box, especially if installed in the head or sides of the mixing vessel. Vessel heating systems should be designed in such a way that local overheating cannot occur.

All metal surfaces coming into contact with pharmaceutical products should be chosen with care and special attention paid to the quality of welds and the standard of polish achieved. Solid austenitic stainless steel may be preferred to nickel-coated mild steel if the metal surface is subject to metal-against metal impact during use.

Filling of the bulk solution

The objective behind the design and function of a filling zone is primarily to protect the product from viable and non-viable particulate contamination. This is best achieved by conducting the process not only in a clean room area but also within a laminar flow unit. The further away that personnel can be kept from the exposed product, the quicker the speed of operations and shorter the distance of the filling line, the less likelihood there is of such contamination entering the product. The laminar flow unit should be installed at the required working height and in such a position that all rinsed containers are protected within the unit from the time and point at which they are rinsed to the point at which they are effectively sealed. The manipulations undertaken in the laminar flow unit may or may not involve a final container rinse with IGW but will involve filling and bunging, and possibly capping, if the bungs are not of the type that fit firmly into the bottle neck. The decision as to which type of laminar flow unit to choose will depend on the geometry of the manipulations being carried out during these latter stages, bearing in mind the configurations of the bottles and bungs relevant to the operator and the machines. Obviously, if the filling machine is of such a design that it effectively shields the exposed bottles from a horizontal laminar flow air stream then a vertical flow system is more appropriate. The placing of equipment and containers in the laminar flow unit should be carefully considered before deciding whether to choose a horizontal or vertical system. The filling machine design and bunging system will have to be related to their compatibility with the laminar flow unit and the operator's actions. The laminar flow unit should contain the minimum of equipment at any one time, and consequently the flow pattern of bottles should be examined especially in light of fluctuations in operator output, in order that a laminar flow unit of the necessary size is purchased. With the most modest output (e.g. 200×1 litre bottles/batch per half day) a 6 feet by 2 feet HEPA filter installed in a horizontal unit would be satisfactory.

Certain factors should be considered before choosing a filling machine. Those parts of the filling machine which come into contact with the solution should be easily dismantled for cleaning and subsequent sterilisation, preferably wrapped to maintain sterility. The material used in the construction of the machine should be compatible with the products. Filling machines with 'blind corners', inaccessible valves and other complications in design make for difficult cleaning and should be avoided. The type of filling machine chosen should obviously be related to the output rate of the unit and the type of container being filled; it should be possible to instal terminal bacteria-retentive membrane filters on the filling nozzle of the machine. Before choosing sophisticated automatic machines it is important to bear in mind the fact that such machines can be a burden and a menace unless tight control is exercised over the geometrical specifications of the glass containers, and adequate engineering skill is available for its maintenancc or repair at the time needed (with the small batch size of ampoules, for example, which are generally required to be made in hospitals, it will often be cheaper and quicker to fill and seal these batches by hand). Generally speaking, the faster the machine and lower the volume fill, the greater will be the problems associated with machine-component performance in terms of output rate and fill-volume control.

The vessel containing the bungs should be sited in such a position that it does not reduce the effectiveness of the laminar flow unit. If a screw-cap system is used then for large batch sizes, the tightening torque should be established for that particular container and the bottle closure tightened on an automatic tightener outside but adjacent to the laminar flow unit. Reaming or spinning machines should be similarly placed where appropriate. All tubing coming into contact with the solution should be dismantled, cleaned and autoclaved after each usage.

For small-scale production it is normal to use membrane filters with a maximum pore size of 0.45 µm for filtration of the solution immediately before it passes into the containers from the filling machine. With larger batch sizes it is necessary to use cartridge type filters with similar retention characteristics, and in all cases the assembled filter must be subjected to a performance test. This performance test must be the one recommended by the manufacturer of the filter material and take account of the nature of the solution and its conditions of use. The technique may vary between manufacturers but will involve either a 'bubble point test', a 'gas diffusion rate test' or a 'forward flow test'. All of these tests rely on a correlation established during product development by filter manufacturers between maximum pore size as determined by a microbiological challenge test and a gas permeability test (Pall 1975).

Preparation, storage and distribution of injectable grade water (IGW)

Injectable grade water is the major constituent of the majority of parenteral products, and can easily become contaminated by chemical or microbiological agents. Consequently the preparation, storage and distribution of such water will be considered in some detail below.

In practical terms the objective is to produce water which, after sterilisation, complies with the monograph for Water for Injections of the *European Pharmacopoeia* (1973). Such water must be produced in sufficient quantity that it can be used and sterilised within 6 hours (in exceptional circumstances water can be stored at elevated temperatures, normally 80°C).

Water pretreatment and steam quality

The majority of stills will fail to produce water of the required quality consistently if impurities are present in the feed water or steam. In addition, impurities may cause extensive damage to the still. Consequently, it is important to establish with the still manufacturer that the local feed water and steam qualities are of an acceptable standard, and if not, what measures must be taken to provide services of the correct quality before deciding on which still to purchase. The vast majority of problems arising out of the use of stills are primarily due to poor quality feed water and/or steam services, resulting in priming, corrosion and the presence of dissolved gases in the distillate. Stills are available which either boil return condensate (water 'trapped' from the hospital steam lines) or boil local feed water followed by subsequent condensation and collection. Stills of the former type should not be installed in hospitals since steam-volatile additives (e.g. filming amines) may be introduced into

Table 5.1 Common factors which can affect the performance and structure of a still

Effect	Feed water/steam contaminant	Remedy
Corrosion and priming	Temporary or permanent hard water	Boil feed water or deionise/soften feed water
Corrosion pitting and stress corrosion	Chloride in water	Deionise water
Contamination of distillate	Filming amines in steam	Do not use return condensate steam
Corrosion and low pH of distillate	Carbon dioxide in water	Deionise; heat feed water above 80°C
Corrosion	Carbon dioxide in steam	Improve steam generation
Reduced efficiency of heat exchangers and corrosion of heating elements due to deposition of scale	Temporary or permanent hard water	Deionise feed water

the steam line at the boiler house. These cannot be removed by passing the return condensate through an ion exchange or adsorbent column system. Table 5.1 summarises factors that can influence the working of a still with consequences for the product.

A routine maintenance schedule for the still and its feeds (water and steam) should be established between quality assurance, production and engineering staffs, since it is only a combination of such surveillances with physical (e.g. steam pressure, conductivity, pH) and biological (pyrogen testing) monitoring that can give a satisfactory pattern of retrospective acceptability.

Distillation

When deciding on the required output of a still, the simplest method is to calculate the volume of water required for the manufacture of the bulk solution and double this volume to arrive at the quantity required for all the manufacturing processes necessary. Subsequent decisions as to which still is most suitable will then be mainly economic and a cost/benefit exercise should be undertaken. The economic factors are as follows:

1.   The volume and cost of cooling water, which can vary from 0.25 to 10 times the volume of distillate produced.
2.   The heating costs.
3.   Depreciation on capital costs and routine maintenance costs.
4.   Additional costs due, for example, to the need for deionisation of the feed water or installation of header tank systems.
5.   Any additional costs of equipping the still with an automatic warning and dumping device which operates if and when the conductivity of the distillate rises above a predetermined value (probably indicating that a fault has arisen in the functioning of the still) and also rejects the first quantity of distillate if an automatic start-up is required.

The use of a recording conductivity meter provides an ongoing record of the still performance, and should be seriously considered as an aid to QC. The importance of running the initial output of the still to waste must not be ignored; the time required for this will vary with the design of the still. Those stills which are designed in such a way that distilled water remains within the equipment at room temperature after closedown will require a longer period of flushing in order to remove any water contaminated due to the growth of microorganisms during this period. Functional factors should also be included. These include the quality and output rate of the distillate, complexity of operation (or automatic), complexity of maintenance by both hospital staff and contractors, physical dimensions including the 'take-off' points, noise levels and heat output, temperature of distillate (up to 80°C), delivery schedules and lag time prior to distillation commencing after switch-on.

Storage and distribution

It is possible to design a system whereby water of the correct quality can be made available 'on tap' by running the still on a semicontinuous basis and collecting a large volume of IGW heated and held at an elevated temperature (80°C or higher). The installation of such a system does introduce further hazards into the manufacturing procedure, which should be considered carefully. The still distillate must be fed directly into the heated tank and the pipe system from the still should not allow water to be trapped in 'dead legs', bends or rises. The installation of pumps and complicated piping systems should be avoided by siting the storage tank as near as possible to the point of use. Long delivery lengths are also a disincentive to adequate cleaning. Piping leading from the storage tank to the point of use should be as straight as possible, have a gradual fall and be lagged. If a 'T' junction with the necessary taps is installed at the tank connection point then the entire length of pipe can be isolated from the tank and drained at the end of each shift, thus enabling the line to be flushed with hot water (80°C) daily and left in a dry condition overnight. This avoids a build-up of organisms in this potential reservoir.

An alternative system is to instal a pump and ring main system whereby all of the IGW is continually cycled to and from the heated tank and thus at the correct elevated temperature throughout. The system should be lagged and easily dismantled. The pipework is best constructed from a pharmaceutical grade of stainless steel incorporating ISS type fittings in preference to screw threads, which are more difficult to disconnect and may contain undesirable crevices. The water in the circulation system can be maintained at a positive pressure by allowing the pump (normally a stainless steel centrifugal pump with non-contact impellers and Teflon or ceramic seals) to operate against a throttle valve at the tank return inlet. The number of take-off points should be minimal. In most units, two taps, one installed in the final rinse area and one in the bulk solution area, should be sufficient. A continuous temperature recording chart system should be installed together with a direct reading mercury-in-glass thermometer fitted to the vessel. The storage tank pumps and piping systems should be designed so as to prevent contamination of water due to corrosion of metal structures as a result of poor finish or mechanical wear of surfaces. The tank should be equipped with a system whereby air entering the vessel during emptying can be filtered through a bacteria-retentive filter.

The advantages of using a heated tank system for the storage of IGW are that the water is always instantly available, a still with a lower output can be installed and more efficient use made of the still since it will be operating for longer periods. Routine and other maintenance can thus be performed on the still without immediately affecting the availability of IGW. However, the system may not, in fact, be any more economical than to have a larger still capacity and two disadvantages apply. A hazard is introduced since there are more opportunities for human and mechanical error and the calibration of tanks and vessels will have to be corrected to the temperature of the water in use at the time, unless an inline cooler is used.

Socially clean areas
Storage of used bottles

Used bottles should be inspected on receipt into the unit and those showing signs of damage and gross contamination should be rejected. All bungs and seals should be discarded and the bottles drained, rinsed and stored inverted in their crates. The crates should be washed so as to be in a socially clean condition awaiting reuse. The layout and procedures should be such that the possibility of physical contamination or mix-up between those bottles which have been returned for reuse and those which have been delabelled, emptied and inspected for damage etc. is reduced to a minimum. Rejected bottles should be discarded from the unit immediately.

Storage of new bottles and closures

The packaging materials used for new components are quite often the major sources of particulate contamination of the final product. To reduce this problem new components which have been approved by QC should be removed from their outer wrappings and cardboard boxes away from the final washing zone and stored in suitable containers which are not a source of particulate contamination and which protect the components from adverse conditions. It may be necessary to prewash these bottles if the packing system produces excessive amounts of particulate matter.

Prerinse and delabelling of reused bottles

This process is designed to remove from the bottle any heavy contamination which can be easily removed (e.g. dust as opposed to clotted blood) and the labels. Various machines are available for this purpose, some of which combine this stage with the next stage which is the final washing and rinsing prior to delivery to the filling zone. However this procedure is undertaken, it is important to prevent the large number of fibres generated when removing the labels from being carried through the process such that they present difficulties at the final rinse stage and result in a high rejection rate of the final product.

It is an advantage to organise the work flow in such a way that delabelling, crate washing and bung and cap removal take place in a segregated area (Fig. 5.3). This should be adjacent to, and leading into the zone in which the bottles

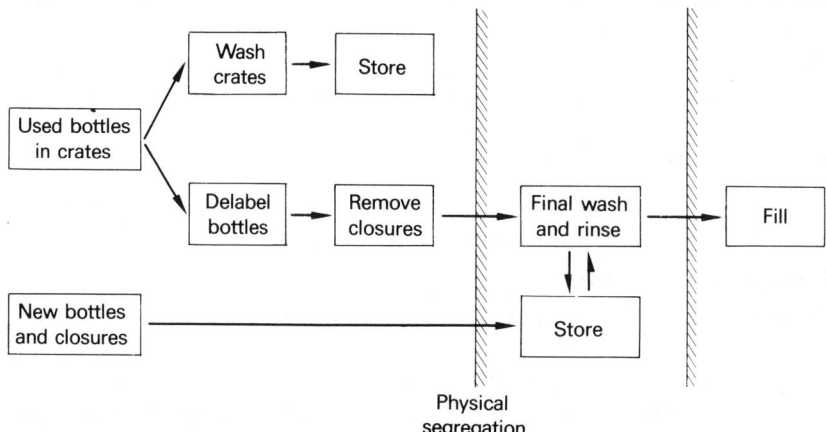

Fig. 5.3   Organisation of work flow in the reuse of bottles.

are given their final wash (and inspection for damage) and in which new bungs and caps are cleaned. Rewashed bottles which are not required for immediate use may be stored inverted and dried in a clean area. They must be rewashed prior to use in the filling area.

Washing of bottles and closure

The final washing and rinsing process should expose the bottles to powerful jets of hot aqueous detergent followed by cold water and finally IGW which has passed through a bacteria-retentive membrane filter. The filter assembly and piping from the water tank to the machine should be designed so that it can be removed for cleaning and sterilsation. It is important that certain parts of the machine, including tanks, pipes, pumps and filters through which cleaning fluids travel, are easily dismantled, cleaned and inspected on a regular basis. Where relevant, a device should be installed which operates a visual warning if the detergent supply falls below the working level.

The system should be drained at the end of each shift and disinfection achieved by the use of steam, hot distilled water or 75% v/v ethanol or iso-propyl alcohol. The header tank, normally made from suitable stainless steel, should have a well-fitted lid and a protective air bleed. Level control systems should be readily cleaned, disinfected and left to dry quickly. The contents should be subject to routine microbiological surveillance. The final rinse stage should take place as near to the access point for entry of rinsed containers into the clean room filling zone as possible to reduce the possibility of contamination of the container. If a conveyor-belt system is used then the system should be designed so that the clean room filling zone belt stops short of the component washing room and vice versa. Alternatively, the bottles can be transferred by hand into the filling zone through a small purpose-built hatch. Bottles entering the filling zone should be held inverted where possible until reaching the laminar flow filling zone, which should be immediately adjacent to the components entry point.

The method of pretreatment of the rubber or synthetic closure will vary depending on the type of bung and its application. Some will require heating in an autoclave whilst immersed in an aqueous system (with or without a specified antimicrobial substance) whereas others will require washing with a non-foaming detergent followed by rinsing with IGW. It is, however, difficult to remove particles by boiling bungs in water and detergent and then allowing the water to drain from a base stopcock. The equipment used for this process should not cause excessive damage to the bungs due to mutual attrition which would cause the continuous shedding of fibrous material adhering to the bungs. Having washed away any undesirable material adhering to the bung surfaces, the next problem is to remove, by successive rinsing, the considerable quantity of fibrous material suspended in the detergent solution. If the aqueous layer is drained away from the bungs by simple downward flow through the bed of bungs then the latter will act as a filter bed for the fibres and consequently even many washings will give little improvement in the situation. This is why various systems have been devised for the continuous rinsing of rubber components by passing filtered IGW up through a moving bed of bungs and away to waste by the use of an adapted rotary horizontal drum washing machine, or by rapid sucking of the supernatant water after each rinsing activity. The final rinsing water should be filtered through a bacteria-retentive membrane filter and the type and number of cycles documented for each bung system. The rinsed bungs should be left immersed in IGW in a suitable covered container. Some bungs may be difficult to insert into the bottle neck unless moist. Rinsed bungs should be used and the sealed containers sterilised within 6 hours of processing or be reprocessed. The metal caps and seals used in conjunction with the bung system should be washed separately from the bungs. If attempts are made to wash closures in their assembled form metallic particles produced by mutual attrition will adhere to the seal surfaces and are difficult to remove.

Sterilisation zone

User area

A number of factors should be considered. Physically segregated bays should be provided for the short-term holding of batches before and after sterilisation and the content of each bay should be adequately labelled, including the sterilising cycle number where relevant. In addition a colour indicator system may be adopted so that visible evidence is provided that the batch has been subjected to a heat process (Medicines Commission 1972). Where possible, however, no more than one sterilising cycle load should be present in the zone at any one time. Sufficient space must be planned to allow for the manœuvring of trolleys, transfer of cages and pallets, and the flooring should withstand the wearing effect of such movements. It should also be self-draining and easily cleaned in case of spillage. Adequate lighting must be provided so that instruments and temperature–time charts can be read easily. Access should be provided to the steriliser thermocouple boss by means of a hatch or port in the steriliser façade; this also assists verbal communication with maintenance staff in the service zone. A convenient power point should be provided for test instruments and inspection lamps etc. If a double-ended steriliser is installed then physical segregation between batches, before and after sterilisation, is made easier to achieve. However, considerable experience indicates that such machines are difficult to justify both in terms of cost and maintenance problems in this kind of hospital situation. Ventilation should be provided above the sterilisers to assist in the dispersion of heat generated in the user area.

Service area

This area should be designed to allow routine access (and removal of the steriliser when necessary) without entering or disturbing other sections of the department. It should be large enough to allow access to all parts of the steriliser during maintenance and removal of the chamber lagging for routine insurance survey purposes. A well-illuminated work bench should be provided for use by the maintenance engineer. Adequate ventilation is critical, and ten air changes per hour should be regarded as minimal. Modern electronic control systems, whilst normally of high reliability, are very sensitive to excessive temperatures, and in no circumstances should the temperature exceed 27°C (80°F). Steam, water and compressed air services should be lagged where appropriate, clearly marked, and installed with a view to ease of access during maintenance. Essential steriliser spares, test instruments and tools should be kept in a locked enclosure within the area. Components and services must be sited with particular regard to the unusual temperature distribution often experienced with this type of installation.

Further guidance on the layout and organisation of these zones is given in Hospital Technical Memorandum (HTM) 10 (DHSS 1968).

Inspection and labelling zone

The major objectives to be considered when designing the inspection and labelling zone are that the batch being processed in this area should be safely isolated from other batches of product within the department at all times, and that the overall services should be designed to suit the type of inspection, mechanical aids or viewers which are to be used.

If more than one batch of product is to be inspected and labelled at any one time, then the cubicle system can be adopted. A number of basic principles apply to this product handling area. Labels, whether as cut labels or self-adhesive roll labels, should be delivered to the zone normally previously batch numbered, expiry dated etc. (unless this is done during an automatic labelling sequence) and counted; they should be sealed in a suitable package or other container and be accompanied by a document describing the contents. The inspection and labelling process should follow a defined series of events as described in agreed protocols and the relevant documentation completed. At the end of this activity the supervisor reconciles the number of labels remaining and used against the number delivered and also reconciles the number of rejects and accepted products against the number of containers delivered. Rejects and excess labels are then destroyed. After sampling by QC, the labelled bulk containers containing the accepted product are stamped as in 'quarantine under test' and sealed using a 'pilfer proof' device by the QC inspector and the batch transported to the quarantine zone awaiting QC approval prior to delivery to the approved products store.

The lighting system should not only allow for optimum detection of visible particulate contamination but should also allow for adequate inspection of the outer surfaces of the bottle and seal for cracks or distortions. This will mean providing a lighting system which throws sufficient light at the product for adequate execution of the latter inspection without reducing the efficiency of the viewer used for the detection of particles. The ergonomics of the inspection and labelling system should be studied carefully so that operator fatigue is reduced and product security and efficient manipulations are not impaired. Bench height must be related to the seating position and location of the viewer. The provision of 'reject bins' such that rejects of differing categories can be segregated (in case management wish to assess not only the total number of rejects, but also the cause) should be such that rejects can be immediately removed from the flow line so as to prevent the rejects being mixed with accepted products.

Label bureau and overprinting

Labels should be stored in an area physically segregated from other production zones, and with facilities whereby product labels can be stored in suitable identified and separate cabinets or boxes. This label bureau should be locked and access restricted to a nominated person. Batch numbering and overprinting of labels should also take place in this area, and all labels issued from this area should be placed in sealed containers. Each distribution of labels should be recorded in a log book or on a file sheet, and a second document completed which accompanies the sealed labels to the relevant production area. Labels should be issued in this way to nominated responsible persons only.

Adequate space is necessary for the installation of overprinting devices and the label bureau designed so that loose labels cannot fall undetected between cupboards or machines. Only one type of product label should be processed at any one time. All deliveries of labels from the printers should be checked for printing faults and rogue labels. The QC section must have agreed both the circumstances under which labels are received into the bureau from the printers and also their issue to production areas. A code-edge marking system may be adopted to aid the detection of rogue labels.

Quarantine store

The purpose behind the establishment of a quarantine area is that batches can be stored physically segregated from either 'in process' batches or approved batches in a locked store to which access is restricted to a responsible person. Facilities should be available for segregation between batches and the storage system designed so that easy access to each batch of product can be made by an approved person in case the need for resampling arises. The quarantine store will have many features in common with the drugs store (see Chapter 3).

Changing facilities and cleaning for socially clean areas

The changing facilities for personnel working in the socially clean areas should provide the necessary locker space for personal belongings along with facilities for toilet and personal hygiene. Certain installations such as toilet-flush mechanisms, locks, taps and hot air hand dryers, when equipped with foot controls, are convenient ways of reducing cross contamination. Washing facilities should be installed between the toilet area and its exit point. The necessary equipment and its use for cleaning the area must be documented and a copy held in the possession of the person delegated as responsible for the procedures. A cleaning programme indicating the daily, weekly, monthly etc. tasks must be drawn up indicating not only the sequence of procedures but also outlining in detail how these procedures are carried out. A suitable enclosed area must be set aside for the storage of the cleaner's equipment and documents. The equipment and documents stored in this area may serve other facilities in addition to the component washing area, but it is important that all cleaning equipment used in the pharmacy follows the classification and segregation principles already outlined. Many of the basic principles discussed later for the cleaning of clean areas and aseptic facilities apply also to socially clean areas.

MANUFACTURE OF PARENTERAL PRODUCTS MADE ASEPTICALLY

The objectives behind the design and operation of an aseptic area are similar in many ways to those discussed for a clean room area with the additional requirement that all materials and equipment brought into the area should be sterile, which is best achieved by the use of a heat process (see below). The air supply into the aseptic room will be terminally filtered to a higher minimum standard (i.e. filters that are 99.97% efficient with test dust no. 1, British Standard 2831 : 1971) and a higher air change rate will be expected (15–20 changes per hour) to give a Class 10 000 Federal Standard 209B Clean Room (1973). A pressure differential of 0.05–0.10 inches water gauge above that of the adjacent interconnecting areas should be achieved and all manipulations whereby the product is exposed to the environment should take place in a laminar flow work station (see p. 107). Obviously all items which are brought into an aseptic area should be designed to undergo an acceptable sterilising process during the entrance procedures, and personnel should change into previously sterilised clothing. The area itself may require, in addition to regular cleaning, disinfection by fumigation to ensure that all vegetative forms and most spores present on wall surfaces and machines (but not porous absorbent surfaces) are killed. This means that the aseptic area and its associated equipment must be designed to withstand the high humidity and formaldehyde gas concentrations used to effect this disinfection.

An aseptic room, if properly equipped and used, will go a considerable way towards providing a 'sterile environment' for the preparation of medicinal products; however, even in the best designed areas viable organisms will be found from time to time. It is folly to assume that a batch of product prepared using an aseptic technique has the same level of assurance of sterility as a product terminally heat sterilized in a sealed final container.

Batch sterility testing (on the basis that each day's fill or shift represents a batch) will only show up a situation where gross contamination has occurred; the majority of single unit contamination events will go undetected by this procedure. This is why continual environmental monitoring and surveillance, during which a pattern of 'retrospective acceptability' emerges, is a far greater assurance than is a terminal sterility test.

The cost of building and running an aseptic area with all the necessary features to fulfil the ambitions mentioned above will be very high, and in the case of small-scale activities (e.g. intravenous additives and single patient prescriptions for immediate use within a period of hours), techniques similar to those adopted in some operating theatres may be more relevant, where sterilised items are brought into a controlled environment using a double-wrap pack technique, the contents of the pack having been previously sterilised in this form elsewhere. Since the actual facilities required will vary from hospital to hospital depending on the type and number of products, it would be impracticable to attempt to categorise the design of the necessary facilities into product numbers and types. Therefore, features and procedures additional to those in the clean room (white) area required for an aseptic area equipped to do medium-scale aseptic manufacture and filling of parenteral products will now be considered. It is assumed that the aseptic room is built adjacent to the bulk manufacture and filling (white) area. In this circumstance, aqueous or oily solutions made in the latter zone can be brought into the aseptic area through suitable sterilised tubing connected to a sterile 0.22 μm bacteria-retentive membrane filter leading to a sterile vessel sited within the aseptic room (A performance test should be done prior to the product being exposed to the aseptic environment, see p. 80).

The aseptic area should be designed so as to be interconnected with the adjacent white areas by four double-doored interlocked access routes: the changing room, the hot air sterilising oven, the double-doored steam steriliser, and the product interchange zone.

Changing room

Before entering this changing room, personnel will have gone through the black to white changing room procedure and should have to remove white area clothing only prior to donning sterile garments. The lockers and cupboards provided in this changing room should have transparent doors (if fitted) to aid surveillance. The number of people using the changing room at any one time should be strictly controlled, and sterile garments should be worn each time. The number of air changes per hour may be higher than for the aseptic room which may necessitate the installation of suitably placed terminal filters in the changing room. The sink U-bend drains should be fitted with heating devices, or, better still, avoided by the installation of an air break in the drain which is designed to drain dry, and can easily be cleaned and inspected. Procedures can be adopted to decrease or eliminate the microbial contamination levels of the water supply by filtration or chlorination disinfection. These, together with the water itself, will require frequent scheduled and documented checks. The changing room will be equipped with two sinks, one on each side of the boot barrier, with foot-operated tap controls. There are advantages in the use of hot air dryers operated by foot or elbow control. Facilities must be provided for easy access to and disposal of face masks and disposable gloves since these will be required not only on entry into the area, but also intermittently during the time the operator is working in the aseptic area. A full-length mirror should be installed so that personnel can correctly adjust clothing after donning sterile garments.

Double-ended hot air sterilising oven

The decision as to whether this should be of the floor loading type or not will depend to some extent on the weight and size of materials to be handled. It is preferable to avoid such ovens if possible since difficulties can arise due to the control of heat dissipation and the achievement of a tight seal at floor level. The oven should conform to the performance specification of the British Standard 3421: 1961, which, for practical purposes, requires a circulation fan.

A small vent may be installed on the aseptic side of the oven connecting the inside of the oven to the positive pressure of the aseptic room such that air from the aseptic room can flow through the oven and out via an automatically controlled valve. This valve can then be automatically switched to the open position at the end of the sterilising cycle, thus speeding up the cooling rate of the contents and preventing the ingress of air into the oven from the white area side. It should not be possible to open both doors of the oven at the same time. It may be considered wise to arrange that the non-aseptic (white area) door cannot be opened from the white area side, unless a person in the aseptic room pushes a control button first. The oven should operate on a semi-automatic cycle, the effect of which has been related to a knowledge of the oven temperature–time characteristics for each load type by the use of a multi-channel temperature recorder.

If the oven is to be charged with large loads of, for example, glass bottles, then the cooling time will be considerable (several hours) and this may necessitate installing an overnight automatically controlled cycle. The additional requirement of frequent inspection by the security staff will be necessary and this problem may be aggravated by the need to arrange a black to white area change each time the oven is viewed. In addition the facility should be designed so that the oven is visible on its aseptic side from the white area. The oven should be designed to operate a cut out and indicate an aborted cycle if, for example, the recirculation fan or the ventilation valve fails to operate. It should be designed in such a way that it fits flush to the aseptic room wall. The inner furniture of the oven (e.g. racks, heating elements) should be so designed as to facilitate safe and easy cleaning; corners should be rounded off. If the oven is operated during the day then the additional thermal gain must be allowed for when designing the air conditioning plant on both sides of the oven. An access point should be installed on the white area side of the oven for the introduction of thermocouple leads.

Double-ended steam steriliser

Many of the principles outlined above apply equally as well to a double-ended steam steriliser as to a double-ended sterilising oven. There will probably be more frequent demands for maintenance visits to the autoclave by the engineering staff than would be the case with an oven (e.g. renewal of door seal gaskets) and this should be accommodated for in terms of training and clothing requirements. A set of tools should be retained within the aseptic area for use by the engineer and they should be cleaned and sterilised after each use. In general, multicycle sterilisers (e.g. those with different cycles for bottled fluids, porous loads, ethylene oxide etc.) are not recommended but if such facilities are chosen, much greater demands are placed on both the person operating the machine and on those responsible for their management.

Product interchange zone

The object of this zone is to provide an exit route for finished products and equipment from the aseptic room to the adjacent white area. If this involves the transportation of products on trolleys, the procedure adopted will necessitate the use of two trolleys, one designed and clearly marked as the aseptic area trolley and the other as the white area trolley with each stored in its appropriate area. A low-level physical stop board at the floor interjunctions is a useful means of delineating a white zone from an aseptic zone in an air lock.

General points regarding aseptic areas

Speak panels should be installed, and carefully sited, to allow for ease of communication; they are easier to clean and control than are telephones. Intercom devices, if used, should be of the type which operate by the push of a button (using the elbow) and which will withstand formaldehyde gassing programmes and other cleaning and disinfection procedures. It is important to bear in mind the fact that a device handled or used by several people will represent a means of microbial cross contamination. Piped gases (e.g. pneumatic airlines, nitrogen, propane) should be passed through an inline sterilising membrane filter before being fed into the aseptic area. Sprinklers should be avoided where possible, but if the authorities insist on their installation, care should be taken to ensure that they do not 'weep' and thus introduce microbial contamination into the aspetic room.

Personnel using the area must be subject to routine microbial screening to ensure that they are not carriers of infectious diseases or represent a hazard above that normally accepted. Personnel should be encouraged to report any conditions which might put at risk the aseptic environment such as throat infections, skin lesions or a condition which necessitates the operator leaving the area more frequently than usual.

Whenever a new plant is installed in the aseptic area or a major clean down is completed, the area must be completely disinfected as efficiently as possible. One of the most convenient methods of achieving a reasonable disinfection is to generate, in the aseptic zone, formaldehyde gas at as high a relative humidity and temperature as possible (80% RH and 85°F) (Taylor 1974). If correctly used this method can be relied upon to kill all vegetative forms and most of the common spores remaining after the room has been cleaned to clean room standard and as long as there are no absorbent surfaces within the installation.

The adjacent white area should be equipped to handle the various pieces of equipment used in the aseptic zone which require washing and drying after use and prior to re-entry into the aseptic zone through one of the interlocked systems described above.

CLEAN ROOMS AND ASEPTIC AREAS: CLEANING AND CLOTHING

It is comparatively simple to maintain a correctly designed clean room or aseptic area within its performance specification so long as people and materials are not brought into contact with the controlled environment (Austin 1970). However, people are an inevitable part of the manufacturing process, and since they may account for some 85% of the contamination potential, it is obviously important to restrict their number and movements to a minimum, and to protect the environment from those who must gain access, by the adoption of well-designed protective clothing. The generation and distribution of contamination brought about by the introduction to the clean room or aseptic area of people and materials makes frequent cleaning a vital necessity, and raises the importance of having a clearly defined schedule performed by a competent person.

Cleaning

The objective is to remove contamination which has been generated within the area without putting the product at risk. It is important not to perform any cleaning until operatives have left the area, and production has been suspended with the product suitably protected from the environment. Empty containers and components awaiting processing should be removed from the filling zone or, better still, the line run to an empty status to coincide with the shift change. Some basic points should be considered. Firstly, all cleaning equipment required for a designated area should be clearly identified by a visual indicator as belonging to a specific area. All cleaning equipment should be sterilised by heat whenever possible after use, and before being introduced into an aseptic area (Maurer 1978). Vacuum cleaners should be avoided in aseptic areas and clean rooms and use made of a piped system to a remote vacuum plant through $1\frac{1}{2}$-2-inch diameter pipes. The hoses and attachments can then be sterilised using a heat process when necessary. All cleaning equipment should be stored in a dry condition. Possible inactivation of detergents by inadvertencies, such as the mixing of incompatible ions, should be avoided by exercising control over the distribution, use and purchase of such products within the hospital, similarly, if disinfectants are used (and it is difficult to substantiate their use outside aseptic areas) then careful control is also necessary (Maurer 1978). Aqueous cleaning fluids should be discarded when they fall below 60°C during use due to the rapid growth of microorganisms that may otherwise occur (Ayliffe *et al* 1967). Any schedule will be limited in its effectiveness by the design constraints of the area. Consequently, whenever an area is being designed, it is vitally important to consider the ease with which the area and its equipment can be cleaned. As previously mentioned, product security (good pharmaceutical manufacturing practice) should be built into the design, not merely 'tagged on' as an incidental afterthought after the unit has been constructed. Cleaning and asepsis are inseparable companions; if it is difficult to carry out the former then it is probably impossible to achieve the latter.

Day cleaning

This schedule is best undertaken immediately after the last operative has left the area and the product and components have been suitably protected. The cleaning activities are principally concerned with benches, floors and all working surfaces, and may involve the use of clean room vacuum cleaners (or central suction points) and hot aqueous detergents.

Weekly cleaning

This schedule may consist of the day procedures with additional activities such as the emptying of cupboards and lockers. An aqueous detergent rinse followed by a rinse with water is required. Such cleaning is best undertaken after the last shift each week.

Closedown cleaning

This schedule is often a 4-weekly event, and should also coincide with any major events (e.g. introduction of new equipment) which could put at risk the environmental standards. This cleaning schedule will involve preliminary removal of gross contamination prior to the normal weekly schedule. The final stage of such a programme in the case of an aseptic zone is disinfection by the use of a chemical agent such as water/formaldehyde vapour (Taylor 1974). However, porous materials can only be reliably treated by heat sterilisation.

Clothing

The major difference between the clothing required for use in a clean room and that required in an aseptic area is that in the case of the latter, the garments must withstand heat sterilisation. The most satisfactory sterilising cycle is that achieved in a porous load steriliser, of a type conforming to British Standard 3970: 1966 (part I) at 134°C for 3 minutes, since there may be less degradation of some fabrics during this short time period (Medical Research Council 1959). Resterilised clothing should be worn each time an operator enters the aseptic area.

Considerable experience has been gained during the last decade by the pharmaceutical industry and the clean room garment manufacturers on the adaptation of clean room clothing for pharmaceutical purposes. The choice of design and materials is well documented (Austin 1970). The material should be of a tight weave, retain its properties under in-use conditions and be non-linting. Nylon and terylene fabrics with calendered finish made from monofilament yarns yield very little particulate matter in use. It is essential that the fabric is porous to water vapour and antistatic so as not to lead to operator discomfort. The porosity of garments may fall off rapidly after successive laundry treatments and careful surveillance should be undertaken. It is important that the air conditioning plant is designed in conjunction with the clothing system to be adopted so that operatives will not become uncomfortable whilst wearing such garments.

Suits

The most convenient and effective design of suit is probably the one-piece coverall with ribbed cuff fittings at the ankles and wrists. Sufficient excess should be allowed in the length of the sleeves to prevent the sleeve from 'working up' the arm during use; raglan sleeves may offer greater freedom of movement. The use of 'Velcro' fastenings makes it easier for the operator to fit the garment, allows greater variation in fit between operatives and effects a better seal but may degrade in use and generate particles with ageing. A fold-over flap either over or under the zip gives additional protection from particle emission.

A one-piece coverall that fits very loosely will allow areas over chest and abdomen to balloon when bending down. This air is squeezed out by standing erect, or using the arms, or by pressure against a work bench etc. This is likely to force fine skin and textile particles through the cloth or out from loose sleeve ends, trouser bottoms or jacket necks etc. The garments worn should filter out particles cast off by the skin or underclothing. Two-piece garments may be found to fit more closely and reduce the bellows action that takes place when the garment round the arms and chest is compressed. The lower part of the jacket should be tucked into the trousers and the trouser bottoms should be tucked into the tops of the long bootees. The garments should be rendered antistatic, to prevent them attracting particles. The antistatic agents increase the surface conductivity of the fabric. The charges then move more freely across the surface and dissipate to the cloth below. The build-up of static electricity can be reduced by increasing the moisture content of the atmosphere to 65–70% relative humidity. An equally important thing is an adequate fit whatever system is adopted, and the garment must be easily put on and taken off. Body exhaust system suits, however, offer the best form of protection (Charnley & Eftekhar 1969), but their use in pharmaceutical practice has only recently been established.

Head covers

These should be elasticated to fit snugly around the face just above the eyebrows, down past the eyes and fastening under the tip of the chin and down the neck, preferably by means of a 'Velcro' strip or zip. It should fall into a continuous cape fitting over the shoulders and falling down the chest and back by approximately 6 inches. This head cover is worn underneath the boiler suit. Too much elasticity can cause discomfort around the neck and face.

Foot covers

The foot cover should be designed to fit over the top of suitable plimsolls or shoes. The base should be firm, hard-wearing and not readily cut if the wearer treads on glass spicules. The base should curve upwards from the flat sole (to prevent the foot from sliding off this base) before being firmly attached to the leg and upper foot section. This section is best designed so that it extends just below the knee but above the calf, where it is fixed using tags, 'Velcro' or elastication. The clean room or aseptic area plimsolls or shoes worn underneath this foot cover should be donned immediately before the operator places on the foot covers. These should be capable of being cleaned and sterilised frequently if aseptic conditions apply.

Face mask

In aseptic areas a face mask is of course worn and this should be designed from a material with a minimum of linting property. The face mask must not become moistened during use, and consequently may need to be changed periodically during a shift. In general cloth masks are only 50% efficient and if higher efficiency is needed, then synthetic fibre masks should be used.

Disposable gloves

The effectiveness or otherwise of the gloves worn by an aseptic area operator may have a considerable influence on the cross-infection potential between the person and the product. Since it is impossible to sterilise a process worker's hands by scrubbing and use of antiseptics, any object which is handled will always present a gross contamination risk. Consequently, it is important that the glove is chosen with due regard to its important role. The glove should be elasticised and sufficiently strong to prevent puncture during use, yet allow sensitivity of touch. They should be packaged in such a way as to facilitate an aseptic technique during removal from the pack and putting on. The gloves should be lubricated such that donning and removal are readily accomplished using an aseptic technique, but they should not generate excess lubricating powders into the environment; they should not significantly reduce the sensitivity of the fingers or cause unacceptable discomfort to the wearer after continual use during a shift. Gloves should extend up the forearm over the outer garment sleeve by at least 3 inches, thus providing a seal between the inner atmosphere of the garment and that part of the environment which is most likely to be close to the exposed product.

Packaging of clothing

A convenient procedure is to pack the garments into double-sealed bags with zip-fastenings, each containing a head cover, a pair of foot covers and suit immediately after laundering and prior to sterilisation of the packs in a porous load steriliser. Paper wrappings should be used with discretion for the packaging of clean room clothing and a double-bag system should be adopted if the clothing cannot be brought into the aseptic area using a double-ended steriliser. In all cases a 'pilfer proof' or 'telltale' tape or tag system should be adopted to indicate that the product has been subject to a heat process and that the package has remained unopened until used.

Laundry

Clean room clothes should ideally be laundered in special facilities but this is probably not an economic possibility in the hospital service. However, it is important that certain basic procedures should be considered when laundering garments. The garments should not be washed during the same cycle as linting materials (e.g. cotton gowns), and at all stages precautions should be taken to prevent such cross contamination of the garment. The garments may be monitored periodically after the laundry process for the presence of particulate contamination (ASTM–FSI–65T 1964). The garments should be treated with any necessary antistatic products. The washing cycle should not result in the garments shedding detergent or soap particles when in use due to oversoaping or the choice of an unsuitable detergent for the type of fabric involved. Such contamination can be assessed by using a suction/membrane filter testing technique (ASTM–FSI–65T 1964). Garments must be checked carefully before and after processing for holes and faulty seams and any repairs which are undertaken should give due regard to the special function of the garments.

Changing procedure

The sequence of events followed by an operator entering an aseptic area from a street condition should be clearly defined. It is an advantage to display a written brief abstract of this procedure at relevant places in the changing rooms in order to remind staff of the required sequences.

Changing procedure for an operative entering an aseptic area

Having wiped the feet, enter the 'black' side of the 'black-to-white' changing room and store belongings not required within the manufacturing areas (including clothing etc. that will not be worn beneath the aseptic area sterile garments). Sit on the boot barrier and swivel over to the 'white' side, removing street shoes and donning 'white' area shoes, the street shoes being placed under the boot barrier on the 'black' side, during this movement. Wash the hands and dry (e.g. the hot air dryer). Don the 'white' area hair net, head cover and coat or overall and leave the changing room, entering the 'white' zone preferably by stepping on to a 'tacky' mat. Enter the 'white' side of the 'white-to-aseptic' changing room through the interlocked door and change into the sterile clothing in the following sequence:

1.   Remove the 'white' area coat and head cover and place in the 'white' area locker.
2.   Wash the hands in the 'white' side sink and dry.
3.   Sit on the boot barrier and swivel over to the aseptic side, donning the sterile foot covers during this movement.
4.   Don the sterile head cover followed by sterile face mask and sterile suit, ensuring that all fastenings and overlaps are adequate and checking that the garments are not torn or damaged.
5.   Wash the hands using the aseptic side sink and dry.
6.   Don the sterile disposable gloves ensuring that an aseptic technique is adopted.
7.   Swab the gloved hands with 75% v/v aqueous ethanol immediately on entering the room, and change into new sterile gloves within the changing room after contacting focal points such as door handles.

Mirror facilities should be provided whenever possible in the changing room so that each operator can inspect both the front and rear aspects of his or her appearance before confirming to themselves that they have donned the clothing in a proper manner.

COMMISSIONING, MAINTENANCE AND MONITORING OF PRODUCTION AREAS

Commissioning procedures relating to environmental control will be considered for an aseptic area only; clean rooms and socially clean areas will require only some of these procedures.

Commissioning may be regarded as a three-stage procedure (Fig. 5.4). In the first stage the objective is to confirm, by the use of physical instruments, that the air supply into the area including that passing through laminar flow work stations is filtered to the required standard, feeds into the area at the specified rate, leaves the area by a satisfactory route, provides the necessary positive pressure within the aseptic area and achieves the required airborne particle standard. The second stage is concerned with the effect that equipment and machines have on the air flow patterns and the airborne particle count. Finally the effect of people working in the environment is assessed since this may influence air flow patterns and will certainly affect the airborne particle count and the microbiological condition of the area. The tests undertaken during the commissioning stages will be considered in turn.

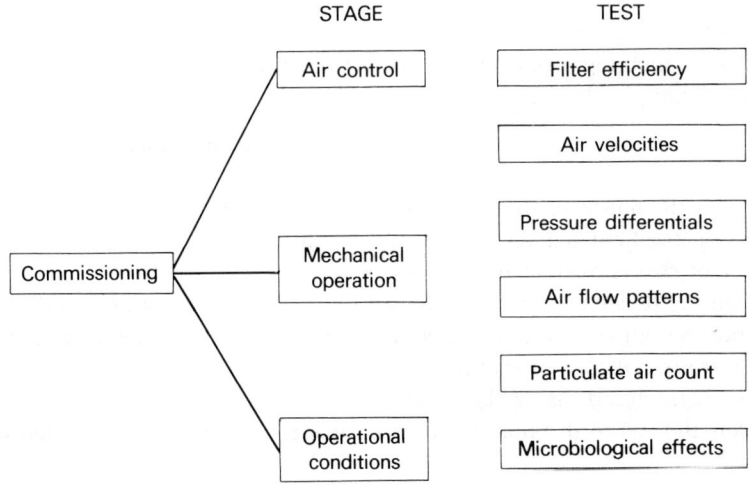

Fig. 5.4   Commissioning of aseptic areas.

Filter efficiency

The object of this test is to challenge the filter with a known concentration of particles of a controlled size at a fixed air flow rate and establish by the use of a physical instrument the ratio of particles which pass through the filter assembly including any which bypass its gasket systems. Consequently, the challenge particles are generated upstream to the filter and fan and the filter face scanned for the emergence of particles at a fixed distance from the filter installation, in the aseptic area. There are two official test methods for this type of commissioning, one of which involves the generation and detection of dioctylphthalate smoke (*Tentative Standard for Laminar Clean Air Devices, AACC—Designate CS—2T*) and the other the generation and detection of sodium chloride crystals (Chemical Defence Establishment, Porton Down, Wiltshire). The efficiency of the filter can also be assessed using a microscopic technique involving the evaluation of a sample of the filtered air collected on a special membrane (British Standard 5295: 1976); however this method does not provide instantaneous results and unlike the other two techniques cannot be used for the precise location of leaks in a filter or gasket system.

Air velocities

The air velocity across each filter must be within set limits, and these figures are laid down by the manufacturers of the filters, or, in the case of laminar flow work stations or laminar flow rooms, in official standards (British Standard 5295: 1976; Federal Standard 209B, 1973). The values normally used for HEPA filters are 27 m ± 6 m per minute. Anemometers of various types may be used to establish the performance velocity of a filter, and it is important that a rate is measured at several points across the filter face in order to ensure that the plenum characteristics (i.e. the size and shape of the ducting from the fan) are technically correct, thus giving an even flow rate across the entire face of the filter.

Pressure differential

The pressure differential obtained between the aseptic room and adjacent areas should be measured using a manometer, and the minimum pressure under the worst case conditions (i.e. with the outer doors of both access air locks and hatches open together) established.

Either a recording manometer or a direct reading manometer will have been fitted to the aseptic area and this should be calibrated and checked at this stage.

Air flow patterns

The air flow pattern achieved throughout the area should be observed by the use of smoke tubes (Mines Safety Appliances, Maidenhead). Special attention must be paid to places where convection currents are likely to be found (e.g. near sterilisers and ovens). Entrance and exit air locks and hatches should be examined with great care and air flow patterns examined at all heights.

Particulate air counts

This test is designed to determine the number and size distribution of particles present in samples of the air in the aseptic area. There are two ways of performing this test, one of which is a microscopic technique (British Standard 5295: 1976) and the other a direct reading apparatus which computes the number of particles in various size ranges using a photometer (Federal Standard 209B 1973). The former method can be undertaken with much less capital equipment cost, whereas the latter method offers the considerable advantage of an instantaneous reading.

Microbiological effects

These tests are much less specific since they rely on sampling procedures and the uncertainties of microbiological methods (Kelsey 1972).

The object of this procedure is to monitor the microbiological flora which results from the introduction of people into the area. Several methods may be used, and the final conclusion from such tests will rely on correlation among the different techniques and the number, type and likely source of the organisms detected. Variations in the results of tests undertaken on different occasions are to be expected and considerable experience is required for effective and practicable interpretation. The tests undertaken should include the following:

Finger touch plates and swabs

The object here is to establish the range and number, if any, of organisms to be detected on operators' gloved hands and critical surfaces such as door handles and bench surfaces. The technique usually involves the use of poured nutrient agar plates.

Settle plates

Airborne particles are collected on an exposed nutrient agar plate by either natural displacement or active sampling using a suction system for a predetermined period (e.g. half an hour) at specific places in the area (e.g. adjacent to a filling machine, on a boot barrier in a changing room) under operational conditions and preferably during the first hour of production.

Challenge trials

In order to establish the likely incidence of contamination for a product the material is substituted by a formulation of similar consistency and appearance but which is known to be a good growth medium for the more common types of organisms. The maximum batch size for the most difficult process should be chosen for this test, and the maximum number of people allowed in the area should be present. A contamination rate of 0.3% may be regarded as a very good result. Reservations have been expressed by some concerning the potential hazard of introducing into an aseptic area a nutrient medium; however, if there is uncertainty regarding effective cleaning and removal of any spillage of such a nutrient then clearly the area is badly designed and should not be used.

Sterility tests

Since sterility of an aseptically prepared product cannot be confirmed by the use of process monitoring instruments alone and since contamination of the sterile bulk solution is a possible occurrence, sterility testing of the product is necessary and must be performed on each batch. However, the sterility test has serious limitations (Kelsey 1972) and is a potential source of disillusion unless account is taken of all other physical and microbiological tests before releasing a batch for use (*Dear Pharmacist Letter* 132/R 227/25).

Maintenance and monitoring

When the tests necessary for the commissioning of an aseptic area have been completed to the satisfaction of all those responsible for its future use, a detailed record must be made summarising the data obtained. This data will then be used as a reference whenever the results of in-process monitoring and maintenance tests are evaluated. Consequently production and quality control staff

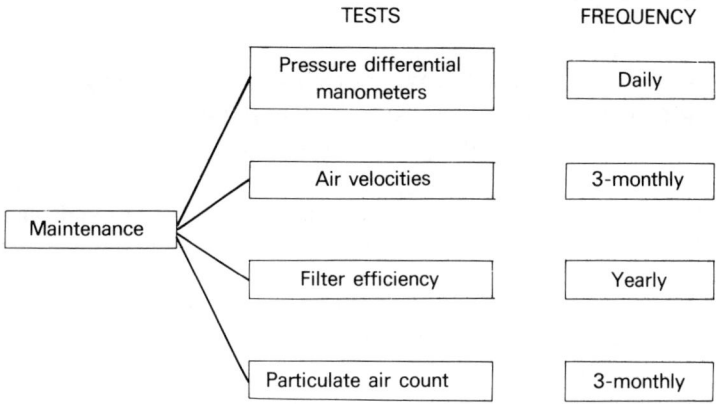

Fig. 5.5 Maintenance of aseptic areas.

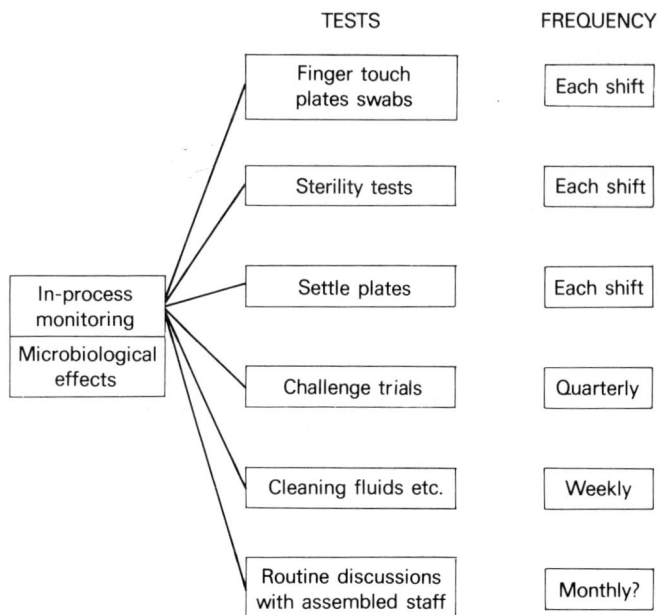

Fig. 5.6 Microbiological monitoring of aseptic areas.

will gradually build up a detailed dossier as records are made, and this will provide considerable retrospective reassurance if satisfactory results are achieved. An example of a maintenance schedule for the air control plant is shown in Fig. 5.5 and for microbiological monitoring in Fig. 5.6. The tests undertaken are identical to those used at the commissioning stage (Fig. 5.4.).

To conclude, aseptic manufacture is an act of faith in the effectiveness of training methods and the job integrity of personnel, enhanced by effective maintenance of plant and microbiological monitoring.

COMMISSIONING AND MAINTENANCE OF HOT AIR STERILISERS, STEAM STERILISERS AND LAMINAR FLOW WORK STATIONS

The vast majority of terminally sterilised products in the hospital pharmacy unit will involve bottled aqueous fluids in sealed containers to be sterilised by autoclaving. In order to ensure sterility, it is essential that each unit of production is of a low order of contamination prior to autoclaving, and is held at the correct temperature for the necessary time (*British Pharmacopoeia* 1973; Medical Research Council 1959). The temperature distribution for a load of bottled fluids during a sterilisation cycle will vary, not only from machine to machine, but also within load type and size within any one machine. Consequently, the relationship between the temperatures throughout the load and the temperature recorded in the chamber drain must be correlated to the temperature recorder chart characteristics for each different load condition. Thus, a 'fingerprint' representing the necessary chart record print for each type of load for a given steriliser can be established and used as confirmation that each batch has been processed correctly. Such a 'fingerprint' system, however, will not be practicable without the necessary commissioning and maintenance controls being routinely carried out and due regard taken of the guidance and standards shown as references in Fig. 5.7. Sterilisation procedures are considered in greater detail in Chapter 6.

When using a steriliser equipped with an accelerated cooling system those responsible for approving the final product should take due regard of the fact that, before a technique such as spray-cooling is adopted, the container and closure systems used should have been proven capable of withstanding the extreme physical conditions to which the closure system will be exposed. In the case of ampoules, where the integrity of the seal is an accepted defect possibility, the use of dye solution leak testing is necessary (Brizell & Shatwell 1973). If a certain percentage of seals are likely to become defective during a production run then some means must be adopted to identify these defectives so that they can be rejected. The most sensible approach is not to subject containers and closures to conditions for which they were not designed (for a detailed discussion of containers see Chapter 6.

Hot air sterilisers

A hot air sterilising oven is generally so deceptively simple a piece of equipment as to be easily overlooked. They should be regularly cleaned since baked-on residues can affect temperature distribution. The door sealing arrangements should be routinely checked and adjusted where necessary, since this aspect of oven design is of paramount importance in effective performance. The quality control of sterilising processes is dealt with in Appendix 1 to this chapter.

Purchase, installation, commissioning and maintenance

Each steriliser must be subjected to a documented planned programme of installation, commissioning and routine maintenance. This must be carried out by either experienced health service staff and/or the steriliser manufacturer's staff under the terms of a maintenance contract. Complete records must be maintained of all such checks. In view of the specialised knowledge required by those responsible within the Health Service for the purchase, installation, commissioning and maintenance of sterilisers, and the high cost for the purchase and maintenance of the necessary test equipment, some Regional Health Authorities have found a three-tier system of delegated responsibility to be a satisfactory means of exerting the necessary control.

The three tiers are: a Regional Steriliser Engineer; a maintenance engineer; the operator. The duties of each tier are considered below (Fig. 5.7).

Regional Steriliser Engineer

This person will be an officer of the Regional Health Authority (RHA) (e.g. an Assistant Regional Engineer). His team will be involved in the following functions:

1. Approval of the choice of steriliser in conjunction with the appropriate health authority staff and agreeing the contract details and specifications in accordance with DHSS recommendations.
2. Supervising and/or performing commissioning tests.
3. Carrying out the routine test schedules which have not been delegated to the district or hospital engineer (e.g. temperature/time profile checks for each load condition, calibration of gauges and temperature recording devices) (see Appendix 1).
4. Undertaking surveillance of the district or hospital engineer's duties and providing him with a job schedule and training assistance.
5. Approving any maintenance contract with the suppliers and checking that it is complied with.
6. Keeping records for each steriliser of the documents arising from all maintenance checks, such as recorder charts, thermocouple recorders, a test report

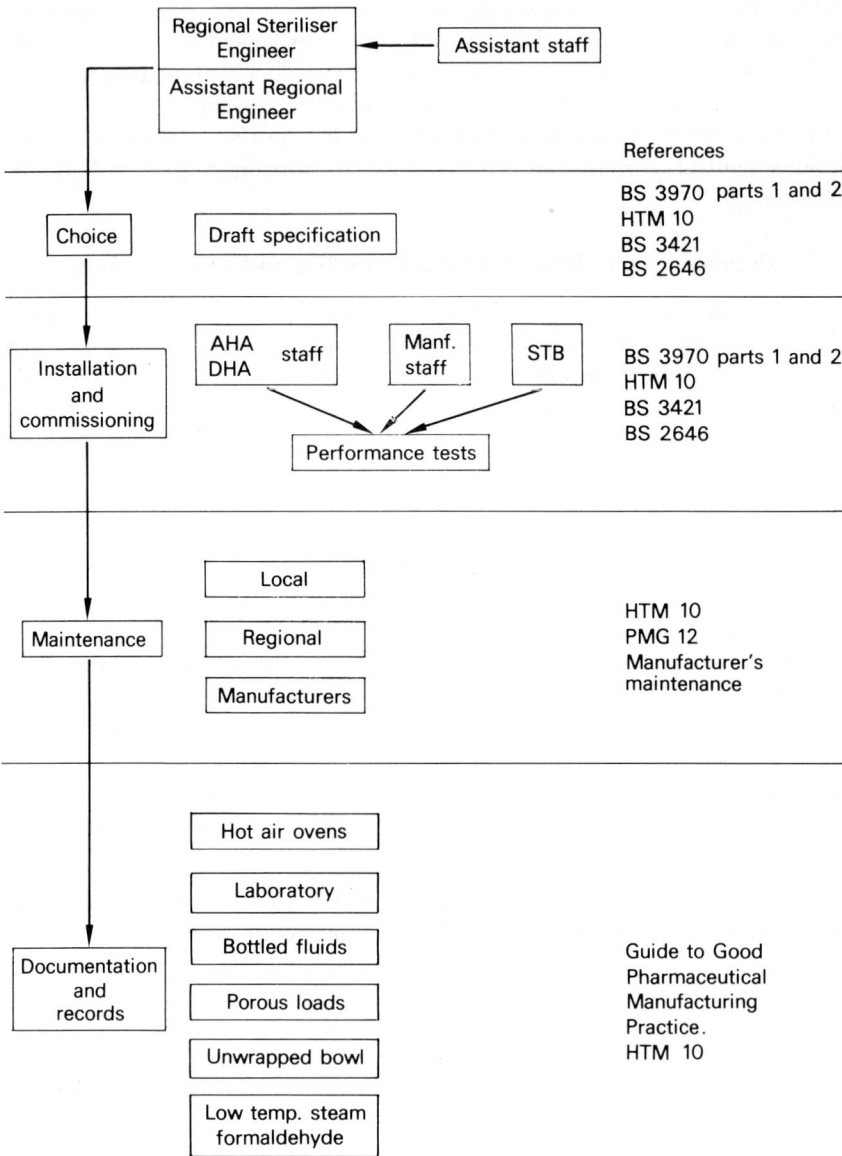

Fig. 5.7 Diagrammatic representation of responsibilities for the purchase, installation, commissioning and maintenance of sterilisers in the Health Service. BS, British Standard; HTM, Hospital Technical Memorandum; PMG, Planned Maintenance Guides; STB, Scientific and Technical Branch; AHA, Area Health Authority; DHA, District Health Authority.

sheet, insurance reports, general reports, maintenance contract reports and unscheduled investigation reports.

7.   Checking the plant history records and ensuring that the agreed procedures have been undertaken.

8.   Communicating routinely with the relevant quality controller to confirm in writing that the steriliser is being adequately monitored and that the performance of the steriliser complies with the specification laid down during the commissioning trials. (If faults arise in the performance of the steriliser then the equipment must be withdrawn from service and the quality controller informed immediately in writing. The equipment must not be used until it has been repaired to the original specification.)

Maintenance engineer

This officer supervises routine maintenance tasks approved by the Regional Steriliser Engineer. He keeps records on the approved test report sheets and the plant history records. He will communicate routinely with the quality controller according to an agreed protocol.

The operator

The operator must be trained in the correct loading and operation of the steriliser and the use of the necessary documents and tests. Each steriliser must be subjected to normal housekeeping procedures by the operator; for example, regular cleaning of door joints and seals, removal of broken glass, labels etc. from drain filters. Since the temperature chart recorder from the steriliser forms an important part of the documentation, care must be exercised when handling the recorder to avoid damage, especially when changing the charts or replenishing an ink supply. Responsibility for such tasks should be given to a nominated person who shall hold the key of the locking device of the recorder. (Hospital Technical Memorandum 10 on sterilisers (DHSS 1968) contains considerable detailed guidance relating to the commissioning, operation and maintenance of all sterilisers used in the Health Service.)

Laminar flow work stations

Design

The following aspects should be considered prior to choosing laminar flow work stations:

1.   The choice of prefilter (normally with a minimum collection efficiency of 95% on British Standard 2831 : 1971 test dust number 2) and its frequency of routine cleaning or replacement should be stated by the manufacturer, upon due consideration of local environmental conditions. The filter should be easily accessible and removable for cleaning and/or replacement.

2. Terminal filters should be of the High Efficiency Particulate Air type (HEPA) (i.e. at least 99.97% retention of test dust no. 1, British Standard 3928: 1965) and should be certified by the manufacturer as complying with this British Standard test.

3. Adequate lighting (i.e. between 850 and 1000 lux) should be provided at the work surface and steps taken to avoid glare.

4. Surfaces within the work space of the work station should be fabricated from impervious materials (e.g. stainless steel) and so designed to facilitate cleaning (e.g. coved corners). The work top of a horizontal laminar flow work station should be designed with a coved lip at the filter-to-filter frame interface to prevent soiling of the filter in the case of accidental spillage of fluids on the work top.

5. Operator comfort is an important consideration when purchasing a work station. The height of the work surface (e.g. is the operator going to be sitting, standing etc.), vibration, noise etc. are aspects which should be considered.

6. Work stations should be fitted with suitable filter screens to protect the HEPA filters against accidental damage.

7. A manometer or similar device should be fitted to indicate the pressure difference across the filter bank. Also, a warning light and/or audible indicator should be incorporated to operate should the differential pressure go outside the recommended range.

8. It is an advantage to equip work stations with fan speed control devices to allow adjustment of the air pressures to compensate for soiling of the HEPA filter. Where a work station has such a facility to vary air flow rate, the control should not be capable of indiscriminate adjustment.

Installation and commissioning (including replacement of the HEPA filter)

The unit should be tested thoroughly after installation and during commissioning by personnel having knowledge and experience in the use of the necessary equipment required. Special attention should be paid to the following:

1. The efficiency of the HEPA filter and the gasket sealing system should be confirmed using a dioctylphthalate smoke generator in conjunction with a suitable detector (*Tentative Standard for Laminar Clean Air Devices, AACC— Designate CS–2T*). Alternatively a sodium chloride thermal generator operated in conjunction with a portable detector unit may be used (Chemical Defence Establishment, Porton Down, Wiltshire).

2. The air velocity measured at right angles to and 10–12.5 cm (4–5 inches) from the HEPA filter face should be 27.35 m (90 feet) per minute plus or minus 6.08 m (20 feet) per minute *across* the filter.

3. The environment of the work station should be monitored using a continuous monitoring particle photometer and the level of particulate contami-

Table 5.2 Comparison of the test methods of British Standard 5295: 1976 and Federal Standard 209B

Test	BS 5296	Fed. Std. 209B
Air quality	(a) Microscopic method all classes (b) Aerosol photometer	(a) Microscopic method for particles 5 µm and above (b) Aerosol photometer for particles 0.5–5 µm
Filter integrity (*in situ*)	(a) Test aerosol $\left\{\begin{array}{l}\text{DOP}\\\text{NaCl}\end{array}\right\}$ all classes (b) No aerosol needed if upfield count is high enough (work stations *only*)	Test aerosol using DOP
Integrity of construction joints	Test aerosol $\left\{\begin{array}{l}\text{DOP}\\\text{NaCl}\end{array}\right\}$	None
Filter retention characteristics	BS 3928 99.95% BS 2331 (test dust no. 1) 99.997%	AACC CS–2T
Fan and motor capacity	Baffle plate test	None
Uniformity of air flow	(a) Air velocity at different points (b) Smoke tests ($\not>10\%$ divergence over 2 metres)	None

Table 5.3 Comparison of the environments specified by British Standard 5295: 1976 and Federal Standard 209B

Aspect	BS 5296	Fed. Std. 209B
Class of environment	Class one $\not>85$ per ft³ @ 0.5 µm + Class two $\not>8500$ per ft³ @ 0.5 µm	Class 100 $\not>100$ per ft³ @ 0.5 µm + Class 10 000 $\not>10\,000$ per ft³ @ 0.5 µm +
Air change rate	$\not<20$ per hour	$\not<20$ per hour
Pressure differentials	$\not<0.06$ inches w.g.	$\not<0.05$ inches w.g.
Air velocity	Horizontal 105 ft/min Vertical 70 ft/min	90 ft/min

nation must be within the required standard for a class 100 environment (Federal Standard 209B 1973) or class 1 environment (BS 5295: 1976). Alternatively, a microscopic technique described in BS 5295: 1976 may be used, in which case the work station must comply with this standard. Although some minor deviations between BS 5295: 1976 and Federal Standard 209B may be found, it is not expected that they will conflict in practice. The two standards are compared in Tables 5.2 and 5.3.

4.   The calibration of the pressure differential manometer or equivalent device should be checked and the warning light and/or audible indicator tested to ensure that it would indicate a fail condition.

5.   A signed certificate should be provided by the tester (who may be the manufacturer) to indicate that the equipment has been installed and commissoned to meet the required specification.

Routine maintenance tests

Routine maintenance and checks should be carried out by personnel having knowledge and experience on the use of the necessary equipment to test this type of work station. A suggested protocol is set out below:

1.   The pressure difference across the filter bank should be recorded daily by the user. The pressure differential manometer or equivalent device should be checked and the warning light and/or audible indicator tested every 3 months to ensure that it would indicate a fail condition.

2.   The air velocity should be monitored every 3 months (see above, installation and commissioning, **2**).

3.   The HEPA filter and its gasket sealing should be checked for integrity every 6 months (see above, installation and commissioning, **1**).

4.   The prefiltration system must be checked, cleaned and if necessary replaced at a fixed frequency. The interval between cleaning and/or replacement of prefilters will vary from several weeks to several months, according to local conditions; a frequency must be established for each site.

5.   The environment of the work station should be monitored every 12 months (see above, installation and commissioning, **3**).

MANUFACTURE OF OINTMENTS, LIQUIDS AND CREAMS

During the last decade there has been an increasing desire that all medicinal products should be manufactured or prepared in such a way that they do not become vehicles of infection (Medicines Commission 1972). This has led some authorities to stipulate a minimum level of microbial contamination by certain organisms per unit weight of product, with a total absence of other specified organisms; other authorities have required that certain products conform to various tests for sterility. The consequence of this trend is that hospital pharmacists will need to manufacture and prepare products under more sophisticated environmental control conditions which, in some cases, will have close similarities to those required for the manufacture of sterile products. If the product is required free of viable organisms and can be subjected to a terminal heat sterilisation process in its final sealed container (e.g. some ointments and liquids) then the facilities required will be less expensive and sophisticated since, unlike parenteral products, freedom from submicron particulate contamination and pyrogens is not normally a part of the product specification. However, it is important that the product is processed in such a way that it does not become grossly infected prior to terminal heat sterilisation. Other products will present greater difficulties. Some will require bulk manufacture in clean conditions followed by sterilisation of the bulk product by membrane filtration and then aseptic filling into previously sterilised components or containers.

In even more complicated cases, the product will be manufactured in two or more parts which are sterilised separately by heat or membrane filtration followed by aseptic blending and/or homogenisation and then aseptic filling. The bulk material may require continuous stirring and warming during the filling procedure. It is unlikely that hospitals will be called upon to provide facilities for the complicated, and thus expensive, process of manufacturing the items described in this paragraph, but will be concerned mainly with the dispensing of such products in small quantities to meet individual prescriptions. A detailed account of the design factors and operational functions required for the manufacture of such products will not be relevant to this book. Discussion will, therefore, be restricted to the design factors and operational functions within a unit in which the following two categories of products are made:

1. Products that can be terminally sterilised by heat in their final sealed containers or products that are not required to pass the test for sterility.
2. Products that must be sterilised either at, or before, the bulk preparation stage by heat or filtration prior to an aseptic fill into sterile containers.

Terminally sterilised products and products not required sterile

The products which present the greatest difficulties in terms of microbial growth are, of course, aqueous systems. During the manufacture and filling of such products, the sources of microbial contamination are numerous. For instance, the storage of distilled water before use in open tanks or vessels which are not adequately microbiologically monitored; the intermittent use of long piping systems for the delivery of distilled or deionised water to the site of use; badly designed plant fitted with inaccessible pipe work or crevices where water may remain trapped and inadequate cleaning of the manufacturing environment. Inadequate ventilation, overcrowding by products and personnel, inadequate hygiene procedures, the use of contaminated disinfectants or deionisation plant infected with microorganisms and insufficient space and facilities for cleaning and proper storage of equipment can also increase the risks of microbial contamination of the product.

The objective behind the design of a unit for terminally sterilised products or products not required sterile is to provide a consistent and controlled environment equipped with access zones through which materials and equipment on the one hand, and personnel on the other, can enter or leave the socially clean area. Such access zones will be used as changing rooms (where operatives can change from street clothes to protective clothes) or as decontamination areas (where equipment or materials can be cleaned prior to entry into the working area). Each access zone should be equipped with self-closing doors and the work area should be ventilated in such a way that the air entering the area is subjected to a purification system. Routine environmental control surveys should be undertaken to provide evidence that the area is conforming to a set standard. Extraction plant will be required in certain parts of the area to remove heat and odours. This should be designed in such a way that the ducting climbing vertically above the appliance can be easily dismantled for routine cleaning. The air conditioning system must take account of both the heat output levels of certain plant and the air loss due to extraction plant. The extraction system should be protected against contamination and blow back. The principles of cleaning and personnel hygiene apply as previously discussed for certain sterile product activities.

The considerations concerning the design of the area (floors, ceilings, services etc.) have already been discussed. Since it is very likely that more than one product may be at different stages of manufacture within the unit at any one time, as certain operations may require extended periods of time, then it may be convenient to separate the filling area from the bulk manufacture zone by a floor to ceiling physical barrier. If this barrier is half glazed then supervision will be made easier, and the environment will be pleasanter to work in. If this type of unit is chosen, then a specific facility must be available for the safe storage of bulk products awaiting filling or intermediate QC approval prior to filling. Before a new batch is started, the bulk manufacture or filling area should be inspected by a responsible person to confirm by signature that the area has been cleared of all items remaining from the previous batch, that it is clean and that batch accountability has been established.

If QC-approved raw materials are to be stored permanently in the area then steps should be taken to ensure that materials are used in their proper sequence, and that the storage area conforms to the requirements of an approved raw materials store. This storage area should be inspected frequently by both QC and production supervisory staff. All raw material containers should be thoroughly cleaned in the access zone prior to admission to the area. An alternative system to having raw materials stored in the area is to have materials delivered to the area from the dispensary weighed, labelled and sealed in suitable containers accompanied by the necessary documentation.

Final product containers, such as collapsible tubes, glass bottles and jars, will require pretreatment prior to use in the filling zone. This pretreatment area is best sited adjacent to the filling zone, and the facilities provided should be similar in principle to those provided for the washing of sterile fluid bottles and other components, except that the final rinsing with IGW may be omitted. After washing, it may be necessary to dry containers and seals in a drying oven, possibly designed as a double-ended facility leading into the filling zone. If products are to be sterilised by dry heat in their final containers a second oven should be provided for this purpose. If a steam-sterilising process is required then exactly the same conditions relating to sterilisers apply as previously discussed.

If it is necessary to allow the products to cool for several hours after filling and before labelling and further batches are to be filled during this period, then the area should be equipped with a quarantine zone in which the batch can be stored and identified in a safe, segregated manner. Label security should follow the guidelines set out previously.

Products sterilised at or before the bulk stage

When preparing products of this type, one of the objectives is to reduce to a minimum the time during which the sterilised materials are exposed to an aseptic environment, and to use heat as a means of sterilising materials brought into the aseptic area whenever possible. The principles behind the choice of facilities and procedures are basically a combination of the points already made and with the added restrictions and controls covered in an earlier section dealing with aseptically processed parenteral products. The technique involves the siting of suitable vessels (e.g. stainless steel jacket-heated pressure vessels) adjacent to the aseptic area which are connected to receiving vessels in the aseptic area. The entire system is so designed that it can be steam-sterilised throughout prior to use. After this sterilisation the piping system is closed off and the materials to be sterilised placed in the pressure vessels on the non-sterile side. After sealing of the vessel, the contents are sterilised by heat, and can then be fed into sterile receiving vessels by opening the isolation valves. The receiving vessel in the aseptic area will be equipped with the necessary blending and homogenising devices so that the product does not become exposed to the aseptic environment until it is a final bulk product. This approach is expensive in terms of plant and machinery and would almost certainly not be practicable in the majority of hospital situations. Therefore, it will probably be more usual practice to introduce liquids into the aseptic area by the use of terminal sterilisation by membrane filtration (see p. 90). Materials which are difficult to filter, even at above ambient temperature, can be introduced into the area by sterilisation in a double-ended oven system (this is both time consuming and expensive; in certain situations it may be feasible to use a double wrap system in conjunction with a single-ended oven and a hatch). The most critical procedures which are likely to take place in the aseptic area concerning the product itself are the blending of previously sterilised fluids, the addition of a sterile solid to a sterile base and the filling process. Since most of these activities on a hospital scale can be undertaken by one or at the most two people, the economics may favour the installation of a horizontal laminar flow room wherein all the critical activities mentioned above take place against the filter bank, with the operator downfield. Such a system has economic advantages only if large laminar flow units would be necessary to protect bulky equipment sited in the alternative system, a conventional clean room designed as an aseptic area. If the scale of operation is small and the batches to be processed involve the use of bench mounted equipment, then a cost-benefit analysis may favour the design of a traditional aseptic area in conjunction with small bench-mounted laminar flow cabinets. The installation of extraction plant in the aseptic area should, if possible, be avoided because of the increased risks of contamination.

MANUFACTURE OF TABLETS, CAPSULES, GRANULES AND POWDERS (DRY PRODUCTS)

It is most unlikely that hospitals will be engaged in the large- or medium-scale preparation of such products, but as regional organisation proceeds, a small number of units could be envisaged in each region with modest capacity for the preparation of tablets, capsules, granules and powders. No attempt will be made to consider formulation factors and only a general consideration of the design of facilities and the broad principles for their use and control will be discussed. The environmental standards including the provision of adequate ventilation, access points for personnel and materials, cleaning and routine monitoring, should be similar to those outlined for the preparation of ointments, liquids and creams which are not required sterile (i.e. a socially clean area). Additional factors which should be taken into account when designing a unit are described in the following stepwise account of the preparation of a small batch of tablets coated with an enteric barrier since all the points relevant to granules and powders will be covered by this example. The tabletting process can be split into five stages and, on the hospital scale, it is assumed that only one batch will be processed at a time (otherwise a cubicle system is necessary).

Dispensing

If approved raw materials are to be kept within the dry products area they should be stored in a locked cupboard or other physically intact storage facility, and only one raw material removed at a time for weighing and checking into a second labelled container. The alternative procedure is to use a central dispensary for all raw materials used in the pharmacy (see Chapter 3). Dust extraction points will be required at each weighing station so that fine powder which becomes airborne can be removed at source.

Granulation

During this stage the dispensed materials, after any necessary preliminary treatment, are blended together according to the batch document, and the dry mass moistened with the granulation fluid and a suitable moist mass prepared. This mass is then, in most cases, passed through a sieve and the resulting moist granules dried to a fixed moisture limit. Assuming that the batch size will not exceed 15 kg, then this stage may be accomplished by the use of a small blade mixer or by hand. However, it should be borne in mind that the use of machinery helps to reduce operator to operator variation for a given process, especially during the moist granulation stage where not only batch size but, in the case of hand processes, the physical technique of the operator during the moist massing or kneading can affect not only the physical characteristics of the tablet but, by inference, its physiological effects.

If materials are to be mixed by hand then the mixing tray should have extended sides (e.g. 6–8 inches high) and rounded corners, and be sufficiently large to prevent spillage of its contents. It should be designed so that the product can be scooped out from the tray without significant loss of material or contamination of the product. If a mechanised process is adopted, then the equipment should be easily cleaned down between batches, should not cause a loss of material in the form of dust during the mixing stages, should be made of material compatible with the material to be handled and should not allow lubricating oils to gain contact with the product. Bearing seals are particularly difficult in this respect. The machine should comply with safety requirements.

Dust extraction will be required during the dry mixing and early stages of granulation. This is probably best achieved by the installation of a small free-standing dedusting unit which can also be used as a vacuum cleaner during clean-down exercises. Facilities will be required for the preparation of granulation fluids and control must be exercised over the water supply to ensure that it does not become grossly contaminated with microorganisms or other foreign material. The water supplied to this unit may be recently distilled or deionised, and the pitfalls previously mentioned must be avoided. Sieving of both raw materials and the moistened granulation mass prior to drying may be required, and in most cases this is probably more conveniently performed by hand than by the use of machinery since the setting-up and clean-down times required for the latter will be disproportionate to the length of the machine run. Sieves are best stored in racked cupboards, and should be checked for damage both immediately before and after use. Facilities will be required in the dry products area for the washing of all equipment such as sieves, trays and other containers. The sink should be sufficiently deep to allow adequate immersion of larger items, and should be designed with rounded corners. Overflow systems should be avoided and plug drains should be constructed in such a way that they can be frequently cleaned and disinfected using hot (80°C) water.

After the moist granulation, the moist granules are dried using either a small fluid bed dryer or fan-assisted hot air oven, and in either case the equipment must be easily cleaned down after each batch. Fluid bed dryers lend themselves more easily to control of the drying process on a weight basis than do ovens. The drying time is reduced considerably by the use of fluid bed dryers, it being feasible to dry 15 kg of moist granules in less than 30 minutes, compared to 3–4 hours in a good hot air oven. Consequently it may well be more convenient to adopt fluid bed drying as the method of choice even on a small scale; however, a hot air oven will still be required for the drying of equipment and for very small batches of product which may be required on occasions. Facilities will be required on which to weigh the product at various stages including the fluid bed drying cycle, since yield accountability will be necessary at various stages during the overall production process. If the fluid bed drying process is to be controlled on a weight basis then the scales should have sufficient capacity to weigh the tared bowl and its moist contents. Dust extraction facilities should be available adjacent to all weighing equipment, and sensitive weighing facilities which may be affected by air turbulence will require special siting and protection if installed in the dry products area. Ease of cleaning must be borne in mind when choosing or siting weighing equipment.

Dry blending

The dried granules are screened next, using a hand or mechanical process similar to that described for moist granules above, and it is at this stage that fine powders become airborne, with the attendant risks to both the operator and the environment and thus other products. Consequently, the operator must be protected by suitable clothing in the case of oestrogenic and cytotoxic products, for example, requiring such investment and house experience as to preclude the preparation of this type of product from the hospital scene on all but a very small scale of activity and batch size. The dry sieving stage may not be practicable until after the granules have cooled and hardened (e.g. products granulated with strong gelatin solution), and consequently facilities will be required for the storage of the product, correctly identified in all aspects, overnight in a suitable environment. The final dry blending stage generally requires the addition of dry powders to the granules, and the mixing of these may be achieved using a manual or mechanical system similar to those discussed for the wet granulation stage, and again dust control and personnel protection are necessary.

Compression

The compression of the final blend granules into tablets will take place on either a hand or a mechanically driven press, and it is difficult to envisage the need for high-speed tabletting machinery in the hospital unit. Most units will find a mechanically operated single-punch machine adequate for their purposes, since the introduction of a rotary press into a unit raises considerable additional problems. These include the high cost of punches and dies of differing diameters and concavities. Routine maintenance is expensive and demands considerable training for both the polishing and examination of tools, and the servicing of the machine itself, and the risk of permanent damage to the operator and/or the machine if inexperienced personnel operate or maintain it. A large proportion of the product is required during set-up and run-off periods of small batches (e.g. 1.5 kg for a sixteen-station rotary press). Floor loading restrictions due to the weight and vibrations, and the high capital cost of the machine and associated hardware, also create problems. Hand-operated presses should not be used for the preparation of tablets in larger quantities than can be produced in a reasonable time, since operator fatigue may affect the running speed of the machine, the feed properties of the granules and consequently the tablet. A tabletting machine should be stripped down for cleaning after each batch, and the tools examined and polished when necessary. A cost analysis may indicate that it is cheaper to send tools away for polishing when necessary and have duplicate sets in stock. During the compression stage facilities will be required for the performance of various physical tests by the machine setter/operator, including, hardness, thickness and weight determinations, and such facilities must be provided adjacent to the machine. Other measurements such as disintegration and friability would be performed industrially by the machine setter/operator, but in the case of a small hospital unit these measurements could be carried out using the adjacent QC laboratory facilities. (Before the start and at the final stages of compression QC staff must be informed, since they will have to approve the initial product against its specification and may wish to take more frequent samples during the run-off stage.)

Tablet dedusting facilities and dust extraction also will be required during the compression stage. The compression weight may be predetermined by granule assay or the tablets made to the theoretical weight; in either case the product must be held in quarantine bond after the compression stage until QC approval has been documented. The containers used for the transportation and short-term storage of granules and tablets should be preferably of the 'one trip' type; if the containers are of the reusable type then they should be designed in such a way that they can be safely decontaminated between batches, and a system must be developed whereby decontaminated containers are safely stored separately from those awaiting decontamination. A further problem which will arise with the reuse of containers is the delabelling process during the decontamination stage; if this is overlooked then obvious and serious consequences could arise. The containers should be designed in such a way that the product is protected from the atmosphere, including light and dust, and facilities should be available for each container to be sealed and labelled appropriately to the product's status in the production cycle. The containers should not be so large that physical damage might occur to the product due to the mass of material above the lower strata of the contents. Female operators are likely to have difficulties lifting quantities of materials in excess of 10 kg. The containers should be tared so that yield accountability can be readily confirmed by weight.

Coating

If the small batches of tablets likely to be made in the hospital unit are required to be coated then it is probably impracticable to think in terms of achieving a sugar-coated or film-coated product with the high-quality finish achieved in industry. The best that can be expected is an uneven coating using, preferably, a chloroform-soluble coating polymer with the required physical properties, and dusting the product at the end of each application with talcum powder, using a hair dryer for example, to remove the solvent. Suitable steps must be taken to remove the solvent vapours from the working area during this process. A small bench-mounted coating pan can be purchased for this type of exercise, but the final product will not have a very pleasing appearance. However, in case of need, and using the modern synthetic films, a reliable product having the required properties and fit for its intended use can be made.

The packaging of tablets and other medicinal products is dealt with in Chapter 10.

PROTOCOL AND DOCUMENTATION SYSTEMS

Before discussing protocol and documentation systems (PDS), a brief note on the subject of quality control (QC) is appropriate, since many people may still regard QC as analytical control and not in its real broad sense, which is the management responsibility for three key areas:

1. Analytical control laboratory.
2. Microbiological control laboratory.
3. In-process quality control.

This section will deal only with in-process quality control (IPQC) since laboratory activities are covered in Chapter 8. IPQC should be designed to give assurance to senior management that the assigned standards and methods built into the unit are being observed and undertaken. However, it is the responsibility of the production team to ensure that the correct quality standards are adhered to, since most IPQC checks are dependent on a sampling procedure and any sampling procedure has limitations regarding its implications on the quality of any one batch and environment which it represents at that time. A continuing record of satisfactory IPQC checks will build up into a reassuring dossier of information, and a change in the pattern may be recognised when routinely reviewing a record. This change may otherwise not have been detected until the problem became serious, that is affecting the product to such an extent that it becomes unacceptable and apparent only during final product testing. Such 'fall-offs' can be brought to the attention of the production manager who can discuss these records with the supervisor and operatives who, if trained and managed correctly, will appreciate the warning and improve this aspect of their performance. IPQC is a useful tool to production management, but it is not in itself an authorisation that all is well at any one time. It gives additional assurance only if staff are trained to use correctly designed facilities and documentation systems in a manner compatible with good pharmaceutical manufacturing practice.

The protocol and documentation system (PDS) outlined below is one example; the principles which require consideration are common to any of the several other systems which can be adopted.

Basic philosophy of PDS

Fig. 5.8 explains diagrammatically how a PDS serves as the life blood of a manufacture or preparation facility. It is a means of ensuring that the subject

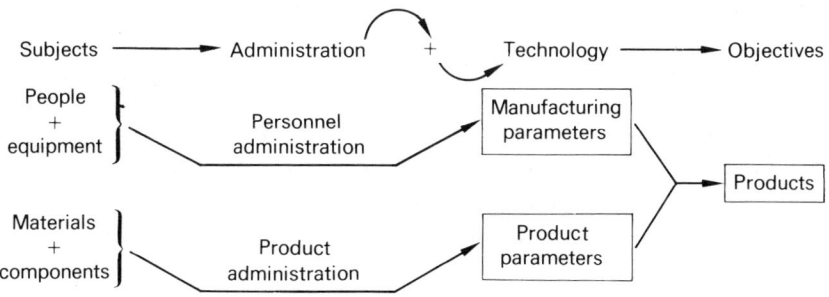

Fig. 5.8 Protocol and documentation.

matter (people and equipment on the one hand and materials and components on the other hand) produce the objective (products) by undergoing the necessary 'interactions', so resulting in a safe and defined product processed under controlled conditions.

For these interactions to be reproduced from batch to batch, year to year, manager to manager, both the administration techniques and the technology must be clearly defined and rigidly applied. A PDS can therefore be split into two groups, one relating to administration matters (such as personnel and product administration) and the other dealing with the technology aspects concerning manufacturing and product parameters.

Administration matters basically cover personnel and product administration and can be subdivided as shown in Fig. 5.9.

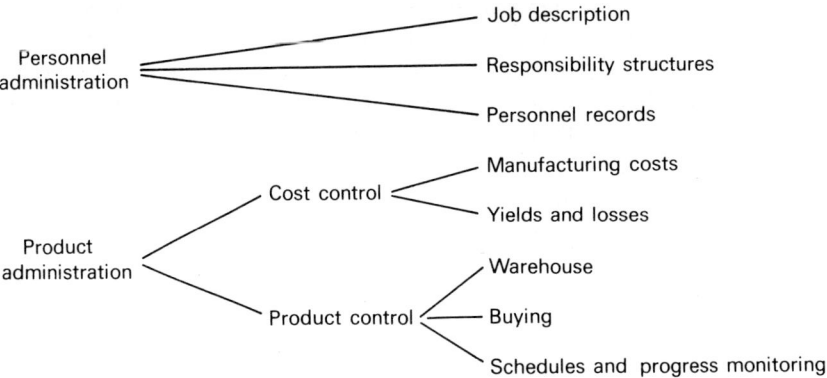

Fig. 5.9   Subdivision of personnel and product administration.

Technology aspects are a means of defining what materials, components and intermediate and final products (product parameters) are required and how people use the equipment to turn these materials and components into the intermediate and final products required (manufacturing parameters). These two parameters can be subdivided as shown in Fig. 5.10.

By product parameters are meant both the product specification in terms of raw materials, intermediate and final products and components and the achieved parameters obtained during the manufacture of a particular batch. By manufacturing parameters are meant firstly the protocols describing the facilities in which any particular product may be handled, in terms of design factors and flow patterns, and secondly PDS covering the processes and procedures adopted for training, maintenance, identification (for example machine and product labels), and the manufacture of products.

The subdivision between product parameters and manufacturing parameters is illustrated in Fig. 5.11. Many of the same raw materials and components (each described by a specification with relevant control documents)

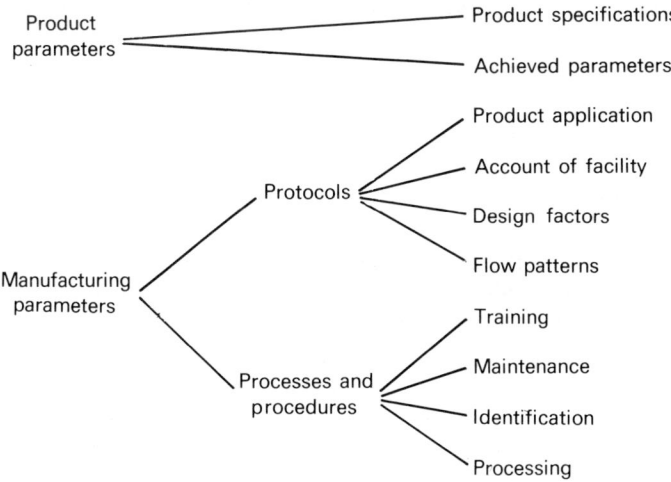

Fig. 5.10 Subdivision of product and manufacturing parameters.

can be used for the production of a variety of products. During the production of these products exactly the same techniques may be used at certain stages and these will be covered by an operational specification used in conjunction with previously applied training documents covering the use of both the equipment and the documentation systems. The operator's techniques will be

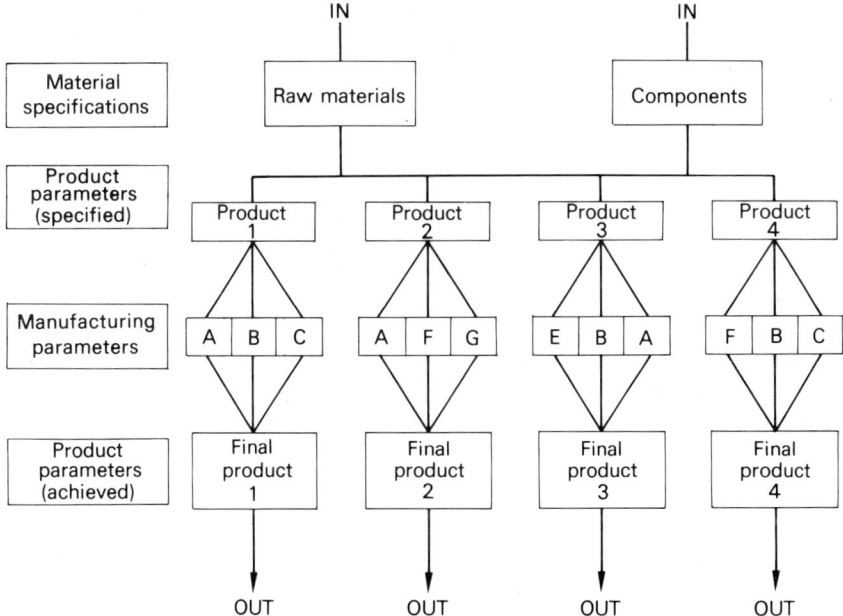

Fig. 5.11 The relationship between product and manufacturing parameters.

similar regardless of the product, and will thus be covered by an operational specification. However, certain parameters or techniques will be specific to the product itself (for example mixing times, sieve sizes, quantities of materials) and these would therefore appear on the product parameter document which will be a unique document for each batch or sub-batch of product. This document therefore serves as a written 'feed-in feed-out' system for the operator who in addition has permanent possession, and a full understanding, of the operational specifications. Product specifications are fed in and achieved parameters are fed out on the product parameters document which accompanies the product throughout its processing life. Thus the PDS for a manufacturing process requires (Fig. 5.11) an operational specification indicating how to carry out certain basic manipulations, and a product parameter document laying down those specifications required for the particular batch in question, and providing a facility for the written feedback in terms of the achieved parameters recorded on the document at this time (IPQC is included in this latter aspect).

Having split PDS relative to the technology of manufacturing into these two groups, each will now be considered in general terms and then in specific relationship to the three major manufacturing activities.

Manufacturing parameters

This is the larger of the two groups and can only be successful if all aspects of the manufacturing process have been analysed and the correct judgements made. Product security can be influenced at this stage.

Protocols

Protocols are a fairly straightforward concept aimed at giving all persons coming into contact with the facilities a broad knowledge of their function and purpose. Before any operator can be trained and supervised so as to gain experience and confidence, he or she must be aware of the significance behind various design concepts of the departments with which he or she comes into contact. Hence the need for a written account describing in simple language how the facility is designed to meet the special requirements of the products met during his or her working life. Such a protocol should describe in general terms the facilities and their use, any special factors or systems, how materials and documents flow through the departments, and in broad terms what the products are and how their safe use may be prejudiced by operator errors during the manufacturing stage.

Processes and procedures

The processes and procedures carried out in a manufacturing unit become more complicated and difficult to describe as the size of the unit and number of staff employed increases. In order to consider this extensive subject in a logical manner, the activities in this area can be broken down into four groups: training documents, identification systems, maintenance documents and processing documents. Training documents and identification systems are not within the scope of this chapter.

Maintenance documents

In the hospital service the majority of the maintenance engineering staff do not come under the control of the person responsible for manufacturing or preparing medicinal products. Consequently, it is even more important that all services provided by the engineering section should be fully documented and accurate records of the actions taken during routine or remedial maintenance retained. Certain of these activities should only be undertaken with the prior approval of both the production and quality assurance staff, and it is important that a written account is available signed by the senior engineer, the head of production and the quality assurance manager describing the restrictions to be imposed and the checks to be made.

Processing documents

As previously mentioned processing documents can be split into two types, operational specifications describing the manipulative procedures required for the satisfactory operation of the equipment, and document specifications laying down the manner in which the documentation system is to be used by all concerned.

An operational specification is a detailed and succinct description giving the trained and experienced operator the information needed to operate the equipment or perform a technique. Such specifications should be explicit and objective and not simply represent a descriptive commentary on what might be expected to happen. This point is illustrated in the following abstract (Baker 1974, reprinted with permission).

'At this point the ... is added, which has previously been dissolved in freshly boiled and cooled distilled water and filtered using kieselguhr as filter aid.' The difficulty about criticising such a statement is only one of deciding where to stop. How much distilled water? How long does the still take to produce it? Boil it in what? How long does that take? Cool it how? And time for doing so? Dissolve by what means? What filtration apparatus? How much kieselguhr? What grade? Does the factory stock anything called kieselguhr or only something under some other, proprietary name? Can this solution and filter step be carried on alongside the other parts of the process or not? Or must it begin the day before?

As a further example, take this step from an autoclave operating procedure: 'At this point the temperature should be 115°.' What does this mean? 115 degrees on what scale? Does it mean that it will read 115°? Or that it might read 115°? If it does not read 115°, what should be done? If it read 115° some time ago and is now at 120° and still rising, then what? Clearly, instructions should be given in numbered steps, and begin, in the first case, 'Distil 50 litres of water' or even more basically, 'Turn on the still', and continue with the other steps in order.

Operational specifications, like all PDS, should be reviewed regularly to ensure that they are still fulfilling their objectives, and an identification system should be developed so that obsolete specifications can be recalled and accounted for before the new specifications are issued. This distribution and control should be the clearly delegated responsibility of one person.

Documentation specifications give a detailed account of the use of the documentation systems, indicating which data the operator must report back, and which data are relevant to each stage in the production procedure. The specification must be written in a language which can readily be understood by all process workers likely to be employed in the unit and should be related closely to the training programme. Such specifications must be reviewed and revised when necessary, and an identification system should be developed for the recall and accountability of obsolete specifications.

Product data and achieved parameters

The general function of a product data and achieved parameters document(s) for each batch of product has already been described. The relevant data required for each of the three types of products are described firstly in general terms and then in specific terms (see Appendix 2) relative to the data to be issued to, and the data to be recorded by personnel.

The record and documentation systems required will vary from unit to unit, and consequently a general account of the parameters which should be covered will be given, but no attempt will be made to suggest form layouts or discuss the basic principles of form design. All individual batch documents can be issued and reassembled into a batch document envelope. Each batch document envelope should accompany the product from stage to stage. Such envelopes can be printed so that the product title, strength, batch number, etc. appear on the outside of the envelope. The issuing of data specific for each batch of product is best reproduced from a master document using a photographic technique. The master document must be checked carefully for error, and identified with a code number so that documents reproduced from it can be identified as having originated from the correct master. A recording and recall system should be developed so that an amended master can be issued and the outdated master and all copies issued from it recalled if in circulation. A record should also be kept of the reason for any changes to master documents.

The same photocopy can also serve as the batch document on to which achieved parameters (e.g. yield of product) are recorded. (It is important that full titles are used to describe raw materials and products and that a standard title is used throughout the pharmacy department for each material. A dictionary may be compiled to indicate the 'house title' of each raw material. If a raw material is supplied labelled with an alternative title, then the 'house title' may be affixed to the material before the delivery is sampled by QC.) Other records which are made during the processing of a product (e.g. environmental checks) may be more conveniently recorded in log books or files, rather than dispersed throughout individual batch documents. A cross-reference system must be operated in order to correlate individual batch documents with such separate records. Record systems must be inspected regularly and signed by both QC and production authorities.

The data required will now be considered in terms of that which is issued and that which is recorded for each stage of the production process. It may not be necessary to provide a separate document for each stage of production, especially if the entire production run is completed up to the final quarantine store within the same day. Separate documents may be required if two or more processes are being undertaken in separate areas.

Examples of the types of documents required for various processes are given in Appendix 2.

APPENDIX 1

Sterilising processes: quality control

The quality controller should confirm that records of routine maintenance and other checks are made and obtain assurance that the professional staff responsible for this work are exercising their duties in a satisfactory manner. Records will be considered for four types of steriliser:

1. Automatic bottled fluid sterilisers.
2. Laboratory autoclaves.
3. Porous load sterilisers.
4. Hot air sterilising ovens.

The necessary records will vary according to the type of steriliser and the format of the records may vary from one health authority to another. The data set out below must be recorded at the relevant time and records retained (DHSS 1977). Biological indicators, chemical indicators and sterility tests are not acceptable as evidence that a steriliser of the above types has functioned correctly.

Automatic bottled fluid sterilisers

These sterilisers should be purchased to conform to the requirements of British Standard 3970: 1966 and include those sterilisers used for the sterilisation of fluids in sealed containers.

Six records are required:

1. Temperature recorder charts (TRC).
2. Plant history records.
3. Steriliser processing logs.
4. Maintenance contracts and insurance surveyor's reports.
5. Commissioning data.
6. Quarterly monitoring data.

Temperature recorder charts

The following data must be recorded (on each recorder chart) by the nominated person responsible for the production process. A separate circular chart must be used for each load.

1. Product title and batch size or description of load.
2. Batch number.
3. Steriliser cycle number.
4. Both the operator's and quality controller's signatures and date to confirm that the TRC matches the master TRC for the product and batch size, or type of equipment (see below, commissioning data).

Plant history record

This document will carry the plant reference number for the individual steriliser and the date of installation and commissioning. It will also record that the minimum of maintenance check tests and examinations as cited in the relevant *Planned Maintenance Guide* have been undertaken by the nominated engineer. It should be noted, however, that the maintenance schedules may be modified to suit any particular steriliser in accordance with the maker's recommended maintenance schedules, such variations being noted in the plant history record.

The following entries signed and dated, must be recorded by the nominated engineer for each steriliser at the minimum frequencies stated:

1. Records of test results for accuracy of the indicating thermometer and the pressure gauge: *weekly*.
2. Records of pressure gauge, indicating thermometer and TRC readings under steady state conditions and confirmation that they correlate: *weekly*.
3. Confirmation that all TRCs have been examined: *weekly*.
4. Records of periodic tests carried out on the automatic thermostatic controller: *6-weekly*.

5. Records of the results of quarterly monitoring tests (see below, quarterly monitoring data): *quarterly*.
6. Every week all entries must be examined by the quality controller and the record signed and dated. Any faults found by the operator, or quality controller or nominated engineer must be recorded. Details of remedial action and subsequent performance checks must also be recorded. The quality controller's signature of approval must be obtained before the equipment is put back into service: *weekly*.

Steriliser processing log

This document will carry the plant reference number of the steriliser and will contain the following entires, all of which must be made by the nominated person responsible for this production process, and for every load sterilised.

1. Product title and batch size or description of load.
2. Batch number.
3. Steriliser cycle number.
4. Indicating thermometer, TRC and pressure gauge reading at 'steady state'.
5. Time at sterilising temperature, from TRC.
6. Operator's signature that temperature and pressure readings correlate and that the TRC matches the master TRC for that batch or equipment.
7. Quality controller's and nominated engineer's signatures and relevant comments to confirm that they have examined the entries at least weekly.

Maintenance contract and insurance surveyor's report

Certification documents must be submitted to the quality controller at agreed fixed intervals by the nominated engineer, stating that the necessary surveys and schedules of contract maintenance tasks have been satisfactorily completed (a detailed entry must have been made, in the plant history record, see above). It will be the task of the quality controller to obtain certification documents from the engineer's department at the stated intervals.

Commissioning Data

This must be provided to cover all batch sizes and types of product to be sterilised. Evidence must be provided of correlation between TRCs and multichannel temperature recorder charts, sensing from bottles throughout the load and chamber drain described in British Standard 3970: 1966, and Hospital Technical Memorandum 10 (1968).
A TRC is obtained simultaneously to the above commissioning record for each batch size or type of equipment and forms the master TRC for the load.

It should be given a specific reference number and be signed and dated by the quality controller. Each multichannel record should be accompanied by a Health Authority engineer's report and be clearly marked with the following data:

1. Sterilizer plant reference number.
2. Number and size of containers, product title and distribution pattern in steriliser chamber.
3. Confirmation that all monitor bottles in the load reached the required temperature and maintained this for the necessary time.
4. Date of test.
5. Signature of the quality controller and the nominated engineer.

The Health Authority engineer's report must be in the form of a test report sheet and in addition may include specific entries for safety device checks (e.g. temperature lock on door mechanism, function of safety valve etc.) (see HTM 10).

Quarterly monitoring data

Quarterly monitoring must be carried out using a multichannel temperature recorder with a minimum of three channels. When a three-channel system is used, one temperature sensing probe shall be inserted into the chamber drain, and the other two within the bottles representing the two extreme worst case conditions. These will be determined by taking into account the report of the thermocouple tests performed at the commissioning stage (see above, commissioning data) where those parts of the challenge load subjected to the greatest temperature lags (i.e. the bottle slowest to heat up and the slowest to cool down) have been determined for each batch size and type of product or load. Only one batch size need be checked each quarter, each batch size may then be tested in rotation. Following major overhaul or modification, however, full commissioning tests should be carried out and the master TRC revised. All superseded master TRCs must be recalled by the quality controller and formally marked 'cancelled'.

Quarterly test results should be countersigned by both quality control and Health Authority engineering staff and similar records made to those described for the original commissioning tests (see above, commissioning data).

Laboratory autoclaves

These types of steriliser vary in size from bench-top models to those comparable with automatically controlled bottled fluids sterilisers. Construction and instrumentation are covered by British Standard 2646: 1955. These machines are manually controlled. It may not be practicable to equip smaller autoclaves with mechanical interlocks to prevent the doors or lids opening with the loads above a safe temperature or when the sterilisation cycle has not been performed satisfactorily. It is imperative that the operating procedures, determined from the commissioning data, are strictly adhered to since both product integrity and staff safety are at risk.

The following basic records are required:

1. Temperature recorder charts (TRCs).
2. Plant history record.
3. Steriliser processing log.
4. Maintenance contract and insurance surveyor's report.
5. Commissioning data.
6. Quarterly monitoring data.

Temperature recorder charts

As with automatically controlled bottled fluid sterilisers described above, a temperature recorder is essential. For bench-top machines there is practical merit in choosing an electronic instrument in preference to the Bourdon tube type. The latter is subject to damage of the capillary system due to constant flexing. Each TRC should carry the following information recorded by the nominated person responsible for this production process:

1. Product title, batch size and description of load.
2. Batch number.
3. Steriliser cycle number.
4. The operator's and quality controller's signatures and data to confirm that the TRC matches the master TRC for that particular product and batch size or type of equipment (see below, commissioning data).

Plant history record

Although laboratory autoclaves are mechanically simpler than automatic bottled fluid sterilisers, it is equally important to maintain adequate records. These will include the data described under automatic bottled fluid sterilisers.

Steriliser processing log

The data described under automatic bottled fluid sterilisers is also required when laboratory autoclaves are used.

Maintenance contracts and insurance surveyor's reports

Certification must be agreed between the quality controller and the engineering department. This must follow the principle described for automatic bottled fluid sterilisers.

Commissioning data

In smaller sizes of autoclaves it may be possible to monitor all bottles in a challenge load and yet use less than twelve temperature probes. In all other respects documentation and certification must follow that described under automatic bottled fluid sterilisers. In the case of sterilizers which generate steam within their chambers, there will not be a chamber drain from which to sense temperatures.

Quarterly monitoring data

The data required is that described under automatic bottled fluid sterilisers.

Porous load sterilisers

These should be purchased to conform to British Standard 3970: 1966. The operations described below are based on guidance which has been available to the health services for many years. These operations should be normal practice for the purchase, installation, commissioning, maintenance and use of any porous load steriliser regardless of its siting within the Health Service (e.g. CSSD, HSDU, pharmacy) or its use (e.g. theatre packs, the processing of equipment used in the assembly of medicinal products etc.). The sterilisers must be used and maintained to the standards described and the following records made:

1. Temperature recorder charts (TRC).
2. Plant history records/steriliser processing logs.
3. Maintenance contract and insurance surveyor's reports.
4. Commissioning data.
5. Quarterly monitoring data.

Temperature recorder charts

If of the circular type, it may record several cycles on one chart, each of which must be so marked to identify the cycle number of the load processed. All stages of the cycle must be shown on the chart including the air removal stages, the sterilising stage and the vacuum stage. The inclusion of all stages of the operating cycle on the TRC is of importance in checking the ability of the steriliser to deal adequately with air which otherwise may remain in the load; malfunction of the steriliser control system with missed or inadequate steam and vacuum pulses may seriously impair the performance of the steriliser.

Plant history record/steriliser processing log

The nature of the work makes the combination of these two records possible in the majority of cases. This document will carry the plant reference number and the date of installation and commissioning along with records of the maintenance tasks and insurance surveys. The maintenance schedules (*Planned Maintenance Guides*) may be modified to suit any particular steriliser in accordance with the maker's recommended maintenance schedules, such variations being noted in the log. The following information must be stated and each entry signed and dated by the supervisor for **1** and **2** and the nominated engineer for **3** to **5**.

1. Bowie and Dick tape test: *daily*.
2. Confirmation that the TRCs are satisfactory: *daily*.
3. Calibration of indicating thermometer, recording thermometer and the pressure gauge: *weekly*.
4. Air leak rate test: *weekly*.
5. Air detector system: *quarterly*.

The importance of the correct functioning of the air detector system and the satisfactory performance of the Bowie and Dick tape test is emphasised (for an explanation of these tests, see BS3970 and HTM 10). Whenever maintenance is carried out which may affect the functioning of the air detector the machine shall not be used until satisfactory commissioning data have been obtained. If the steriliser cycle number is identifiable on each package within a steriliser load then a recall procedure can be adopted.

Maintenance contract and insurance surveyor's report

The documents required are described under automatic bottled fluid sterilisers.

Commissioning data

Performance tests are described in BS 3970 and HTM 10; they are based on both single pack and full load challenge tests, sensing temperatures at test pack centres and relating these to the temperature in the chamber drain. A record of these tests is obtained using a multichannel potentiometric recorder sensing from thermocouples in the test pack and the chamber drain. Satisfactory performance of the air detector system must be demonstrated by the test method described in HTM 10 and BS 3970.

Two master TRCs are prepared, one relating to the single pack test and the other to the full load test. Both are related to their appropriate multichannel TRC. Each pair of master TRCs must be given a specific reference number and be signed and dated by a responsible person; all superseded master charts must be recalled and formally marked 'cancelled'.

Quarterly monitoring data

This must be a repeat of the commissioning tests described above and similar records must be made.

Hot air sterilising ovens

These should be purchased, installed, commissioned and maintained to the requirements of British Standard 3421: 1961. The following records must be maintained:

1.   Temperature recorder charts (TRC).
2.   Plant history records.
3.   Processing logs.
4.   Maintenance contracts (insurance surveyor's reports are not required).
5.   Commissioning data.
6.   Six-monthly monitoring data.

Temperature recorder charts

When fitting a temperature recorder to an oven not previously so equipped, care must be taken to site the probe in the coolest part of the oven. This position should be established by precommissioning tests (see later). On each TRC the following data must be noted, for every load sterilised (and a separate circular chart used for each load), by the nominated person responsible for this production process:

1.   Product title and batch size or description of equipment.
2.   Batch number.
3.   Operating cycle number.
4.   Operator's and quality controller's signatures and date to confirm that the TRC matches the master TRC for the product and batch size or type of equipment (see later and commissioning data).

Plant history record

This document will carry the plant reference number for the individual steriliser and the date of installation and commissioning. The following entries, signed and dated, must be recorded by the nominated engineer for each steriliser at the minimum frequencies stated:

1.   Records of test results for the accuracy of the indicating thermometer: *weekly.*
2.   Confirmation that the indicating thermometer and the temperature recorder correlate at ready state condition (i.e. 160–162°C): *weekly.*
3.   Confirmation that the door seal has been examined and is satisfactory: *weekly.*
4.   Confirmation that all temperature recorder charts have been examined: *weekly.*
5.   Records of any faults found by the operator, or quality controller or nominated engineer. Details of remedial action and subsequent performance checks

must also be recorded, and the quality controller's signature of approval obtained before the equipment is put back into service.

6. Every week all entries must be examined by the quality controller and the record signed and dated.

Processing log book

This will carry the plant reference number and will contain the following entries made by the nominated person responsible for this production process:

1. Product title and batch size or description of load.
2. Batch number.
3. Cycle number.
4. Indicating thermometer and temperature recorder chart readings at steady state.
5. Time at temperature from TRC.
6. Operator's signature that both temperature readings correlate and that the TRC matches the master TRC for that batch or load.
7. Quality controller's signature, at least weekly, to confirm that the log has been examined: *weekly*.
8. Nominated engineer's signature weekly to confirm that the log has been examined: *weekly*.

Maintenance contract

Certification must be submitted to the quality controller at stated intervals by the nominated engineer, confirming that the agreed schedules of contract maintenance tasks have been undertaken satisfactorily.

Commissioning data

The oven must meet the performance specification of BS 3421: 1961. The use of a multichannel temperature recorder is essential for commissioning. Sensing probes which may be thermocouples, or resistance elements or thermistors are placed in challenge load containers distributed throughout the oven. A specific operating instruction for each batch size, type and loading pattern, using thermocouples to determine the necessary temperature–time relationships, must be established before any master temperature recorder chart can be considered specific to that batch. Each master TRC must be signed and dated by the quality controller. It should be given a specific reference number and related to its multichannel temperature recorder chart.

Each multichannel TRC should be accompanied by the Health Authority engineer's report and be clearly marked with the following data:

1. Steriliser plant reference number.

2.   Number and size of containers, product title or description of load and distribution pattern in steriliser chamber.

3.   Confirmation that the batch or load reached the required temperature and maintained this for the necessary time.

4.   Date of test.

5.   Signatures of the quality controller and the nominated engineer.

The Health Authority engineer's report must be in the form of a test report sheet.

Six-monthly monitoring data

This must be a repeat of that data obtained during commissioning, but may, however, be restricted to one batch or load type only.

APPENDIX 2: DOCUMENTATION SYSTEMS

Parenteral products

Bulk manufacture

Data issued

⎧ Product name and strength
⎪ Batch number
⎨ Order number
⎩ Batch size

Ingredient types
Ingredient quantities
Manufacturing method (e.g. mixing times, methods)
Precautions for the product
Precautions for the operator (e.g. wear face mask)
Intermediate QC tests
Pretreatment before sampling
Volume of sample
Document reference number
Master document check signatures

Data recorded

Raw material control numbers (if not allocated above)
Intermediate QC check results*
Signature of dispenser
Signature of checker

* completed by QC staff

Signature of operator at each stage and date
Bubble test on membrane filtrations (check signatures and pressure recorded)*
Reference numbers to equipment used
Number of containers filled, volume per container and total volume
QC release stamp, signature and date*
Expiry date of bulk approval
Signature of supervisor on completion
Steriliser cycle numbers of sterilised equipment

Note. Requisition sheets may be required as separate documents for withdrawal of raw materials and components

Component preparation

Data issued

Product name and strength
Batch number
Order number
Batch size
Document reference number
Number of components to be issued
Description of components
Master document check signature
Specialised treatment (e.g., pretreatment of rubber bungs with bacteriocide)
Washing procedures
Sterilisation procedures
QC sample requirements

Data recorded

Number of units received from store
Control numbers of units
Number of units prepared
Reference numbers of equipment used
Signatures of operators and date
Expiry date of sterilised packs
QC approval, signature and date*
Number of packs and number of components per pack prepared
Signature of supervisor on completion

* completed by QC staff

Filling and sterilisation

Data issued

{ Product name and strength
Batch number
Order number
Batch size
Document reference number

Master document check signatures
Filling data: aseptic or clean room; volume or weight limits; tightening torques; seal length; stirring speed; gas (e.g. CO_2, N_2); inline terminal filtration
Precautions for product
Precautions for personnel
Pretreatment of bulk solution
Terminal sterilisation procedure
Component types
Sampling procedures
Dye test methods for seal integrity

Data recorded

Date of run and time
Production area used
Periodic volume or weight checks
Machine or line reference numbers
Sterilisation cycle numbers of sterilised equipment used
Operators' signatures
Record of line stops including extent and reason
Number of components used
Number of components filled
Number of components returned to store
Number of containers of filled components produced and total yield
QC approval, signature and date of filled products*
QC start checks*
Signature of supervisor on completion
Terminal sterilisation cycle data
Number of containers of filled components sampled by QC*

* completed by QC staff

Inspection and labelling

Data issued

Product name and strength
Batch number
Order number
Batch size
Document reference number
Master document check signatures
Number of labels required
Number of samples required
Expiry data
Labelling procedure

Data recorded

Number of labels issued
Number of units labelled
Number of rejects
Number rejected under each category
Number of labels unused
Label accountability achieved*
Operator's signature, date and time
Bay identity (work area)
Number of samples taken by QC*
Number of containers of filled components received
Product accountability achieved*

Yield summary

Data recorded

Total components issued by store; washed/prepared; returned to wash; filled; destroyed during filling; inspected; labelled; sampled by QC
Percentage gain or loss

Additional records

All additional records should be checked regularly by QC and production authorities. Examples of such records are:
Environmental control log book (see above)
Steriliser data (see above)
IGW production plant log books

* completed by QC staff

Processing log books. These are an ongoing record of each batch of product produced in each area and include the batch number, the volume of product or number of units produced, the date of manufacture and the signature of the operator. Such log books are a useful means of identifying which batches of product were processed during a particular period if troubleshooting has to be undertaken. Thus, log books can be kept for bulk manufacture, component preparation, filling and inspection/labelling activities.

Ointments, liquids and creams

In general there is a close similarity between those parameters required for parenteral products, and ointments, liquids and creams.

Bulk manufacture

As for parenteral (sterile) products

Component preparation

As for parenteral products

Filling

Data issued

As for parenteral (sterile) products but add:
Collapsible tube crimp detail
Maximum and minimum temperature of bulk

Data recorded

As for parenteral (sterile) products but add:
Operator and QC checks of batch number impressed on to the tube

Inspection and labelling
Yield accountability   } all as for parenteral products
Additional records

Tablets, granules and powders

An account of the parameters which should be covered during the preparation of a batch of tablets coated with an enteric film will serve as a general example for this class of product. These parameters will be considered stepwise throughout the production process.

Moist granulation

Data issued

Product name and strength
Batch number
Order number
Batch size
Document reference number
Master document check signatures
Ingredient types and quantities
Pretreatment of ingredients
Precautions for product
Precautions for personnel
Mixing machine and settings
Mixing time
Wet sieve method and sieve size
Drying method
Drying temperature
Drying time and/or weight
Theoretical yield of granules
Procedure for treatment of rework materials

Data recorded

Reference numbers of machines used
Signature of dispenser/admixer of materials
Check signature of dispenser/admixer of materials
Control numbers of materials used (unless allocated above)
Signature at each stage by operator
Actual granulation conditions if different from specification
Actual drying conditions if different from specification
Actual yield of granules produced
Quantity of granules per container and total number of containers
Signature of supervisor on completion
Batch number of reworked material and quantity used

Dry blending

Data issued

Product name and strength
Batch number
Order number
Batch size
Document reference number
Master document check signatures
Ingredient types and quantities
Pretreatment of ingredients
Precautions for product
Precautions for personnel
Dry sieve/milling methods (sieve sizes, hammer speeds, etc.)
Theoretical yield of final blend
Blending method, machine type, order of additions
Procedure for treatment of reworked material

Data recorded

Reference numbers of machines used
Signature of dispenser/admixer of materials and check signature
Signature at each stage by operator
Actual dry sieve/milling method used if different from specification
Actual yield of final blend
Number of containers of final blend and quantity per container
Batch numbers of reworked material and quantity
Signature of supervisor on completion
Number of containers received from granulation stage
Samples taken by QC*
QC approval, signature and data*

Compression

Data issued

Product name and strength
Batch number
Order number
Batch size
Document reference number
Master document check signatures
Precautions for products
Precautions for personnel

* completed by QC staff

Theoretical yield of tablets (weight and number)
Tablet weight (bulk weight and single tablet weight)
Tablet thickness; hardness; disintegration (dissolution time); friability; machine and speed; machine tools

Data recorded

Actual tablet weights (bulk and single);† thickness;† hardness;† disintegration (dissolution time);† friability;† machine and speed; machine tools
Signature of operator and date
Start check QC approval, signature and date*
Final run-off check by QC*
Details of machine stops
Number of tablets produced and weight
Quantity of material to be scrapped and accountability established
Number of containers of tablets and weight per container‡
Signature of operator feeding each container of granules
Samples taken by QC*
Check signature for correct granules identity by QC*
Final QC approval, signature and date*
Signature of supervisor on completion

Coating

Data issued

⎧ Product name and strength
⎪ Batch number
⎪ Order number
⎨ Batch size
⎪ Document reference number
⎪ Master document check signatures
⎪ Precautions for product
⎩ Precautions for personnel
Theoretical yield of coated tablets
Type of varnish (reference to a separate standard master formula)
Method of varnishing (e.g. drying temperature and time, number of coats)
Weight of tablet after varnishing
Disintegration/dissolutions times after varnishing
Drying conditions of cores

* completed by QC staff
† This data is recorded as in-process measurements for each batch by production and at less frequent intervals QC staff, in such a way that it can be related to specific containers of granules and tablets by a cross-reference number.
‡ Each container should be identified numerically in cnronological order of production

Type subcoats (reference to separate standard master formula)
Conditions of application of subcoats
Weight of tablets after subcoating
Type of smoothing coat (reference to separate standard master formula)
Weight of tablets after smoothing coats
Type of final coat(s) (reference to separate standard master formula)
Conditions of application of final coating
Weight of tablet after final coats
Type of polishing system

Data recorded

Batch number of each coating material used*
Number of containers of tablets received
Total weight of tablets received
Weight of tablets coated
Number of containers of coated tablets and weight per container
Actual tablet weights at the end of each stage
Signature of operator at each stage
Disintegration/dissolution times at relevant stages
Signature of supervisor on completion
Accountability established†
Samples taken by QC†
QC approval, signature and date†

Yield summary

Weight of blended granules
Weight of uncoated tablets
Weight of coated tablets
Percentage gain/loss

* Each type of coating material can be made up from separate master document copies, each treated as a sub-batch document, on which are recorded raw materials control numbers, etc.
†completed by QC.

REFERENCES

Austin P. R. (1970) *Design and Operation of Clean Rooms*. Business News Publications, Detroit.
Ayliffe G. A. J., Collins B. J. & Lowbury E. J. L. (1967) *Journal of Hygiene (Cambridge)* **65,** 515.
Baker R. (1974) *Pharmaceutical Journal* **213,** 236.
Brizell I. G. & Shatwell J. (1973) *Pharmaceutical Journal* **210,** 73.

CHARNLEY J. & EFTEKHAR N. (1969). *Lancet* i, 172.
DEPARTMENT OF HEALTH AND SOCIAL SECURITY (1977) *Guide to Good Pharmaceutical Manufacturing Practice.* HMSO, London.
DEPARTMENT OF HEALTH AND SOCIAL SECURITY (1968) *Pressure Steam Sterilisers.* Hospital Technical Memorandum 10. HMSO, London.
DIAMOND J. A. (1972) *Journal of the Society of Environmental Engineers,* December 7.
Federal Standard 209B (1973) is published by GSA Business Service Centre, Boston, USA.
KAY J. B. (1978) *Manufacturing Chemist and Aerosol News,* June, July, August.
KELSEY J. C. (1972) *Lancet* i, 1301.
MAURER J. M. (1978) *Hospital Hygiene.* Edward Arnold, London.
MEDICAL RESEARCH COUNCIL WORKING PARTY (1959) *Lancet* i, 425.
MEDICINES COMMISSION (1972) *Interim report on heat sterilized fluids for parenteral administration.* HMSO, London.
PALL D. B. (1975) *Bulletin of the Parenteral Drug Association* **29,** 192.
Planned Maintenance Guides are available from the Department of Health and Social Security, Alexander Fleming House, Elephant and Castle, London SE1 6BY.
TAYLOR R. J. (1974) *Journal of Hygiene (Cambridge)* **72,** 41.
Tentative Standard for Laminar Clear Air Devices, AACC—Designate CS–2T is published by Institute of Environmental Sciences, 940 East Northwest Highway, Mount Prospect, USA.

British Standards referred to in text

BS 2463   *Transfusion equipment for use.*
BS 2646   *Copper laboratory autoclaves.*
BS 2831   *Methods for tests for air filters used in airconditioning and general ventilation.*
BS 3421   *Performance in electrically heat sterilised ovens.*
BS 3928   *Methods for sodium flame tests for air filters other than for air supply to engines and compressors.*
BS 3970   *Steam sterilisers. (1) porous loads; (2) bottled fluids.*
BS 5295   *Environmental cleanliness in enclosed spaces.*

6

Special aspects of sterile fluid production

R. HAMBLETON & J. A. MYERS

The manufacture of pharmaceutical preparations, including sterile fluids, is described in Chapter 5. However, there are aspects of the production of injections and other sterile liquids which are worthy of more detailed consideration, in particular the production of Injectable Grade Water, autoclaves and containers.

PRODUCTION OF INJECTABLE GRADE WATER

Injectable grade water is water free from pyrogens and as free as possible from particles, dissolved solids and gases. An efficient well-maintained still should produce sterile distilled water. Most pharmacists agree that it is necessary for the viable count to be extremely low to avoid pyrogen production. The purer the water, the higher is its solvent power (Thomas & Harvey 1976; Weston 1972). It is very difficult to maintain the purity of distilled water in contact with glass, some stainless steels etc. hence the wide use of inert tin surfaces for water stills (Le Sieur 1976).

The resistivity meter which is purely for measuring the quantity of ionisable material in the distillate is at best only a guide to the chemical condition of the water. Certainly where there may be organic particles in the water it is possible for metallic impurities to be bound up in organic molecules which are not ionised and, therefore, a high resistivity reading is not conclusive evidence of chemically pure water. A resistance of 1 $M\Omega$ is often accepted as evidence of quality. This can be misleading, since pyrogens, dissolved organic matter, and particulate matter may not affect conductivity. It is advisable to have the resistivity meter attached to the still which can be preset to divert all water of less than 1 megaohm resistance to waste. A meter may indicate contamination by tap water or corrosion of metal work yielding ions to the distillate etc. Stills must always be correctly maintained as laid down by the manufacturer. After being serviced, the still should be run hot to wash away any foreign matter. Bacteriological and pyrogen tests should then be carried out on the distilled water delivered by the still, to check that this important raw material is not contaminated at source. If plastic tubing is attached to the still outlet, it should not yield extractive matter to the distilled water and should be autoclaved daily. The stills should be fitted with devices to automatically control the input of water and prevent overheating. If the input falls below the optimum level so that the boiling chamber may overheat, the still should automatically switch itself off. If the hot distilled water (70–85°C) is transferred through stainless steel pipework to storage tanks or mixing vessels the pipes should tilt downwards to the tanks so that they can be drained when hot and so left *dry* if the system is to be closed down for any length of time. On no account should there be any points in the line where stagnant water can accumulate. Such areas may become foci for the growth of pyrogenic organisms. The distilled water in long pipelines should be kept in constant motion. This is achieved by arranging the pipework in a ring round which the water can be continually pumped. Draw-off taps are situated along the pipe. It is prudent to arrange for steam sterilisation of the pipework when fitting in the pipes.

The basic still consists of an evaporating vessel where boiling water evolves steam into a condenser which converts the steam back to water. An appropriate system of baffles is placed between the evaporator and the condenser to prevent water droplets carrying pyrogens and foreign matter over in the water vapour. There are many types of stills producing high quality distilled water. In the simpler types, the heat from the condensing steam is absorbed by 8–9 litres of cold tap water per litre of distilled water produced. This heat and tap water usually run to waste. The high-efficiency stills, like the Mascarini Thermocompressor Stills, Barnstead Ultra-Therm Stills and the Santasalo-Sohlberg Finn-Aqua Stills, ingeniously reuse the same heat from the hot distilled water over and over again to produce more distillate. As a general rule, the cheaper simple types of still produce higher-cost distilled water. Occasionally a faint odour may be detected in the distillate. This may be caused by the presence of algae in tap water, usually derived from reservoir sources. Such deposits of algae disintegrate in boiling water and volatile products may then be carried over in the vapour and cause a slight odour in the product. In order to reduce the build-up of boiler scale and other deposits in the boiling chambers of stills, the raw feed water is pretreated to remove most of the impurities such as salts and organic matter. Deposits in the walls of the boiling chamber reduce the rate of heat transmission and so reduce the output of distilled water. It is essential to use high-purity feed water in stills.

Manesty steam stills (manually controlled)

These iron stills are low priced and, if there is ample cheap water (with low magnesium and calcium salt content) and a good supply of cheap steam, can give good service for 16 or more years. Steam produced in the boiling chamber is freed from water droplets and pyrogens by passing round baffles. It flows down a cluster of vertical stainless steel or tin-lined condenser tubes which are cooled by cold water rising up the iron cylinder surrounding the tubes and so to the boiling chamber. Here a constant level device allows the excess inflowing water (87·5% approximately) to run to waste.

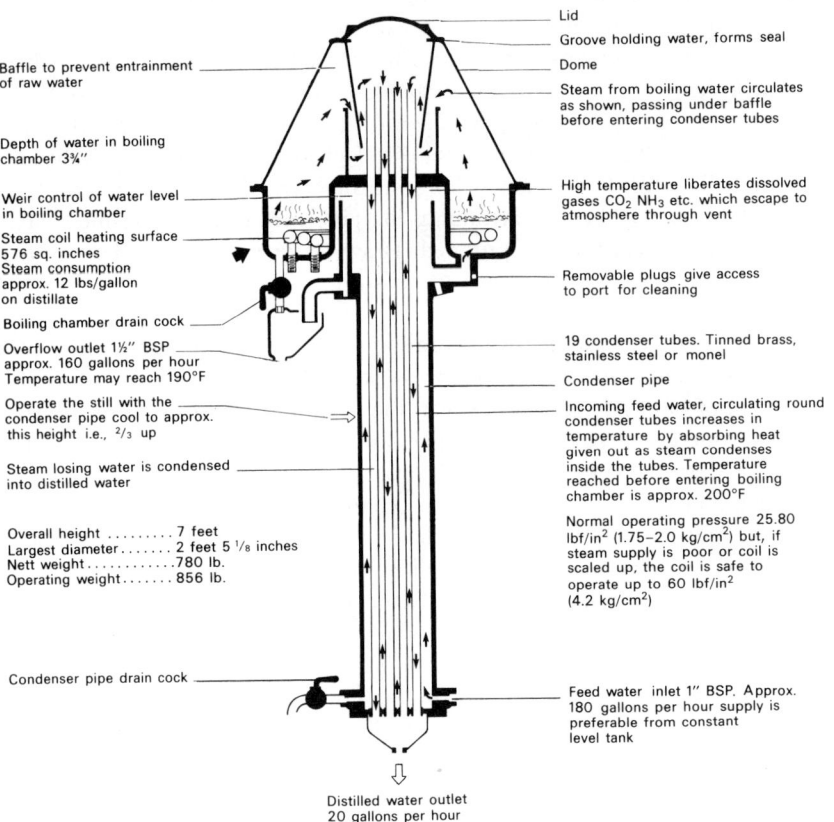

Lid
Groove holding water, forms seal
Dome
Steam from boiling water circulates as shown, passing under baffle before entering condenser tubes

Baffle to prevent entrainment of raw water

Depth of water in boiling chamber 3¾"

High temperature liberates dissolved gases CO_2 NH_3 etc. which escape to atmosphere through vent

Weir control of water level in boiling chamber

Steam coil heating surface 576 sq. inches
Steam consumption approx. 12 lbs/gallon on distillate

Removable plugs give access to port for cleaning

Boiling chamber drain cock

Overflow outlet 1½" BSP approx. 160 gallons per hour Temperature may reach 190°F

19 condenser tubes. Tinned brass, stainless steel or monel

Condenser pipe

Operate the still with the condenser pipe cool to approx. this height i.e., ²/₃ up

Incoming feed water, circulating round condenser tubes increases in temperature by absorbing heat given out as steam condenses inside the tubes. Temperature reached before entering boiling chamber is approx. 200°F

Steam losing water is condensed into distilled water

Overall height . . . . 7 feet
Largest diameter . . . . 2 feet 5 ¹/₈ inches
Nett weight . . . . 780 lb.
Operating weight . . . . 856 lb.

Normal operating pressure 25.80 lbf/in^2 (1.75–2.0 kg/cm^2) but, if steam supply is poor or coil is scaled up, the coil is safe to operate up to 60 lbf/in^2 (4.2 kg/cm^2)

Condenser pipe drain cock

Feed water inlet 1" BSP. Approx. 180 gallons per hour supply is preferable from constant level tank

Distilled water outlet 20 gallons per hour

Fig. 6.1   The Manesty Water Still.

Advantages

These stills are cheap to purchase, install and service.

Disadvantages

They are not normally fitted with compensating devices to deal with fluctuations of water and steam pressure throughout the day. In those hospitals where steam and water pressures fluctuate, the distillate temperature can vary widely and so the still does not constantly work at maximum output. If the water pressure rises rapidly, the water in the still boiling chamber may overflow. It is sometimes difficult to adjust the water input to maintain constant maximum distillate output. Frequently, the outside of the lid joint of the cast-iron boiling chamber becomes coated by an inspissated residue from the boiling water. The conductivity of the water can vary from 0.4 MΩ to 2.65 MΩ. The distillate may have a faint odour if there is algal contamination of the water supply. The running costs are heavy, due to high water and heat wastage in cooling water, run to waste and by radiation. A cooling system whereby the warmed cooling water can be recirculated is now available without any replenishment water being required.

The tinned condensing tubes need removing annually or more frequently for cleaning and examination for leaks. Corrosion of tinned copper tubes may slowly occur at the point where the tubes are held by the base of the iron boiling chamber. Silver nitrate added to a sample of distillate will usually detect leakage of tap water due to corrosion of the collecting tubes.

AMSCO still (American Steriliser Company)

The AMSCO still (Fig. 6.2) is manufactured from passivated stainless steel. The steam from the water boiler in the base passes up through a small orifice which acts as a water droplet baffle, then impinges against a steam-heated bowl surface which literally flash-evaporates any entrained droplets of water containing pyrogens. The steam rises up the outside of the bowl and condenses as it passes over a cooling coil. The distilled water falls into the hot inside of the bowl where dissolved gases are boiled off and rise through the cooling coil to be led away to the outside. The hot distillate flows away through a secondary cooler to the collecting tank.

Advantages

The water boiling tank is easily accessible for cleaning. The whole still is compact and easily kept clean. Automatic control of water levels enables it to be maintained at maximum output. This still can be supplied with automatic controls and safety devices so that it can be left unattended to run continuously. The distillate may be delivered under a pressure of up to 14 lbf/in^2.

Disadvantages

Heat from the distillate and most of the cooling water is run to waste. The constant water level device has been known to jam and feed water then floods into the distillate, hence a diverter should always be fitted to run such contaminated water to waste.

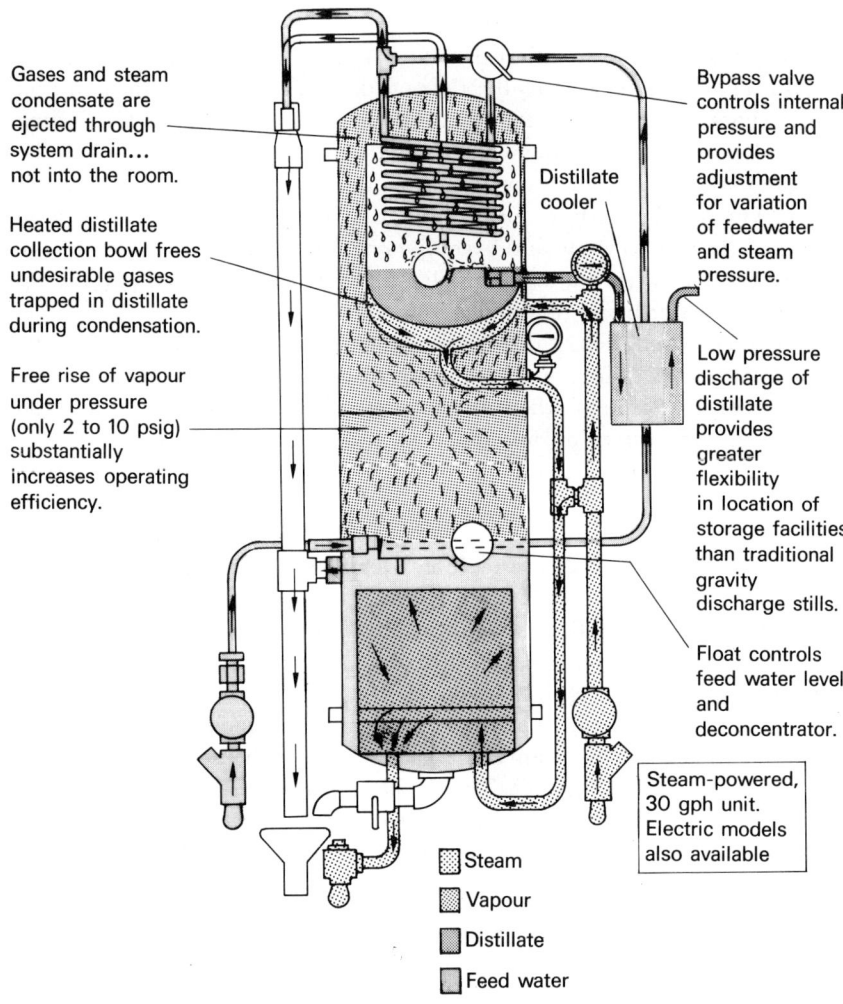

Gases and steam condensate are ejected through system drain... not into the room.

Heated distillate collection bowl frees undesirable gases trapped in distillate during condensation.

Free rise of vapour under pressure (only 2 to 10 psig) substantially increases operating efficiency.

Distillate cooler

Bypass valve controls internal pressure and provides adjustment for variation of feedwater and steam pressure.

Low pressure discharge of distillate provides greater flexibility in location of storage facilities than traditional gravity discharge stills.

Float controls feed water level and deconcentrator.

Steam-powered, 30 gph unit. Electric models also available

Steam

Vapour

Distillate

Feed water

Fig. 6.2   The AMSCO Still.

Drayton Castle thermodrive stills

The thermodrive is a simple evaporator-condenser still (Fig. 6.3). The evaporater and centricyclone are made of mild steel and the condensers, distillate and coolers, baffles, preheaters and all other parts of the unit coming into direct contact with the pure steam or water are made of tin-dipped or lined surfaces.

Thermodrives are supplied in three series with varying outputs:

1.   From 19 to 76 litres per hour (lph).
2.   From 57 to 228 lph.
3.   From 190 to 760 lph.

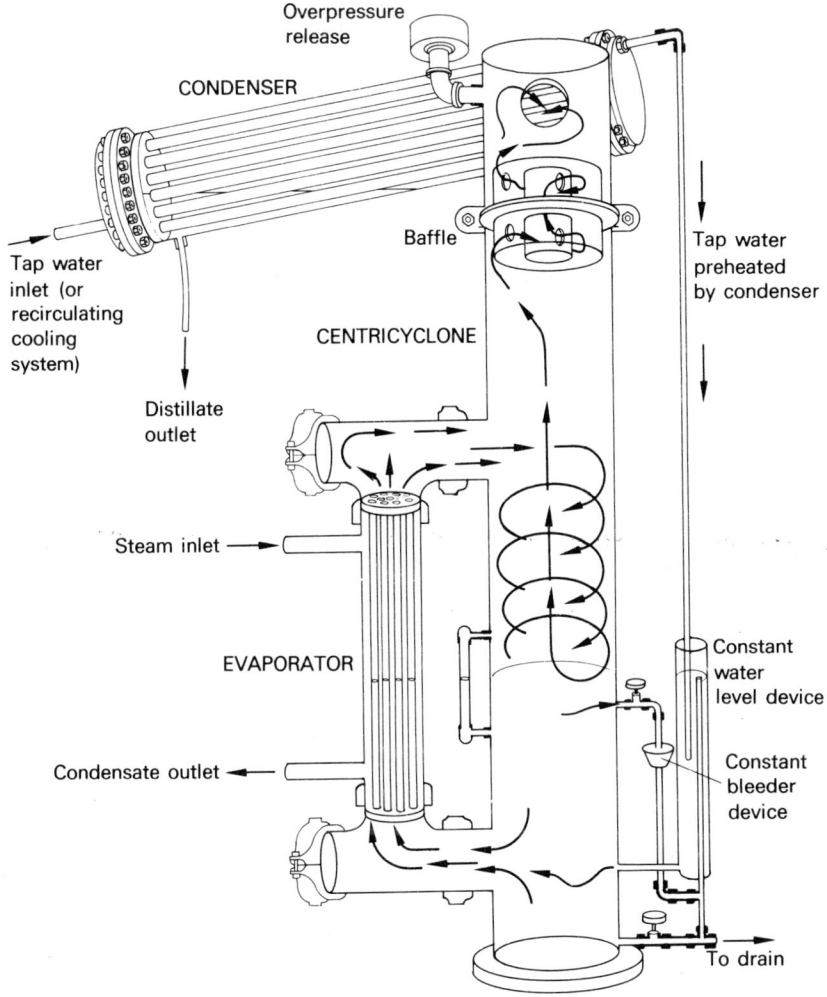

Fig. 6.3   Basic tap water feed thermodrive still (HR series).

Each of these series can be expanded in specific increments of 19, 57 or 190 lph (depending upon the series) by the addition of evaporators, condenser and (with automatically controlled models) automatic valves for the steam inlet to the extra evaporators and cooling water inlet to the extra condensers. Condensers for TD-15 and TD-50 can be initially purchased oversized so that future expansion requirements can be more economical by simply adding on evaporators. Expansion is only possible within the series limits. In the case of the TD-5 series, expansion of capacity is done by the replacement of the smaller-sized steam heating coils located within the evaporator with a larger-sized unit.

All thermodrives can be operated either manually or automatically. Automatic models include valving and tubing to start and stop the still in conjunction with the level of water in the storage tank. They also include an automatic drain valve which will dump all the water in the still every 4 hours to reduce the build-up of scale-forming impurities in the water evaporating chamber. Thermodrives can be equipped with a puromatic diverter to prevent substandard water from going to a storage tank and a high-purity chamber for further elimination of dissolved gaseous impurities, and closed cooling loop condenser for hot cooling water to eliminate the waste of cooling water.

Thermodrives can be fed with pretreated water or with either of two types of a condensate feedback system (utilising the condensed cartridge system). A raw water feed system should not be used in hard water areas and the cartridge feedback return system cannot be used if amines are present in the boiler feed water.

Feed water enters the centricyclone and passes through the evaporator(s) into the tubes located there. Steam to the evaporator(s) circulates round the outside of the feed water tubes. The feed water in the tubes is then almost instantaneously evaporated and passes at high velocity into the connecting centricyclone section. The water vapour is directed downwards in a tight spiral so that even minute particles of impurities are separated out of the water vapour and collected at the base of the centricyclone. A deconcentrating valve constantly draws boiling water from the unit to a waste connection, thereby preventing a build-up of impurities. After the particles have been eliminated by the centrifugal action, the water vapour then rises upwards within the centricyclone through a special pyrogen-removing baffle which strips all the remaining water out of the steam. The pure dry steam is then directed into the condenser section where it is cooled by tap water.

Advantages

The thermodrive design allows for economic flexibility of expansion, eliminating the usual requirement of purchasing additional complete units, at great expense, when more distilled water is required. Having no moving parts, thermodrives are almost noiseless and service problems are minimal. The external evaporator section allows for easy cleaning of the evaporator tubes when necessary, and a spare clean tube bundle can be used to quickly replace one which has become scaled so that production need not be unduly delayed while the dirty bundle is being cleaned. Thermodrives occupy little floor space for the capacity of distilled water produced, and the expansion to greater distilled water production does not significantly alter this feature. Since the design in the evaporator(s) produce an almost instantaneous evaporation of the feedwater, thermodrives have a very quick start-up time, usually within a minute after steam has entered the unit.

Disadvantages

The water and steam consumption is high; a unit with a capacity of 114 litres of distilled water hourly will require 1134 litres an hour of water for both feeding and cooling. Of this amount, about 1020 will be used solely for cooling, to a temperature of 60°C. Cooling water requirements are in direct proportion to the temperature of the cooling water. This same unit will also require 126 kg per hour of steam at a 30lbf/in² pressure. To reduce cooling water use, thermodrives can be connected to a cooling tower or an air-cooled recirculating system which virtually eliminates all cooling water requirements.

Mascarini thermocompressor still

This still is designed to overcome the great expense of wasted heat and cooling water involved in condensing steam by conventional methods (Fig. 6.4). It is fitted with pressure-controlled heaters and a series of safety devices to maintain a constant input of water and constant output of distilled water, so that it can be left to run unattended day and night. The water is heated by electric immersion heaters (Fig. 6.4[8]) or steam (Fig. 6.4[13]) which is regulated by automatic controls to compensate the loss of heat by radiation etc. or to turn off the heat to prevent the still boiling dry. The compressor (Fig. 6.4[4]) acts as a vacuum pump by drawing vapour from the evaporating space (Fig. 6.4[1]). The vapour at 105°C is compressed by this pump which causes the temperature to rise to 120°C (approx) before it passes to the condenser up which the cooling water flows in narrow-bore high-conductivity tinned tubes. The high temperature difference between compressed steam (120°C) and hot cooling water within the tubes causes the compressed steam to quickly pass the latent heat of vaporisation and sensitive heat to the cooling water within the tubes and so condense as distillate.

The hot distillate then passes to the lower heat exchange (Fig. 6.4[3]) and transfers the greater part of its residual heat to the feed water flowing countercurrent through the tubes. The distillate leaves the apparatus by the outlet weir (Fig. 6.4[7]) at 22°C (approx) (i.e. the sensitive heat and latent heat of the steam has been passed back into the still to be used again). Incondensable gases are removed from the system via a special vent (Fig. 6.4[6]).

Advantages

These stills produce very low cost high-purity, pyrogen-free distilled water (resistant greater than 1 MΩ) and are indicated in hospitals where steam and water pressures tend to fluctuate. They are economical in the use of heat and water and can be left to run unattended day and night. The unit is designed to reduce heat loss by radiation to a minimum.

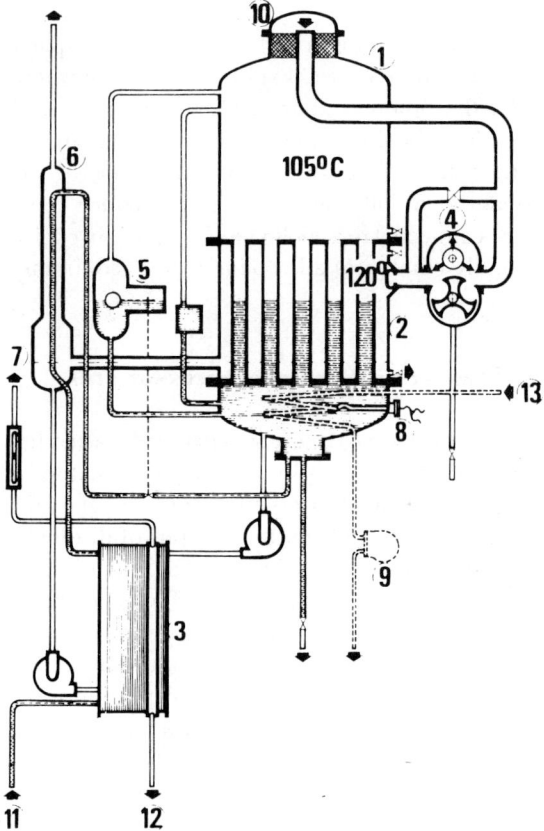

Fig. 6.4 The Mascarini Thermocompressor Still. 1. Evaporator; 2. condenser; 3. exchanger; 4. compressor; 5. level governor; 6. gas discharge; 7. distilled water; 8. electric heaters; 9. condensate discharger; 10. demister; 11. water inlet; 12. concentrate discharge; 13. steam.

Disadvantages

The initial purchase price is high, but this is quickly recovered by savings in heat and water used per litre of distillate produced. The moving parts need routine lubrication and the stuffing boxes in the compressor body require new gland packs at intervals.

Santasalo-Sohlberg AB Finn-Aqua pyrogen-free water still

These stills are manufactured from acid-proof stainless steel. The heat-emitting portions are well insulated to reduce heat losses throughout the system. To reduce the consumption of energy and cooling water, multieffect distillation methods are employed (i.e. the vapour produced by evaporation in one column is condensed in the next column and gives off its heat of evaporation to be taken up by the water evaporating in this next column). The boiler steam used to heat the first column is returned as condensate to the boiler supply, thus there is no contact with the feed water in any way. The feed water vapour generated in the first column passes to the top of the second column, as the heat energy source, and condenses at the base into the first distilled water. Feed water for the second column comes from the bottom of the first column

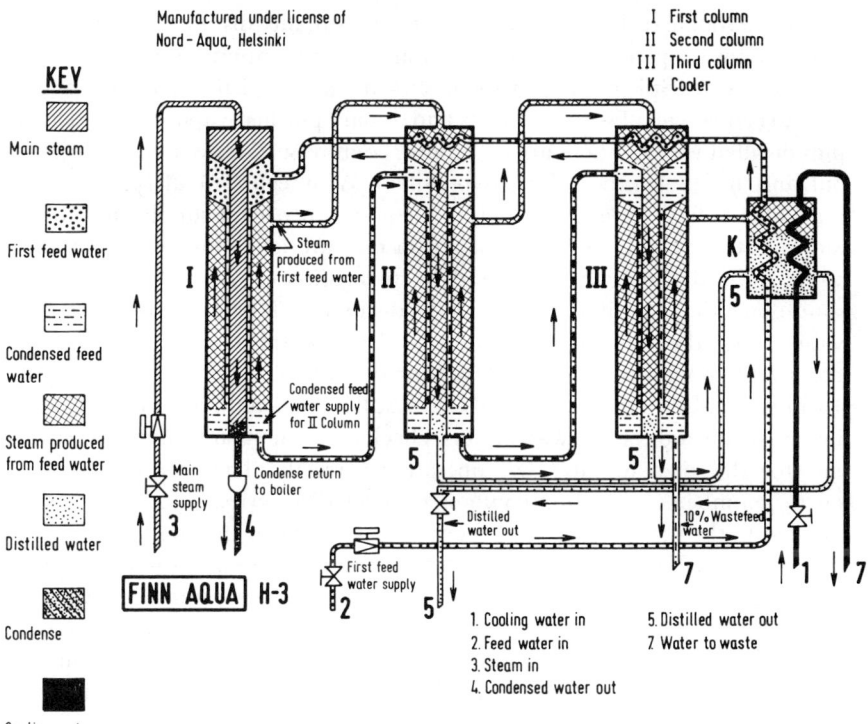

Fig. 6.5   The Santasalo-Sohlberg Finn-Aqua Still.

under pressure from the vapour. The same procedure is repeated to supply column three. The pressure decreases stepwise from the first column to the last. The distilled water from columns two and three, plus the vapour from column three, then goes into the cooling chamber for final cooling. The cooling is carried out by two coils in this chamber, one connected to mains water, or a recirculating cooled supply, the second by the incoming feed water supply, thus commencing the preheating of the feed water. The feed water passes first through the cooler, on through column three, through column two, to supply the feed water for the first column. The feed water temperature reached at this point is 130°C or higher. This hot feed water now passes down tubes as a thin film through the steam energy section to the lower section of the column. The feed water flash-vaporises with high velocity downwards and then it rises in a spiral direction assisted by a fixed spiral inside the column up to the outlet. This tremendous centrifugal force, which is of the order of 500 times the force of gravity, spins out the entrained water droplets and particles, which pass through the perforated wall liner. They then drop to the bottom of the column; this action takes place in all three columns. In the third column only, any remaining feed water plus the impurities are now removed to waste. This is approximately 10% of the incoming feed water. Very high vapour velocity in a conventional still is an impediment to high-quality distillate; it mechanically entrains droplets of raw feed water and so contaminates the distillate. In the Finn-Aqua Still the high vapour velocity is turned to advantage and is used to centrifuge off water droplets and so only purified vapour is condensed into distilled water. There are no pumps, compressors or float valves to wear out, and the whole process is therefore silent. With regard to safety, if the cooling water or feed water pressure is inadequate, the steam supply shuts down and the still stops. Likewise, if the steam pressure falls short of the designed value, the feed water valve closes and the still again stops. A conductivity meter shuts down the plant if the quality of the distillate falls below the set resistance value. Since the still holds very little feed water, this can be heated to the required temperature very quickly, thus the still is in full operation in 10–15 minutes. Maintenance required on this still is very small, consisting of cleaning the steam and cooling water filters, checking of the steam valves and ensuring that the solenoid valves are operating correctly. The economy depends on the number of distilling columns connected in series, since heat is only applied to the first column and external cold water to the cooling chamber. A five-stage still gives the same output of distilled water as a three-stage still, but requires 43% less energy input and 58% less cooling water. The five-stage still is obviously more expensive to purchase, but produces distilled water at a cheaper unit cost. Thus the purchaser must balance the cheaper unit cost of the distilled water and so the annual savings, against the higher initial cost of the larger unit when deciding which would be the most economic and useful to purchase. One litre of distilled water requires 0.45 kg of steam and 2.2 kg of cooling water using a three-stage still.

Advantages

Produces low-cost, high-purity, pyrogen-free distilled water (resistance 1 MΩ or more). These stills are indicated in hospitals where the steam and water pressure tend to vary. The unit is clean, compact and made of polished stainless steel. There are no moving parts to service and it is silent in operation.

Disadvantages

The initial purchase price is very high.

Barnstead ultra-therm thermocompression stills

This is an alternative design to the previously described modular thermodrive stills. It is designed to overcome the major weakness of high water and steam usage noted with thermodrives, by reusing the latent heat of vaporisation to provide an unusually low operating cost (Fig. 6.6). All Ultra-Therms come in five sizes: 57, 190, 380, 760 and 1136 litres per hour (1ph), they are made of stainless steel and all but the smallest capacity units can be heated with electricity, steam or gas or oil. The 57 1ph size can only be heated with electricity or steam. Ultra-therms must be fed with a good quality silica-free deionised water and they are completely automatic with a 7-day timer which can be manually overridden without disturbing the programme. The thermodynamic cycle is temperate-controlled and therefore completely self-balancing. A built-in puromatic diverter continually monitors distilled water purity, automatically diverting substandard water to waste if necessary. Steam vapours are produced in the calandria section and the steam generator, both of which have been fed with feed water, then pass through a set of pyrogen-removing baffles located at the end of each section. These pure vapours join inside a steam ejector which is located after each set of the baffles. The pure vapours are compressed inside the steam ejector and their temperature and pressure are elevated. The pure vapours are then directed back to the shell side of the calandria at a higher pressure than the feed water. The steam which originally came from the steam generator into the steam ejector created a partial vacuum inside the tube side of the calandria when it drew off the calandria steam. This partial vacuum lowered the boiling point of the feed water inside the calandria to 290°F so that the quantity of pure steam required for a heating medium is greatly reduced.

This compressed pure steam coming into the shell section of the calandria meets the cooler feed water and is condensed into pure distilled water. It is the heat given off by the condensing steam which evaporates the feed water inside the calandria, which had already had its boiling point lowered by the partial vacuum created when the steam from the calandria went into the steam ejector.

Advantages

In principle, the ultra-therm design is similar to the Mascarini unit described above. The major difference lies in the use of the steam ejector instead of the motor-driven mechanical compressor to produce the partial vacuum and thus reduce the boiling point of the feed water.

Disadvantages

High electrical consumption in electrically heated units.

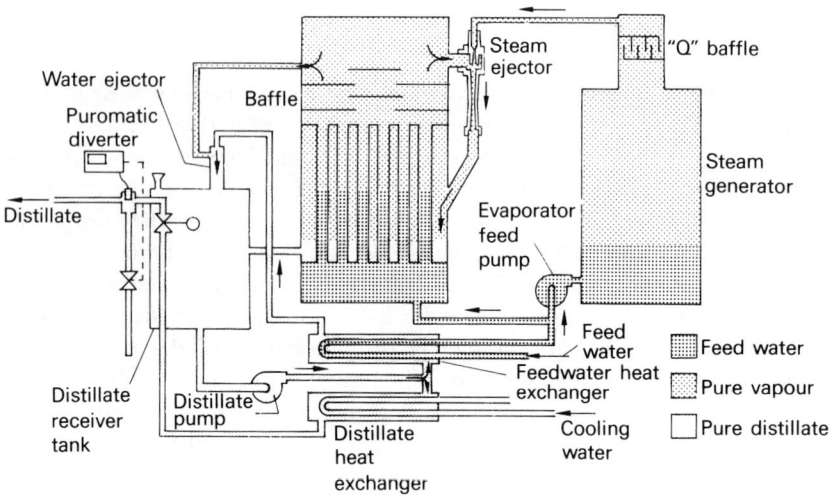

Fig. 6.6   The Barnstead Ultra-Therm Thermocompression Still.

THE STERILISER

The large-scale production of aqueous sterile fluids, whether for injection or topical use, requires the use of moist heat sterilisation as the most practical way of completing the final and possibly most vital stage of this production process. Moist heat sterilisation is eminently suitable for this purpose because it achieves rapid sterilisation of aqueous fluids which are already sealed within their final containers. It is convenient because it employs a medium (steam under pressure) which is often readily available in hospitals. The use of steam is merely to provide a vehicle for heating the fluids.

Staff training

The principles of moist heat sterilisation are learned by every pharmacy student but these principles may be incompletely understood by unqualified staff. This may lead to incorrect processing of fluids and it is essential that the hospital pharmacist ensures that all staff who may have to operate steam sterilisers understand the relationship between the pressure of dry, saturated steam and its temperature and are made to appreciate the function of steam as an agent for transmitting heat energy to the fluids being sterilised. Operators of sterilisers should also be made to understand that the presence of air within the chamber of a steriliser will upset the relationship between steam pressure and temperature, thus leading to a lower chamber temperature for any given pressure. This is important in establishments where fluids may be sterilised both in glass bottles and in plastic containers. In the case of glass bottles the steriliser is operated without air in the chamber but when sterilising plastics containers an air–steam mixture is employed to provide an excess pressure to counteract the tendency of such containers to expand, due to the greater pressure inside the container, and become permanantly distorted.

Having instilled the principles of the process, the pharmacist must then ensure that the operators understand the importance of applying sterilising conditions to all parts of the load itself. It is therefore necessary to show them that the load temperature lags behind that of the chamber during warming up and hence it is necessary to employ a 'fingerprint' of the temperature conditions within the load as a means of monitoring sterilisation (see Chapter 5). This 'fingerprint' may be derived by correlating information from the chamber drain temperature probe, and/or from a simulator, with temperature profiles within test loads during the commissioning of the autoclave.

Modern hospital autoclaves are operated under automatic control. This is necessary as it reduces the time expended in supervising the autoclave during a sterilisation cycle and it should, provided that the controls are adjusted and functioning correctly, ensure that each load processed is given an adequate treatment. However, there is always the danger with such machines that too great a reliance is placed upon the automatic controls and many untrained staff may assume that their responsibility has ended once the chamber has been loaded and the 'start' button has been depressed.

Malfunction of a steriliser is indicated by incorrect pressure and temperature readings and should be indicated on the recorder chart. The British Standard for sterilisers for hospital use (BS 3970: 1966 part 2; currently under revision) specifies controls which should make it difficult for incorrectly processed loads to be issued for use. Nevertheless, it is essential that those responsible for operating sterilisers are instructed to report immediately any incident which might indicate a malfunction of the steriliser.

Monitoring the process

The correct processing of loads during sterilisation has been simplified by the introduction of simulators to control the process. Accurate information about the temperature within the load is an essential part of the quality assurance of sterile fluids. Whilst all large autoclaves have a temperature probe located in the chamber drain, this probe will only indicate temperatures within the chamber and cannot indicate the temperature attained by the load.

Temperature profiles of loads may be obtained by recording the output of thermocouples placed in selected containers in the load. While this may seem to be the most suitable method for determining the temperature profile of a load there are in practice many disadvantages. The repeated insertion of thermocouples into typical containers may lead to eventual damage of the probes. Thermocouples must be placed in the geometric centre of the fluid within the container and it is difficult to ensure that this is always done, especially if the containers are non-rigid or of an opaque material such as polyethylene. Considerable variation is found in the wall thickness of glass containers and some containers of apparently similar design may be available in glasses of different composition. Thus the rate at which containers heat up may vary considerably between different loads. Further disadvantages with the use of thermocouple probes are that it is essential to always locate the probe in that container situated in the coolest part of the chamber, a position which may not be known to the operator. In addition, the insertion of a thermocouple probe destroys the integrity of the closure allowing the leakage of fluid and consequently a different rate of heating than may be true for the remaining containers. Finally the bottle containing the probe may break during the cycle, thus depriving the operator of the information he seeks.

The disadvantages outlined above can be overcome by the use of simulators. A simulator may be a block of metal or plastic located in a fixed position in the chamber or even a selected part of the autoclave chamber wall itself. Being of massive construction, it will heat up more slowly than the chamber void or the chamber drain and will thus follow more closely the temperature characteristics of the load. A thermocouple placed at its geometric centre monitors the temperature within and may be used to activate a timing device controlling the holding time of the cycle. Simulators may only achieve temperature saturation on long cycles for large volume containers. Thus, they may lag behind the temperature of small containers being autoclaved with a short cycle time. This factor does not invalidate the use of the simulator however, as it absorbs heat at a constant reproducible rate on all occasions and the setting of the cycle timer selects that point in the temperature profile for the simulator which is consistent with the achievement of a sterilising temperature by the load. Similarly, the fact that between cycles a simulator may not cool to the temperature of a fresh load before sterilisation does not invalidate its performance. Simulators usually cool to about 40°C between cycles; however, the heating characteristics of the simulator are chosen to take this factor into account at the design stage. The primary function of the simulator is however to control the poststerilisation cooling process. The simulator should operate in conjunction with electrical interlocks on the door mechanism to prevent accidental opening of the autoclave chamber whilst the load is at a dangerously high temperature. The autoclave door should not be openable until the load temperature is less than 80°C.

The simulator must not be considered as a replacement for the drain probe, which is fitted to all autoclaves fed with steam from an external source. The drain probe is effectively in the coolest part of the chamber and has the primary responsibility not only of ensuring that the load reaches the desired temperature before the holding time commences but also of recording this information on the temperature recorder chart. However, in smaller autoclaves of the boiler type in which no drain is fitted the simulator controls both the heating-up and cooling-down processes.

Selection of sterilising plant

The purchase of an autoclave for the hospital pharmacy should not be undertaken lightly, as there are many factors to be considered. The pharmacist must firstly choose an autoclave of a size suitable for the quantity of material to be sterilized in any one working day and secondly he must ensure that the services available within his department (water, compressed air, electricity and steam) are adequate for the plant he intends to purchase. So far as a department producing sterile fluids is concerned, the basic standard for a steriliser is that laid down in BS 3970 (part 2). Sterilisers conforming to this standard have rectangular chambers and are of the downward displacement type, that is, the air from the chamber is displaced via a steam trap in the chamber drain. They are fitted with automatic controls and may or may not have means for rapid cooling of the load with or without an air ballast to maintain equilibrium pressure in the chamber and bottles during cooling. The British Standard specifies the control and sensing devices which should be supplied with the steriliser.

Chamber size

At the time of writing there were 26 different chamber sizes of rectangular form available from British manufacturers. These range from a 20-inch square × 24-inch long chamber to one 72 inches high × 48 inches wide × 82 inches long. With such a variation in chamber sizes it is clear that great attention must be paid to the services, particularly the steam supply, for the efficient operation of the steriliser. Assuming that the services are adequate, the purchaser must choose a chamber size adequate for the intended volume of production of sterile fluids. Thus it is essential to consider how many containers of various sizes and shapes may be loaded into the autoclave in order to assess the total throughput of the steriliser in a given time, say a working day. In considering a particular chamber one must realise that the dimensions quoted by the manufacturer are the total internal dimensions of the closed chamber and the effective useful volume will be less than this. For instance, autoclaves which are fitted with spray cooling devices will offer a reduced effective chamber height. The loading capacity of the chamber will also be less if the purchaser uses a cage type of loading trolley or places the containers in wire crates of an inconvenient size before loading the chamber. The purchaser must also take into account the different sizes of container he intends to sterilise. The number of bottles which may be loaded into a chamber will obviously decrease as the size of the bottles increases. In cases where a chamber and its ancillary equipment were chosen solely on the basis of 1 litre containers it might not be possible to use the chamber to its fullest advantage with smaller containers if the number of shelves in the cage or the crate sizes were fixed. Sterilisers are designed to work with full loads and it is, therefore, inefficient to operate them habitually with a partially filled chamber. Thus, before selecting a chamber size the purchaser must acquaint the manufacturer with such information as the volume of goods to be sterilised in a working day and the sizes of containers used in his establishment, and he should then be in a position to offer advice concerning this point.

Steam supply

In many hospitals, steam is available from a central boiler. The steam pressure in the boiler main may be about 5.5 bar but this may be stepped down by reducing valves before entering different parts of the building. The steam supply to the steriliser must be at pressures adequate to meet the requirements of the manufacturer. BS 3970 (part 2) specifies a supply of dry saturated steam at a pressure of 3.45–4.14 bar. This pressure is reduced immediately before entry to the steriliser and ideally there should be a separate reducing valve between the steam main and each steriliser attached to it. The pressure of the supply should not be too great, as passage through the final reducing valve could lead to superheating of the steam. As well as considering steam pressure one must also consider the quantity of steam which the supply can deliver and the purchaser must ensure that the diameter of the steam supply pipe is sufficient to deliver the weight of steam consumed by the steriliser. This is especially important in areas when more than one steriliser is connected to a single steam supply and where the drain on the supply might at times so reduce its pressure as to make it impossible to operate all the sterilisers simultaneously. Both quantity and quality of the steam may suffer if the length of steam main and supply pipes is excessive, leading to a large amount of condensation.

Where the steam supply is inadequate or not available the purchaser must buy a steam generator at extra cost. In such a situation the provision of an adequate electrical supply is important.

Electrical supply

Some steam sterilisers may require a three-phase electrical supply. Such a supply will normally be available in any hospital pharmacy which has fairly large electrically driven mixers or stills but may otherwise have to be installed at extra cost. Special attention must be paid to the adequacy of the supply if the steriliser operates from a steam generator, as these require a heavy current.

Water supply

Many modern sterilisers employ diaphragm valves which require water at a constant pressure for their proper functioning. The water authority's supply as piped to the pharmacy may be inadequate or, even if quoted as adequate, be subject to local fluctuations depending on the demands of other equipment in the vicinity such as bottle-washing machine, sinks and even WC cisterns. Such fluctuations may lead to intermittent malfunctioning of the steriliser and can be overcome by the installation of a pump to boost the water pressure to the desired level. The additional cost of installing such a pump is usually fairly small in relation to the cost of the steriliser.

Air supply

A supply of compressed air will be necessary for sterilisers which employ an air ballast of the chamber during the sterilisation and/or cooling cycles. Such a supply is usually met by a compressor supplied by the manufacturers but if it is necessary to purchase this separately the pharmacist should ensure that the compressor will satisfy the demands of the steriliser and the steriliser manufacturer's advice should be sought.

Maintenance of sterilisers

Proper maintenance of a steriliser requires a knowledge of mechanical and electrical devices combined with the skills of a plumber and steam engineer. In many instances, staff who are trained in all these skills will not be readily available and may have to be specially trained. Maintenance can, of course, be arranged with the manufacturer on a contractual basis and while this may seem costly initially, it may in the long run be much cheaper to negotiate a contract rather than face the greater cost of calling in the maintenance engineer only when breakdowns occur. Regular maintenance is essential and suitable schedules for maintenance are laid down in HTM 10 (see also Chapter 5). Maintenance carried out according to such a schedule will reduce the instances of equipment failure and lead to the safer production of sterile fluids.

AUTOCLAVEABLE CONTAINERS FOR STERILE SOLUTIONS

Soda-lime glass bottles with aluminium screw cap closures

Ministry of Health aluminium screw bottles for sterile topical water (500 ml and 1000 ml)

Ministry of Health aluminium screw bottles are closed by a flat rubber disc, giving a rim seal. During the heating-up process in an autoclave, air and vapour pressure builds up within the bottle. The aluminium cap expands, may 'back off' and is forced upwards by internal pressures and often allows air and water vapour to escape. At the end of the sterilising process in a spray-cooled autoclave, water and air may be sucked into the bottle. The aluminium cap jams on the bottle neck thread during the cooling-down process and may be difficult to unscrew. There is no metal overseal that has to be broken and so no evidence of tampering with the screw cap. The above flat rubber disc can be replaced by insert type rubber closures to improve the seal (Myers 1974).

MRC bottles (BS 2463: 1962; amended 1963)

These are sealed by an insert rubber stopper. The bung may yield particles to the solution and so is often lacquered. Silicacious flakes can form in some solutions by a reaction involving silicon and magnesium which may originate from the glass or the solution. Threshold levels can be as low as 20 parts/10^6 silica and 1 part/10^6 magnesia. Repeated autoclaving results in the breakdown of the inner bottle surface and glass spicules detach into the solution. Sodium bicarbonate and sodium citrate solutions attack the glass during autoclaving and on storing. Invisible hair cracks can develop by mechanical collisions or other damage in transit. Damage to the bottle lip or inner top centimetre of the neck can spoil the seal. Hence all bottles of solutions must be examined for damage, particulates, haze or fungal growth before use. Aluminium caps deface during autoclaving so a new cap and rubber closure must always be used. The pressure required to screw down the cap on the rubber closure produces a reverse torque in the rubber. During autoclaving the cap expands and the internal pressure of air and water vapour against the cap may raise it slightly and the reverse torque is released and could slightly slacken the cap ('back-off'). There is no tamper-proof overseal.

Borosilicate bottles

Borosilicate glass is more stable than soft soda glass and is of high hydrolytic resistance. This resistance is due to the chemical composition of the glass which is largely composed of oxides of silicon and boron with traces of oxides of other metals (type 1 glass of the *European Pharmacopoeia* 1971). It should be noted that the hydrolytic resistance of borosilicate glass is inherent in the glass and not produced by the treatment of the glass surface (as for example the treatment of soft soda glass containers by SO_2). The greater hydrolytic resistance of borosilicate glass over (soft) glass means that containers may be autoclaved repeatedly with little risk of glass spicules being detached from the inner surface of the containers. They are thus more suitable containers for infusions, especially for the more alkaline solutions, than are soft glass bottles. As well as being more chemically stable, borosilicate bottles have greater mechanical strength. They are thus less liable to damage during handling and this reduction in damage potential, especially at the neck area, contributes to greater safety, since the sealing of the bottle will be more secure. Borosilicate bottles may be reused many times and this facility helps overcome the higher initial cost of these bottles as compared with the soft glass bottles. The problems associated with reuse of glass bottles have already been dealt with in Chapter 5.

A range of bottles for sterile fluids in various sizes is available from manufacturers in a number of EEC countries. These bottles comply with various DIN standards and are freely available in the three grades of glass specified in the *European Pharmacopoeia*. They are designed for plug-insert closures which are secured with aluminium crimp-on seals and all have the same neck size, leading to a useful standardisation of the closures used. The thin wall construction does not detract from the strength of the bottles and has several advantages when sterilising intravenous infusions. A typical 500 ml bottle of this type weighs about half as much as an MRC bottle of equivalent capacity. Thus, infusions will heat up more rapidly in the autoclave and will cool down more rapidly after sterilisation increasing the throughput of the autoclave. Furthermore, the lighter weight assists in loading and unloading the autoclave and in transporting the bottles from the manufacturing area to storage and to the point of use.

AMSCO Square Pak sterile water bottles

These are also made of borosilicate glass (in various sizes up to 2 litres). They are fitted with a neoprene non-drip pouring collar and a bakelite cap which covers the lip and maintains its sterility. The cap allows air and water vapour to escape during heating up in the autoclave. On cooling, the moisture above the sterile water condenses and the vacuum created sucks the cap on tightly, making a vacuum seal. Proof of sealing is established by striking the base of the bottle with a clenched fist. A 'click' denotes a vacuum seal. The neoprene collar must be replaced whenever it shows signs of wear. The bottle cap should only be removed with the bottle in an upright position and immediately before use. Breaking the vacuum with the bottle in an inverted position can lead to an explosion. Square Pak bottles can safely be heated up to 60°C or higher in theatre warming cabinets. If the temperature rises too high, they will not explode because the vapour only fills the vacuum and loosens the cap. The Square Pak bottles are expensive but last many years. They can be fitted with disposable rubber sealing caps.

Glass ampoules for sterile solutions

The glass ampoule may be considered the ideal container for sterile fluids since the method of closure, by fusion of the glass, provides the hermetic seal so necessary for maintaining the sterility of the contents.

Ampoules are available in two types: the open type and the closed type. The open type of ampoule must be washed carefully before use as it can collect much dust during packaging and transportation. The closed type of ampoule is intended to overcome this problem and is supplied by the manufacturer as a sealed unit. Closed type ampoules are blown from glass tubing and sealed by fusion. They may subsequently undergo a heat treatment intended to sterilise them internally. On cooling, these ampoules often develop a pronounced internal vacuum, though some ampoules of German origin are now produced without an internal vacuum. Sealed type ampoules must be opened by the user and this action may lead to the introduction of particulate matter within the ampoule. Prior to filling the ampoules may be cut and broken open, and this action scatters many small glass spicules which may, along with other dirt, be sucked into the ampoule as the vacuum is released. A more suitable method of opening is to heat the ampoules by means of an infra-red heater to raise the internal pressure to a positive level and then use a flame cutter to soften the seal, which will then blow open. Flame cutting produces fewer glass splinters but dirt may still drop into the open ampoule. Machinery is available commercially which utilises both blade- and flame-cutting methods.

Open ampoules and many conventional closed type ampoules require washing before they are filled and sealed. The most efficient washing machines employ ultrasonic agitation as an aid to loosening particles from the inner surface of the ampoule. Ampoules are positioned over needles which inject water inside whilst at the same time the ampoules may be passed through an ultrasonic bath. The washing water is voided from the ampoules by injecting compressed air through the needles. The use of ultrasonic agitation gives much greater washing efficiency than can be obtained with simple jet washing alone. Washing equipment is available which can handle up to 18 000 ampoules per hour.

The filling and sealing of ampoules is essentially the same in both types. The ampoules are filled with predetermined volumes of liquid injected via needles inserted in the necks and the filling machinery often passes the ampoules directly from the filling needle to the sealing jet. Efficient sealing of the glass is achieved by careful adjustment of the burner jets so that the glass is softened adequately to effect a fuse seal and is then annealed to reduce strains in the glass.

The decision as to which type of ampoule is employed may well rest on the availability of suitable washing machinery and adequately trained labour. Closed type ampoules are more costly than the open type but modern machines can open ampoules, fill and seal them again in one continuous operation and hence save labour costs. The more recent vacuum-free ampoules and those heated to a positive pressure before opening may not require washing and this will save the cost of washing equipment.

Plastic containers for sterile fluids

Although historically glass has played a primary role as the material for containers of sterile fluids, plastics seem certain to impinge increasingly on this monopoly. In a number of important centres throughout the world, plastics have to a large extent superseded glass as the material of choice. This is often associated with the adaptation of available facilities or replacement of obsolete plant and machinery. The advantages of plastics are well documented in the Rosenheim Report (1972) and discussed by Groves (1973). In sterile fluid manufacture, plastics are most important in the areas of safety (greater freedom from particles; collapsibility) and, perhaps less significantly, of cost, both direct and indirect (storage; transport; disposability removing the present tendency to recycle glass bottles).

Developments in plastics technology in recent years have provided an enormous range of materials to suit almost any application. When considering suitability for sterile fluid containers, the choice is primarily influenced by the stability of the material when heated. Plastics soften at high temperature, the softening point depending on the nature of the individual plastic. A suitable plastic must have a relatively high softening temperature point. The material, when formed into a sealed container, will be subjected to considerable stresses during sterilisation. The plastic material must be able to withstand increased pressures without seal failure or permanent distortion. The container should at the same time be reasonably flexible at room temperature. These considerations narrow the choice to two important plastics, polyethylene and polyvinyl chloride (PVC).

Polyethylene, of a suitable composition, is sufficiently flexible for use as a sterile fluid container. It is impermeable to water, readily moulded and heat sealed. Unfortunately, polyethylene is to some degree translucent, dependent on composition and thickness. It is also permeable to CO_2 during storage, which may alter the pH of the contents. Pure PVC is a rigid, hard substance; thus grades suitable for use as sterile fluid containers contain added plasticisers to give the desired flexibility to the pack. Suitable grades of PVC are optically clear, may be sealed easily and are strong. However, because some plasticisers are readily extracted from PVC, it is important to ensure the suitability of a particular PVC film for sterile fluid containers. In particular, toxic extractives, such as phthallate salts, should be absent.

Other plastics, particularly laminates, are employed to a limited extent. For example, a nylon–polypropylene combination provides a clear, soft container. However, this material is also permeable to water and is relatively difficult to seal, leading to a high incidence of seal failure during sterilisation.

Many of the Scandinavian hospitals use the 1 litre Haastrup polypropylene plastic container for intravenous fluids. This semirigid container is blown with particle-free air, sealed with a stopper and supplied ready for filling. They require no washing and no rubber closure since they are sealed by fusion of the narrow plastic tube prior to autoclaving. The reject rate is very low because the bottles are sealed almost up to the filling point, immediately after filling. Only a very narrow open orifice is exposed for a second or so during the whole filling process. During autoclaving, these bottles are hung separately on hooks suspended in the autoclave. If they touch each other, the plastic bottles will fuse together. In use, this container does not require an air input filter. Since it does not completely collapse an average of 10% extra fluid must be filled into the containers to enable 1 litre to be removed.

Manufacture of sterile fluids in plastic containers

Source of plastic

Plastic material suitable for sterile fluid packaging must be prepared under far more stringent conditions than are usually found in the plastics industry. Apart from the need to exclude impurities the material should be particle-free. Polyethylene, therefore, is preferably moulded into the final container shape immediately prior to filling (Weiler & Scheider 1966). PVC is obtainable in the form of 'lay-flat' tubing which has been prepared in a particle-free environment. Bags can be moulded into the final shape from this form of tubing by high radiofrequency (RF) or ultrasonic welding. Careful design of the shape, particularly at corners of the PVC bag, is essential to reduce the stress points to a minimum. The most difficult sealing area is between bag and entry port (which must be prepared from separate PVC tubing). This requires an accurately made tool for welding, part of which must comprise an insert within the entry port tubing. Alternatively, PVC bags can be obtained completely welded as a unit. After the filling process, a simple plastic plug with rubber seal is inserted into the inlet port and forms a near-perfect seal provided that the two surfaces are clean.

Filling and sealing

The first striking advantage of plastic containers over glass from the hospital pharmacist's point of view is the elimination of the prefilling washing process. The risk of a particulate contamination in the final product is, therefore, greatly reduced. The filling of non-rigid containers requires relatively sophisticated machinery which must provide rapid filling of the correct volume of fluid through the small inlet port. The air space inside the container after filling should be kept to a minimum to prevent excessive pressure stress within the bag during autoclaving. One feature that requires consideration is the provision of overseals or some other form of cover to protect the entry ports from external contamination after sterilisation. It is essential that all points within the packaging system can be penetrated by steam during autoclaving.

Sterilisation

The process used to autoclave fluids in plastic containers is basically identical to the one used for bottled fluids. Most modern autoclaves can readily be adapted to cope with plastic-packed fluids and some manufacturers are willing to make the necessary modifications. The main additional requirement is for a method of providing an overpressure inside the autoclave chamber to prevent the containers from bursting during sterilisation cycle. The proportion of air and, therefore, the excess pressure, depends on the type and design of container and the amount of residual air remaining inside the container. The latter influences the maximum pressure stress at sterilising temperature. An overpressure of two atmospheres in the autoclave chamber at this temperature is often recommended. The tendency for air to form a layer beneath the steam must be overcome. One method of achieving this is to provide a fan inside the chamber. Alternatively, a continuous spray of hot water through the spray cooling nozzles can provide the necessary agitation of gases. Careful packing of containers in the chamber is essential to ensure an efficient heat distribution. Crazing of the external surfaces of PVC occurs if containers are not placed on clean, non-adhering surfaces. Finally, it is usual to recommend sterilisation at a temperature not exceeding 120°.

Poststerilisation spray cooling must be carried out under an air ballast sufficient to maintain an excess pressure outside the bags. Failure to do this will cause bags to burst. Here again the packing of the load and the form of the cooling spray must permit even cooling throughout the chamber. Handling of plastic containers on removal from the chamber also may pose difficulties, since they will often be at an elevated temperature and therefore soft and misshapen. From the preceding discussion, it should be apparent that the sterilisation of fluids in plastic containers requires very careful monitoring of the process throughout the autoclave cycle to ensure even temperature distribution.

Inspection and quality control

Visual inspection of fluids in PVC containers is feasible provided that the PVC film is of good clarity. Polyethylene is rather more difficult but it is claimed that experienced personnel can detect small particles. All containers should be examined for seal failure, preferably by the application of a standard pressure to the walls of the container for a few seconds (Wikner 1973). Following this inspection, it is normal procedure to overwrap with a water-impermeable plastic, such as polyethylene or polypropylene. This material should not obscure the print of the container. It should be remembered that the inside surfaces of this film will not be sterile unless applied before sterilisation. This procedure is essential for PVC, moisture loss being reduced from approximately 10% per annum to 2% in one study recently reported (Trueman 1973). Overwrapping also helps to protect the pack from damage during handling and aids detection of minute amounts of fluid leaked during storage, indicating the presence of a sealing fault or pinholing.

Clinical aspects of the use of fluids in plastic containers

There are clinical advantages of preparing intravenous infusions in plastic rather than glass containers. Firstly, the reduced particulate contamination has been well documented (Turgo & Davis 1973). Excessive agitation may cause an increase in the amount of particulate matter inside plastic bags (Whitlow et al 1974). Because plastic containers are flexible, they will collapse as infusion proceeds. Consequently, an air filter is unnecessary and microbial contamination from the environmental air is less likely to occur (Hansen & Hepler 1973). Ward staff have also reported a preference for plastic containers, due to reduced weight, their unbreakable property and a reduced danger of touch contamination during the set puncturing procedure (Williams & James, 1973). Nevertheless, some problems do occur, nursing staff have complained of difficulty in inserting giving-set needles fully into bag entry ports and this has in turn resulted in accidental puncturing of the infusion bag wall. It is also claimed that the flow rate tends to fall as infusion proceeds. The examination of the fluid for particles may be difficult due to container opacity and labelling on the surface of the container obscuring the contents, since this often covers a large area of its surface. Staff have also found greater difficulty in reading labels, since plastic packs are often laid flat during ward storage. The release of toxic extractives from PVC, particularly phthalate salts, has been well documented but appears to be insignificant (MacDonald 1974). However, it has been shown that the release of potentially harmful chemicals is significantly enhanced under certain conditions. Chiou and Moorhatch (1973a) have shown that surfactants increase the amount of extractive material in the fluid. Also, some plastics, PVC in particular, absorb certain drugs, for example vitamin A (Chiou & Moorhatch 1974b). This might prove significant when vitamins are added to an infusion as part of treatment. Clinical staff should therefore be made aware of these and other possible adverse effects.

REFERENCES

Chiou W. L. & Moorhatch P. (1973a) Journal of the American Medical Association 224, 1298.
Chiou W. L. & Moorhatch P. (1973b) Ibid. 223, 328.
Department of Health and Social Security (1968) Pressure Steam Sterilizers. Hospital Technical Memorandum 10. HMSO, London.
Groves M. J. (1973) Parenteral Products. Heinemann, London.
Hansen J. S. & Hepler C. D. (1972) American Journal of Hospital Pharmacy 30, 326.
Le Sieur A. (1976) Bulletin of Parenteral Drug Administration 30, 284.
MacDonald A. (1974) Journal of Hospital Pharmacy 32, 70.
Myers J. A. (1974) Pharmaceutical Journal 212, 308.

Rosenheim Report (1972) *Interim Report on Heat-sterilized Fluids for Parenteral Administration.* HMSO, London.
Thomas W. H. & Harvey H. (1976) *Manufacturing Chemist and Aerosol News*, October, 32.
Trueman G. (1973) *Journal of Hospital Pharmacy* **31,** 239.
Turgo S. J. & Davis N. M. (1973) *American Journal of Hospital Pharmacy* **30,** 611.
Weiler H. & Schneider H. (1966) *Die Pharmaceutische Industrie* **28,** 787.
Weston J. H. (1972) *Process Biochemistry* **7,** 17.
Whitlow R. J., Needham K. E. & Luzzi L. A. (1974) *Journal of Pharmaceutical Sciences* **63,** 1610.
Wikner H. (1973) *Svensk farmaceutisk tidskrift* **77,** 773.
Williams H. & James B. (1973) *Journal of Hospital Pharmacy* **31,** 130.

British Standards referred to in text

BS 2463 *Transfusion equipment for use.*
BS 3970 *Steam sterilisers. (1) porous loads; (2) bottled fluids.*

FURTHER READING

Cooper M. S. (1972/3) *Quality Control in the Pharmaceutical Industry*. Vols. I and II. Academic Press, New York.
Department of Health and Social Security (1971) *Guide to Good Pharmaceutical Manufacturing Practice* (Addendum 1974). HMSO, London.
Department of Health and Social Security (1972) *Report of the Committee appointed to Inquire into the Circumstances which Led to the Use of Contaminated Infusion Fluids in the Davenport Section of Plymouth Central Hospital*. HMSO, London.
Department of Health and Social Security (1973) *Report on the Prevention of Microbial Contamination of Medicinal Products*. HMSO, London.
Phillips G. B. & Miller W. S. (1973) *Industrial Sterilisation*. Duke University Press, Durham, N. Carolina.
Secretariat of the European Free Trade Association (1973) *Contamination in the Manufacture of Pharmaceutical Products*. EFTA, Brussels.
Turco S. & King R. E. (1974) *Sterile Dosage Forms*. Lea & Febiger, Philadelphia.

7

Radiopharmaceuticals

W. A. LITTLE

Nuclear medicine is a branch of medicine which is characterised by the observation of nuclear transformations. Although some aspects, notably radioimmunoassays, are undertaken *in vitro*, the larger part of nuclear medicine requires the administration of radioactive substances to the subject. Such substances have to comply with standards of purity and are properly termed radiopharmaceuticals. Since the provision of pharmaceuticals lies within the province of the pharmacist, one might say that radiopharmacy bears to nuclear medicine the same relationship that traditional pharmacy bears to conventional medicine.

All work with radioactive materials is potentially hazardous particularly where chemical and pharmaceutical manipulations are involved. General guidance on radiological protection in hospitals is given in the *Code of Practice for the Protection of Persons against Ionising Radiations arising from Medical and Dental Use* (DHSS 1972).

It should be noted that this Code was designed purely for radiation protection and does not take into account any pharmaceutical aspects. For total design requirements *Guidelines for the Preparation of Radiopharmaceuticals in Hospital* (see Further reading) should be consulted. A laboratory designed for pharmaceutical production to a standard approved by the Medicines Inspectorate will, in fact, meet most of the requirements relating to protection.

A radiopharmaceutical can be defined as any substance prepared for diagnostic or therapeutic use in the human subject, the composition of which has been modified by the introduction into the nucleus of a radionuclide. This process is termed labelling.

LABELLING

If this radionuclide has the same atomic number as one of the nuclides already present in the molecule the addition or substitution is termed 'isotopic labelling' (e.g. sodium *o*-iodohippurate in which some of the iodine-127 atoms have been replaced by iodine-125 atoms). Although the introduction of radioactivity may affect the stability of the preparation, it will usually behave, after administration, in a similar manner to the unlabelled preparation.

On the other hand a substance may be selected as a medium for introducing into the subject a radionuclide having an atomic number which differs from any other nuclide already present in that substance. This is usually termed 'non-isotopic labelling', or sometimes 'foreign labelling'. An example is human serum albumin which has been labelled with technetium-99m, where the purpose is to attach the radionuclide to a blood protein which will remain in the cardiovascular system long enough for blood pool delineation. If suitable gamma-emitting isotopes of all the elements could easily be prepared, there would be less need for foreign labelling. Nevertheless, iodination and chromation of proteins can produce very stable labels which, if not incompatible with the nature of the investigation, might still be acceptable for some studies. However, many natural body constituents are built up from carbon, hydrogen, oxygen, nitrogen and sulphur, and inspection of nuclear tables will show that none of their radioisotopes possess the required characteristics. The choice of label is therefore governed by availability, but this must be qualified by the nature of the investigation. Information regarding iron metabolism must be related to the haemoglobin molecule, which becomes isotopically labelled with iron-59, but red cell volume, survival times and destruction sites are determined by labelling the cells with chromium-51, and are unaffected by the foreign label provided the added chromium does not exceed 0.1 µg/ml of blood. Since some fraction of the label can often be recovered and measured extracorporeally, by sensitive methods such as well crystal or liquid scintillation counting, only small doses need to be administered. Hence, despite a long half-life (12.26 years), hydrogen-3 can be used as an isotopic label for folic acid absorption studies.

In some cases, the chemical form serves only as a vehicle for the introduction of a radionuclide into the body, for radiotherapeutic purposes. Thus gold-198, a beta-emitter, is sometimes used intraperitoneally to control ascites by partial destruction of the epithelial cells of the membrane. A colloidal solution is used to ensure containment; a soluble form would diffuse into the systemic circulation. Conversely, sodium phosphate is used as a vehicle for another beta-emitter, phosphorus-32, occasionally used in the treatment of polycythaemia vera, simply because it is a chemically inert but soluble salt which can reach and destroy red cell production sites in the bone marrow.

SOME RADIOPHARMACEUTICALS OF THE BRITISH PHARMACOPOEIA (1973)

Cyanocobalamin (^{58}Co) Injection (BP); Cyanocobalamin (^{57}Co) Injection (BP)

Cobalt-58 has a half-life of 71.3 days but provides an appreciable radiation dose. Cobalt-57 has a longer half-life of 270 days, but emits only weak gamma photons of 0.123 MeV and the radiation dose is low. The labelled vitamins are produced by biosynthesis in an activated medium (see Selenomethionine (^{75}Se) Injection).

In the Schilling test, an oral dose of 1 μCi of labelled vitamin is given to the fasting subject, followed by an intramuscular flushing dose of 1 mg of un-labelled vitamin and the activity recovered in the urine is measured. Differentiation between malabsorption of vitamin B12 and pernicious anaemia (absence of intrinsic factor) can be made by repeating the procedure in conjunction with an oral dose of intrinsic factor.

To avoid the duplication, Bell's test uses a dual isotope technique. Cyano-cobalamin labelled with cobalt-58 is given simultaneously with cyanocobala-min labelled with cobalt-57 but which is bound to human gastric juice. A flushing dose of inactive cyanocobalamin is followed by urine counting using a well counter as a gamma spectrometer.

Ferric Citrate (^{59}Fe) Injection (BP)

The plasma clearance rate can be plotted by sequential recovery and counting of blood samples, following a 10 μCi intravenous dose. If the plasma iron level has been determined, then the iron turnover rate in the plasma can also be found. Lastly, by collecting blood at intervals over a period of 2 weeks and knowing the red-cell volume (cf. ^{51}Cr), a value can be obtained for iron utilisa-tion.

Sodium Iodide (^{131}I) Solution (BP); Sodium Iodide (^{131}I) Injection (BP) Sodium Iodide (^{125}I) Solution (BP)

Radioiodine tests, which depend upon the rate of accumulation of iodide by the thyroid gland, are used in the assessment of thyroid function. The simple uptake test measures the rate of uptake in the gland by 'neck counting' using two accurately positioned scintillation detectors. A 4-hour uptake can be done with iodine-132, which lessens the radiation dose, but the usual 24-hour uptake requires the use of iodine-131. Evaluation of thyroid function is a complex matter and the many variations include measurement of uptake before and after injection of TSH (thyrotrophin) and T3 (triiodothyronine) suppression tests. Iodine-125 decays by electron capture and the principal emission consists of the 0.027 MeV X-radiation (Kα) of the daughter element, tellurium. Such a soft photon lessens its value for *in vivo* tests because of tissue absorption (unless near the surface as in renography), but it is greatly used for *in vitro* tests using saturation analysis or competitive binding of labelled and unlabelled reagent to the appropriate antisera.

Once production difficulties have been overcome, it is likely that iodine-

123, which provides 0.16 MeV gamma photons with a 13-hour half-life, will assume increasing importance in the field of scintigraphy.

Sodium 2-Iodohippurate (^{131}I) Injection (BP)

In a single renal transit, this substance is eliminated from the plasma almost entirely by proximal tubule secretion without reabsorption. A 50 µCi dose is administered intravenously, and the excretion pattern followed with a gamma camera. Normally the counts accumulate quite rapidly as the nuclide first appears in plasma, then more slowly during the secretory phase, and then fall away as the activity drains into the bladder. Renal dysfunction is indicated by distorted patterns, but a particular dysfunction is not necessarily indicated by a single specific pattern, and interpretation may be a complex matter. Formerly counters were placed individually over each kidney and over the heart, but gamma cameras are now widely used.

L-Selenomethionine (^{75}Se) Injection (BP)

Methionine is a naturally occurring amino acid which has a methylthiol group attached to C4. The only possible radioisotope of sulphur, ^{38}S, has too high a gamma energy (1.9 Mev). Yeast grown on a sulphur-free medium containing traces of sodium selenite (^{75}Se) produces labelled L-methionine by the incorporation of selenium-75 in lieu of sulphur. This can be extracted after hydrolysis. Chemically synthesised material is acceptable if free from the biologically inert D compound. Uptake studies have shown that the short-term behaviours of the labelled and unlabelled molecules are indistinguishable. This may be termed a quasi-isotopic label.

The main use is for pancreatic scintigraphy with a dose of 300 µCi. The pancreas concentrates free amino acids from the blood, but although the pancreas to tissue ratio is favourable for delineation, the liver, which often partially overlies the pancreas, oxidises amino acids and more activity accumulates in the liver, with its greater bulk, than in the pancreas. Hence it is customary also to delineate the liver with technetium-99m sulphur colloid, after which either subtraction techniques, liver shielding or directional scanning can be employed.

Although many interpretations of uptake have been suggested, the main indication is the elimination of advanced pancreatic disease which is evidenced by abnormal visualisation. Another use is complementary to thyroid uptake of radioiodine. Thyroid nodules showing uptake of neither are generally benign, whereas malignant ones often reject iodine, but not selenomethionine.

Sodium Chromate (^{51}Cr) Solution (BP)

Chromate ions readily penetrate the red blood cells and bind to the haemoglobin molecule. After equilibration, the excess chromium(VI) is either removed by washing the cells, or reduced to chromium(III) with ascorbic acid, which equally prevents any further uptake.

Cells so labelled with a 10–15 µCi dose can be used to measure the red cell volume and, if labelled with a 50–100 µCi dose, to estimate the red cell survival time. Large doses of 300–400 µCi were used to label cells which were then denatured, since, following reinjection, such damaged cells were sequestered by the spleen. However, the 0.32 keV gamma radiation is low for scintigraphy, and technetium-99m is a far more satisfactory label.

Iodinated (^{125}I) Human Albumin Injection (BP) Iodinated (^{131}I) Human Albumin Injection (BP)

As a means of finding the plasma volume, $4\,\mu$Ci of either injection is given intravenously. Blood samples are abstracted at regular intervals and the activity compared with a prepared standard. From a knowledge of the packed cell volume, the total blood volume can also be calculated, although it is better to estimate the plasma volume and red cell volume separately. In cases of shock, values obtained in this manner may be misleading. There is a warning in the BP that albumin so labelled is not necessarily suitable for metabolic studies.

Xenon (^{133}Xe) Injection (BP)

This is used for measuring peripheral blood flow in muscle tissue and regional cerebral blood flow. Being an inert gas, it cannot chemically enter into body composition (there may be a slight retention in fat), and is virtually eliminated in a single passage through the lung. It is best purchased in bubble-free cartridges which deliver the stated dose. Dispensing from multidose vials is difficult, since the liquid must be displaced by mercury. The concentration of a dissolved gas is proportional to the partial pressure, and since xenon-133 is a 'carrier-free' radionuclide, it will mainly be present in the gaseous phase if there is any air space over the liquid. The gas itself is used for pulmonary ventilation studies.

Organ imaging

This is a diagnostic procedure which may be regarded as the converse of conventional X-radiography. Instead of using an external source of radiation, a radiating source is distributed in the body organ under survey, and the emitted radiation is collimated, detected, amplified and recorded. It is usual to use a pure gamma emitter (beta radiation would only be absorbed in the tissues), and the amount, while depending upon the energy of the gamma photons, must be such that sufficient is emitted from the body to permit detection and recording. In general this entails the administration of multimillicurie amounts, so that unless the biological life is short, then the radiation-life must be brief so that the absorbed radiation dose is kept within acceptable limits.

SHORT-LIVED RADIONUCLIDES

Although the *British Pharmacopoeia* (1973) includes seventeen monographs on radiopharmaceuticals, these are based upon twelve radionuclides, the iodine radioisotopes having more than one formulation. The radionuclides, together with their half-lives, are listed in Table 7.1. (several more are used infrequently).

Table 7.1   The radionuclides with their half-lives in days (unless stated otherwise)

Radionuclide	Half-life
Cobalt-57	270
Cobalt-58	71
Chromium-51	27.8
Gold-198	2.7
Iron-59	45
Iodine-125	60
Iodine-131	8
Mercury-197	2.7
Phosphorus-32	14.2
Selenium-75	120
Technetium-99m	6 hours
Xenon-133	2.3
Others in common use	
Iodine-132	2.3 hours
Bromine-82	35.4 hours
Indium-113m	100 minutes
Potassium-42	12.4 hours
Sodium-24	15 hours
Strontium-85	65 days
Strontium-87m	2.8 hours

It will be noted that the half-lives vary considerably and that whereas many are measured in days, others are measured in hours. The distinction between short-lived and long-lived radionuclides is a purely arbitrary one. Potassium-40, which occurs naturally with an abundance of 0.0118%, has a half-life of 1.3×10^9 years, whereas the reactor-produced potassium-42 has a half-life of 12.4 hours. If the former is regarded as long lived, as indeed it must be, and the latter as short lived, then by these standards cobalt-60 with a half-life of 5.26 years would also be regarded as short lived. But medically, a bone-seeking beta emitter, which would only decay through 10 half-lives in half a century, can only be regarded as having a dangerously long half-life. In general, the term short-lived radionuclide is dependent upon the application, and in a medical context, is restricted to radionuclides with half-lives measured in hours.

The rate of decay of a radionuclide is proportional to the activity A, i.e. it is a first-order reaction and can be expressed:

$$-\frac{dA}{dt} \propto A; \quad \text{therefore} \quad -\frac{dA}{dt} = \lambda.A$$

where λ is the disintegration constant.

Integrating within the boundary limits A_o (for initial activity) and A_t (for activity at time t), gives:

$$\lambda.t = \log_e \frac{A_o}{A_t} \quad \text{or} \quad A_t = A_o\, e^{-\lambda.t}$$

The activity therefore decreases exponentially with time.

It will be appreciated that if we postulate a radionuclide with a half-life of 2.4 hours, then after 24 hours (i.e. 10 half-lives) the activity would have decayed by a factor of 1024 : 1. This is an order of 3, which is also the relationship between the millicurie (1×10^{-3} Ci) and the microcurie (1×10^{-6} Ci). Thus, an administered dose of 10 millicuries, without making any allowance for excretion, would have been reduced to 10 microcuries in 24 hours, and to 10 nanocuries after a further 24 hours. Such rapid decay exerts an important effect upon calculations of absorbed radiation dose, although other factors are also involved.

Although such radionuclides can be obtained by submitting targets to bombardment in neutron reactors, or particle acceleration, or by extraction from fission products, the time factor renders these methods impracticable unless such facilities are available directly to the user. Recourse is therefore made to separation techniques where the desired radionuclide is produced by decay of another radionuclide which has a longer life. For example strontium-87m can be produced either by neutron irradiation of strontium-86

$$^{86}\text{Sr}(n, \gamma) : {}^{87\text{m}}\text{Sr}$$

or by decay of yttrium-87 which has a half-life of 80 hours:

$$^{85}\text{Rb}(\gamma, 2n) : {}^{87\text{m}}\text{Y} + {}^{87}\text{Y}$$
$$^{87}\text{Y}(\text{EC}) : {}^{87\text{m}}\text{Sr}$$

Separation methods

When the daughter differs from the parent in atomic number, it can be separated by chemical methods. Pertechnetate ion can be separated from molybdate either by acidification and distillation as pertechnic acid, which can be absorbed in sodium hydroxide solution, or by extraction from alkaline solution into methyl ethyl ketone which can then be evaporated. These methods are not convenient, and universal use is made of ion exchange as a means of separation.

The conventional polystyrene resins, which are cross-linked with divinyl benzene and contain quaternary ammonium or nuclear sulphonic groups, are little used since the bonds are liable to radiation destruction. Inorganic materials such as alumina, silica and zirconia, which have greater stability when subjected to radioactivation, are usually employed.

Radionuclide generators

The first commercial application of the principle of ion exchange was the introduction, by the Brookhaven National Laboratory in 1954, of the iodine-132 generator, which makes use of fission-produced tellurium-132 absorbed on to an alumina column. Subsequently, systems producing other useful decay products have been devised, notably that by which technetium-99m is separated from molybdenum-99.

The radionuclide generator can be defined as a convenient means of producing, in the laboratory, a plentiful supply of short-lived radionuclides. Without such sources gamma-scintigraphy could not have developed into a routine examination.

Technetium-99m generator

Molybdenum-99, which in Great Britain is obtained by neutron irradiation of molybdenum-98, as the trioxide, is dissolved in ammonia and the molybdate polyanions absorbed on to alumina contained in a suitable column.

The technetium is produced in its highest oxidation state as the monovalent pertechnetate ion, which can be displaced with another monovalent ion such as chloride. Some of the pertechnetate which is produced may suffer reduction through secondary radiation effects, and become absorbed on the alumina, so it is usual to include a minute quantity of an oxidising agent in the eluate, or else to saturate it with oxygen, to minimise such reduction. The addition of 0.1% chlorocresol will help to maintain the sterility of the column.

A transient equilibrium between technetium-99m and the parent is established after 23 hours, by which time the daughter activity is at its maximum. If however the maximum activity is not required, the exponential character of the growth permits the elution of 25%, 45% and 80% of the maximum at 2, 4 and 10 hours respectively. A rule-of-thumb method predicts that half the final activity will be available after one half-life.

Depending upon the initial loading, the useful life of a generator is about three times the half-life of the parent radionuclide. Although the column cannot be disposed of until the surface dose-rate has fallen to below 20 mrad/hour, if liquid waste can be more easily disposed of, the residual activity can be stripped from the column with strong ammonia solution.

Indium-113m generator

The parent, tin-113, is produced by neutron activation of enriched tin-112, which is dissolved in strong hydrochloric acid and oxidised with chlorine. The anion complex is absorbed on hydrated zirconium oxide.

The indium-113m is eluted with 0.1–0.04% hydrochloric acid to which 0.1% chlorocresol can be added to maintain the sterility of the column. The eluate contains various complexes of indium-111 with chloride ion and has a pH value of about 1.4.

Iodine-132 generator

Tellurium-132 is obtained as a uranium fission product and is absorbed on an alumina column as sodium tellurite.

The generator is eluted with 0.02 mol/l sodium hydroxide solution containing 0.02 mol/l sodium thiosulphate which ensures that all the iodine-132 is obtained as iodide ion and does not contain iodate or periodate.

It will be seen from the decay schemes that if the tellurium-132 is contaminated with tellurium-131 m, the eluate will also contain iodine-131. The column should therefore be eluted upon receipt and the eluate discarded. Provided the column is eluted at least once daily, subsequent elutions will contain much reduced amounts of iodine-131; the longer the interval between elutions, the greater will be the growth of iodine-131.

Other generators

Although many systems have been proposed only a few have actually been introduced. Among them are ^{68}Ge : ^{68}Ga (half-life : 68 minutes) and ^{103}Pd : ^{103m}Rh (half-life : 57 minutes) and the producers of the ultrashort-lived radionuclides, ^{137}Cs : ^{137m}Ba (half-life : 2.5 minutes) and ^{81}Rb : ^{81m}Kr (half-life : 13 seconds).

QUALITY CONTROL OF RADIOPHARMACEUTICALS

Radioactive pharmaceuticals require a higher degree of quality control than inactive ones because additional factors have to be considered.

1. Any initial radionuclidic impurity will not remain constant but will show a variation with time.

2. Radiochemical impurities arising either during preparation, or upon storage, may so alter the body distribution of the radioactive component as to give misleading clinical information and, additionally, may subject a particular organ to an unforeseen radiation dose.

However, from the hospital standpoint, to institute control over all aspects and demand absolute standards of purity is impracticable. In any case such an ideal is usually unnecessary and selective criteria of purity can be established which are appropriate to an individual preparation. The concepts of chemical purity, radionuclidic purity, radiochemical purity, sterility and apyrogenicity should therefore be considered in this context.

Chemical purity

The chemical purity of a radiopharmaceutical is simply the proportion of the substance present in the specified chemical form. Since chemical analysis cannot distinguish between isotopes of the same element, the definition disregards any isotopic substitution. In all but a few instances radiopharmaceuticals are only met with in solution, and if their specific activity is high, it is not possible to isolate and examine the minute amount present. Iodine-131 solutions may be prepared by adding an oxidising agent to a crude solution, distilling in an air stream, collecting in sodium hydroxide solution and neutralising. The BP (1973) also allows the addition of sodium thiosulphate as a reducing agent and up to 0.1 mg/mCi is used. The minimum specific activity permitted by the BP (1973) is 5 mCi/μg, so it will be seen that the weight of active substance is greatly outnumbered by that of the other substances present. Many solutions of radiopharmaceuticals contain, of necessity, carriers and buffers, and the chemical purity of these additives is far more important than the simple chemical purity of the radioactive component. Therefore all reagents used in the preparation of radiopharmaceuticals must comply with Pharmacopoeial standards if such standards exist. In other cases, reagents of analytical standard are usually acceptable, but if any doubt exists, determination of chemical and physical purity must be carried out.

The quality of solute absorbed from a solution of low molarity (10^{-5}) can be significant, and this condition is often achieved with carrier-free solutions. Adsorption can occur on glass surfaces and also on suspended particles. All glassware must therefore be chemically clean and often plastic apparatus is preferable. Since minute impurities may precipitate at a neutral or alkaline pH value, solutions are best kept acid if possible.

Sodium-orthophosphate (^{32}P) is a carrier-free material which keeps well in hydrochloric acid at pH 2–3 but, on neutralisation, losses can be severe, for which reason inactive phosphate is added as a hold-back carrier. However, the buffering power of blood is such that intravenous solutions of low pH can often be injected provided the volume is kept low. Indium-113m is eluted from a generator at pH 1.4 with 0.04M hydrochloric acid. If a protective colloid or complexing agent is added, the pH can be increased without precipitation, but it is usually injected unmodified.

Chemical contamination may also arise in eluates from radionuclide generators, not only because of the ingredients of the eluates, but from dissolution of the ion-exchanger. Soluble aluminium, zirconium or silicon may be present. Considering that the amounts likely to be present are usually of the order of 2–5 parts/10^6 and that the majority of investigations are only carried out on a single occasion, the question is not one of toxicity but of soluble product.

It is often necessary in the course of preparation to add hydroxyl or phosphate resulting in the precipitation of such contaminants as gels, which either effectively scavenge the activity from the solution or alter its body distribution by causing localisation in the liver or lungs.

Radionuclidic purity

The radionuclidic purity of a radioactive material is that proportion of the total activity which is present as the stated radionuclide. Conventionally, the activity due to the presence of decay products is not regarded as constituting an impurity but if equilibrium is not attained until a considerable period of time has elapsed, the activity contributed from such sources will depend significantly upon the extent of growth within that period.

It is evident that in order to give a statement of the radionuclidic purity of a preparation, the activities (and hence the identities) of every radionuclide present must be known. This is a difficult if not impossible task. An examination for radionuclidic purity is usually confined to a determination of such radionuclides as may reasonably be expected to be present after consideration of the nature of the target, and the nuclear transformations which may occur. It will also be qualified by the sensitivity and resolution of the equipment.

In general the radionuclidic purity, as determined by simple gamma-scintillation spectrometry, employing a sodium iodide detector, should not be less than 99% at the time of administration, provided that none of the impurities are alpha emitters. In many cases, however, much closer limits are defined for specific radionuclidic impurities. It will be appreciated that the proportions of contaminating radionuclides which have longer or shorter half-lives than the stated radionuclide will increase or decrease, respectively, with time.

Gold-198

With the high neutron fluxes used today, the nuclear product, which in this case also has a higher neutron activation cross-section, becomes in turn a target for neutron capture.

$$^{197}\text{Au}(n\,\gamma) : {}^{198}\text{Au}(n\,\gamma) : {}^{199}\text{Au}$$

However, the characteristics of gold-198 and gold-199 are not entirely dissimilar, so the BP (1973) allows up to 5% without declaration, and over 5% provided a statement of content is made.

Iodine-125

$$^{124}\text{Xe}(n, \gamma) : {}^{125}\text{Xe}(\text{EC}) — {}^{125}\text{I}(n, \gamma) : {}^{126}\text{I}$$

In this case the contaminant, resulting again from secondary neutron capture, although a beta and hard gamma emitter, has a half-life of only 13 days compared with one of 60 days for iodine-125. After production, the material is allowed to decay until the proportion of impurity is below 1%, which is the BP (1973) limit. After receipt, the proportion will continue to decrease.

Mercury-197

$$^{196}\text{Hg}(n, \gamma) : {}^{197}\text{Hg} \ (\text{half-life: 65 hours})$$
$$^{202}\text{Hg}(n, \gamma) : {}^{203}\text{Hg} \ (\text{half-life: 47 days})$$

Irradiation of natural mercury will result in the production of 2–4% of mercury-203 which, on storing for 7 days, will become 7–14%. An enriched target will greatly reduce this contamination, which, nevertheless will increase with time.

Generator breakthrough

Since the principle of the radionuclide generator is the production of a short-lived radionuclide from a longer-lived parent it is evident that release of the parent from the ion-exchanger could constitute a serious hazard. Provided that the photoelectric peaks are well separated, gamma-scintillation spectrometry using a multichannel analyser and printout, will readily identify and quantify such breakthrough. In fact, in the case of technetium-99m, the BP (1973) gives a simple screening method using 6 mm lead, which enables an ordinary single-channel scintillation counter to be used.

However, where such peaks not only are disproportionate, but also sufficiently close to demand high resolution detectors, it is usual to examine decayed specimens, which necessarily means that the quality control is retrospective. If the breakthrough is of a high order, it may be possible to use chemical spot tests. The potassium ethyl xanthate test for molybdenum and the haematoxyline test for tin(IV) are sufficiently sensitive for these purposes, but are not quantitative.

Radiochemical purity

The radiochemical purity of a radioactive material is the proportion of the total activity which is present in the stated chemical form. If the radionuclidic purity is 100%, it may be regarded as the proportion of the stated radionuclide present in the stated chemical form. The importance of radiochemical purity lies in the alteration which may occur in the biological distribution of the radioactive components. This may result either in misleading clinical results, or in body organs receiving an unforeseen radiation dose.

Radiochemical impurity may arise both in the course of preparation and upon storage.

During preparation

Concomitant labelling of chemical impurities

This may occur either with organic substances such as fluoran derivatives when closely related analogues are often present. Sodium 2-iodohippurate often contains iodobenzoate.

Unreacted labelling agent

This is often present and must be removed, usually by ion-exchange or by dialysis.

After preparation

Radiation effects

Radioactive pharmaceuticals are less likely than inactive ones to retain their initial purity because of their liability to decompose by virtue of self irradiation.

Primary radiation effects include disintegration of a radioactive atom within a molecule (internal effect), and absorption by a substance of some fraction of its own radiation energy resulting in the decomposition of molecules by interaction with the emitted particle or gamma photon (external effect).

Secondary radiation effects are due to primary radiation effects acting upon other substances present such as solvent, preservative, buffer or other additive. Free radicals or other reactive species may be produced which in turn cause or accelerate destruction of the molecule. Many factors are involved including the nature and energy of the radiation, radioactive concentration and storage time. Solutions of 1-triiodothyronine, labelled with iodine-131, undergo radiolytic decomposition, but if the amount of energy absorbed is reduced by substituting iodine-125, then the decomposition also is greatly reduced.

Aromatic solvents such as benzene can dissipate absorbed radiation energy without transferring it to the solute. For most pharmaceutical purposes the solvent will usually be water from which hydroperoxy radicals are produced by secondary radiation effects. The addition of free radical scavengers such as benzyl alcohol may help. Freeze drying into thin films will also facilitate the escape of nuclear particles, but since the molecules are then more tightly packed they are also subject to increased primary (external) radiation effects.

Chemical instability

Chemical decomposition independent of radiation effects will nevertheless cause radiochemical impurity. Halogen bound to aromatic carbon in the ortho position relative to a carbonamide group is activated with regard to nucleophilic substitution. Therefore, in aqueous solutions of sodium 2-iodohippurate, formation of iodide can be expected as a consequence of substitution of iodine by hydroxyl. In such cases substitution of iodine-131 by iodine-125 will not have any effect. Injection of chlormerodrin (^{197}Hg) is sterilised by filtration since autoclaving results in the formation of the 2-hydroxy compound which has a higher uptake and a slower excretion.

Storage

Unless specific limits are imposed, materials containing a radionuclide with a half-life of less than 60 days should not be used after three half-lives have elapsed. When the half-life is 60 days or more then the limit is 6 months.

Determination

Chromatography

Paper and thin-layer chromatography are the commonest methods used for the determination of radiochemical purity. Since the weight of the substance applied is often extremely minute, particular care is required in interpreting results.

The resolved components in the developed chromatogram are identified in the usual manner (i.e. by comparison with standard reference material). Coloured components (e.g. fluorosceins and tetracyclines) can be detected visually and many that are colourless produce coloured complexes if sprayed with a suitable reagent (e.g. gluconates and amino acids). If the amounts present are too low for detection, an inert carrier may have to be added to the test solution (e.g. phosphates). Similarly it may also be necessary to add inert carriers corresponding to anticipated impurities (e.g. iodates in iodides). If the substance being examined is liable to oxidation, the solvents will have to be degassed or purged with nitrogen; in some cases (e.g. selenomethionine) a protective carrier can be added.

The activities associated with these components are then measured radiometrically, most easily by using a radiochromatogram scanner.

If coloured complexes are not formed (e.g. pertechnetate ion and indium) comparison must be made with reference standards. In many cases differential absorption of ultraviolet light will locate colourless compounds on thin-layer plates containing a phosphor. However, once the R_F values are established it is usual to rely upon these for routine examination.

Gel chromatography

This is based upon the permeability of the particular dextran gel selected from materials of different molecular weights. It is particularly useful for examining compounds which have been labelled with technetium-99m. Development of paper chromatograms with alcohols usually results in colloids, chelates, complexes and labelled albumin all remaining at origin. Since reduced technetium bonds to the stationary phase, and also remains at origin, the absence of a second peak at the R_F value associated with a pertechnetate reference developed in the same system, only denotes an absence of that ion; other unbound oxidation states may also be present at origin. These can, however, be resolved by gel chromatography, for, whereas lower oxidation states become bonded to the polysaccharide, free pertechnetate and labelled compounds are eluted in their characteristic volumes.

Electrophoresis

The great advantage of paper electrophoresis is that ionic impurities can be Separated very quickly, using simple electrolytes such as 0.01 mol/1 sodium hydroxide or 0.01 mol/1 sodium chloride. Glass fibre supports effect separation even more rapidly. For blood proteins, barbiturate buffers and cellulose acetate supports are universal.

Dialysis

This method is time consuming and has largely been replaced by gel chromatography.

Sterility

Radiopharmaceuticals are not self sterilising by virtue of their radiation characteristics. While it is recognised that not all radiopharmaceuticals are good growth media for microorganisms, certain preparations, especially those containing proteins and amino acids, are particularly susceptible.

On the other hand Chlormerodrin (^{197}Hg) Injection, which cannot be sterilised by autoclaving because of thermal decomposition, usually contains sufficient mercuric chloride to act as a bacteriostat after the product has been sterilised by filtration. It is not usually feasible to complete sterility tests before release due to the 65-hour half-life of mercury-197.

Most radiopharmaceuticals for injection are supplied in multidose containers. Unfortunately, many bactericides including phenol, chlorocresol, phenyl-mercuric nitrate, thiomersal and chlorbutol are susceptible to radiolytic decomposition. Since bactericides are therefore usually omitted from such solutions, it is necessary, unless a dose has been withdrawn under conditions of complete asepsis, for the contents to be resterilised by autoclaving immediately after such withdrawal. It is then up to the pharmacist to satisfy himself that no chemical decomposition, which adversely affects the characteristics of the material, has occurred as the result of such resterilisation which may, of necessity, be repeated many times.

FORMULATION WITH SHORT-LIVED RADIONUCLIDES

Technetium-99m has by far the greatest medical usage of all short-lived radionuclides, with indium-113m a long way behind. Iodine-132 and strontium-87m are generally used as column eluates without further elaboration and the remainder have no routine or widespread use.

Technetium is a second-row transition element which can exist in all oxidation states from -1 to $+7$. The monovalent pertechnetate oxyanion (TcVII) is quite stable in solution but chemically inert. Reactivity is promoted by reduction of the technetium to a lower oxidation state, often with tin(II) or ascorbic acid. Iron(II) has also been used, although it has a standard oxidation potential of -0.771. Even with an excess of reducing agent the thermodynamic stability of the reduced species is often affected by dissolved oxygen, which can be removed by purging all reagent solutions with nitrogen. Hydrolysis of tin can be a problem and solutions will have to be prepared in strong hydrochloric acid and dilutions purged with nitrogen and filtered through a 100 nm porosity membrane immediately before use.

Solutions containing technetium(IV) tend to hydrolyse until complexed with a ligand and oxidation states V and VI tend to disproportionate, even when complexed. Preferably, reduction and complexation should be effected simultaneously, but even so the two most common radiochemical impurities in technetium-labelled radiopharmaceuticals are insoluble, reduced and hydrolysed technetium which is abstracted by reticuloendothelial (RE) cells and soluble pertechnetate which is found in thyroid and stomach, salivary glands etc.

Indium is eluted from the column as various aquocomplexes of indium(III) and chloride ion. The eluate is very acid (about pH 1.4) but, provided the volume is restricted, can be injected intravenously. Unless protected with acetate or gelatin, raising the pH above 3 results in complexation with hydroxide and colloid formation.

Some labelled compounds will have to be prepared with aseptic technique but even when terminal sterilisation is practised it is recommended that all operations be conducted in a suitable vertical laminar-flow work station. Such a unit must not discharge into the laboratory environment.

Since the pharmacist must be satisfied that the material is suitable for the purpose for which it is intended, some form of quality control must be applied. In view of the rates of decay of these radionuclides this, in many cases, will be retrospective, especially with regard to sterility, but nevertheless must be instituted, since only by such means can an adequate surveillance be maintained over preparative procedures.

Colloids

Intravenously injected colloids are removed from the circulation by RE cells. It has been stated that a differential uptake can be related to the colloid size and that large particles (500–1000 nm) are removed mainly in the spleen whereas small particles (less than 20 nm) are found largely in the bone marrow with intermediate sizes tending to concentrate in the liver (Colombetti *et al* 1969). When the colloid contains a gamma-emitting radionuclide, the uptake by the Kupffer cells of the liver provides a means of visualising that organ. There will always be uptake by the spleen irrespective of particle size but if particulate matter is present in the preparation, it will localize in the lung and prevent clear definition of the upper margin.

A simple and effective method of determining the particle size is to measure the retention of activity by membrane filters of differing porosity. It should be noted that only thin filters such as etched polycarbonate are suitable. Those having a fibrous structure are thicker and are not suitable for this method of differentiation (Davis *et al* 1974).

Technetium-99m-labelled colloids

Technetium-99m is the most commonly used radionuclide for this purpose and a great variety of colloidal preparations have been devised, many of which are based upon the use of colloidal sulphur as a carrier. The most satisfactory and the most stable colloid undoubtedly is that prepared with hydrogen sulphide gas, with which acid solutions of pertechnetate yield the heptasulphide (Harper *et al* 1964; Dunson *et al* 1973). Rhenium has been added as a carrier but is quite unnecessary. However, it has been stated that 'the toxicity of H_2S far exceeds that of HCN' (Cotton & Wilkinson 1972) and therefore care must be taken to ensure that none remains in the final injection. The use can be avoided by substituting thiosulphate, which in acid solution deposits colloidal sulphur, as well as providing sulphide. Theoretically there is no need to continue the reaction beyond conversion of the outer sulphur atom (oxidation state -2 (Szymendera *et al* 1971), but it is found in practice that if the thiosulphate concentration is lowered yields can be improved to 100% by immersing the mixture in a boiling water bath and precipitating all the sulphur. Although many particles will even exceed 1.0 micron in diameter and be visible microscopically, the terminal sterilisation by heating will cause optical clearing and the particle size will then be submicroscopic (Cohen 1970).

Stabilisers are required and included among those that have been proposed are dextran, mannitol, human serum albumin, polyvinylpyrrolidine, carboxymethylcellulose and gelatin, but the latter remains the most popular despite the fact that samples from various suppliers show different characteristics. It has also been blamed for pyrogenic reactions but these should not be encountered if the gelatin granules are kept dry and if solutions are sterilised immediately after preparation.

The preparation must finally be titrated with sodium hydroxide solution but the pH must not be allowed to exceed a value of 6.5 or pertechnetate will be liberated irreversibly (Stern *et al* 1966). It is advisable therefore to add a buffer, and although phosphate is generally used it is necessary to determine that soluble aluminium is absent from the generator eluate or else gelatinous aluminium phosphate will be precipitated. If soluble aluminium is found, it will be necessary to include disodium edetate in the formulation (Haney *et al* 1971), or use sodium citrate solution for neutralisation (Staum 1972).

Colloids other than sulphur can be used and stannous hydroxide is an effective carrier (Lin & Winchell 1972). After admixture with stannous chloride solution, the technetium is coprecipitated by treatment with sodium hydroxide. To produce a colloidal solution, the final tin concentration must be around 10^{-3} mol/l and a dispersing agent such as gelatin must be included. Stannous chloride solutions readily hydrolyse and will have to be prepared and filtered just before required.

Methods have also been devised which involve the addition of eluted pertechnetate to a preformed colloid, followed by heating at 115°C for 30 minutes (Garzon *et al* 1965).

The use of carriers can be avoided by hydrogen reduction of technetium-99m from the $+7$ oxidation state in pertechnetate ion to the $+4$ oxidation state as hydrated dioxide. Although the pertechnetate eluate is simply acidified and treated with sodium borohydride, the preparation has a low stability to oxygen and is easily oxidised to pertechnetate (Johnson & Gollan 1970).

Indium-113m-labelled colloids

As previously indicated these are relatively easy to prepare, since colloidal hydroxide starts to form once the eluate is raised to pH 3.0 and is completed at pH 7·0. A phosphate buffer is often used instead of hydroxide, since the pH is more easily controlled. However, such materials will tend to coalesce and form particles which may become trapped in the lung capillaries. This can be prevented by the prior addition of gelatin as a stabilising colloid, or by complexing with citrate. Again the distribution in the reticuloendothelial system will depend upon particle size, which in turn will depend upon the method used to prepare the colloid.

Chelates

Chelation of reduced technetium with diethylenetriaminepentacetic acid (DTPA) alters the biological distribution and, in contradistinction to pertechnetate anion, activity is absent from the thyroid and parotid glands and the stomach mucosa and is greatly reduced in the choroid plexus. The technetium (VII) is reduced to technetium(IV) with either tin(II) or iron(II), in acid solution to prevent hydrolysis. Even so, in the latter case a kinetically rapid complexing agent such as ascorbic acid must also be present (Brookman & Williams 1970). This preparation exhibits more than one radioactive component and is cleared both by glomerular filtration and tubular excretion. The major portion of the activity is cleared from the plasma and excreted fairly quickly, which makes it useful for brain scintigraphy, but enough is retained by the kidney to enable that organ to be visualised. Tin(II) is a much better reductant provided oxidation and hydrolysis are avoided, and to prevent hydrolysis of the reduced technetium the acid tin solution must be added to the chelating agent before adding the pertechnetate. As well as giving good imaging of brain lesions it is excreted rapidly by glomerular filtration and can be used for the evaluation of kidney function.

Indium is readily chelated by DTPA at low pH values (below pH 3) and the solution can then be titrated to a value suitable for injection, without precipitation occurring. Above pH 3 the rate of reaction with hydroxyl ion or phosphate buffer exceeds that with the DTPA. For chelation at higher pH values, the presence of acetate or tartrate alters the rate constants and single-step procedures can be effected (Hill *et al* 1970).

Many substances are chelating agents, including tetracyclines, amino acids, mercaptosuccinic acids, gluconates etc., and use has been made of them because of their excretion patterns which are mimicked by the labelled counterparts.

Blood pool delineation

Intravenously administered human serum albumin, which has been labelled with a suitable radionuclide, will remain contained within the cardiovascular system and may be used for visualising the heart or a highly vascular organ such as the placenta. All methods of labelling with technetium-99m require the reduction of technetium(VII) to a lower oxidation state, in order to promote reactivity. The mechanisms of the subsequent reactions are obscure but involve, firstly, attachment to a carrier ion such as iron (Stern *et al* 1965), tin (Lin *et al* 1971) or zirconium (Benjamin 1969), followed by the molecular attachment of the albumin, possibly by chelation through vicinal functional groups present in the amino acids. Indium-113m is also used to label plasma protein for these purposes, since intravenous injection produces *in vivo* labelling of a betaglobulin. This is probably transferrin, since prior injection of iron is a contraindication to this use of indium-113m because binding to the plasma protein is low and activity soon appears in the bladder.

Particulate suspensions

Regional blood flow to the lungs can be demonstrated by gamma-scintigraphy, after capillary entrapment of particles of selected size which have been labelled with a suitable radionuclide. Macroaggregates of human albumin, labelled either with technetium-99m or indium-113m, are generally used. Ferric hydroxide particles, which at one time were widely used as a carrier, are now suspect and it is recommended that their use be discontinued.

The *British Pharmacopoeia* (1973) contains a monograph for Macrisalb (^{131}I) Injection which usually is reserved for use only when facilities for labelling with short-lived radionuclides are not available. However the particle size limits for this preparation of 10–100 nm, as determined by microscopy, should continue to be observed for all preparations used for pulmonary perfusion scintigraphy. It is also desirable that they should have a specific activity sufficient to avoid unnecessary blocking of lung capillaries.

A convenient method for the preparation of technetium-99m-labelled particles, is to prepare a labelled sulphur colloid and to add a solution of human albumin while buffering at the isoelectric point. Degrading by heat will coagulate the protein around the colloid (Cragin *et al* 1969).

The preparation of albumin microspheres for labelling with technetium-99m (Zolle *et al* 1970) is possibly stretching the capability of a hospital radiopharmaceutical laboratory, but commercial preparations are now available, although the cost is high.

Indium-113m is most easily incorporated in ferric hydroxide particles, but since these are no longer acceptable, recourse must be made to other materials. Stannous hydroxide and aluminium hydroxide have been used and also human albumin. One method is to precipitate the albumin with strong hydrochloric acid in the presence of thiocyanate. The precipitate is separated and dissolved in saline and after titrating to the isoelectric point, the solution is heat denatured. The particles produced are separated, washed and examined for size. If satisfactory they can be stored and labelled, as required, by the addition of eluted indium-113m at pH 5–7. The hydroxide is adsorbed on to the preformed particles (Ciscato *et al* 1969).

Labelling of red blood cells

Denatured erythrocytes are sequestered by the spleen and if labelled with a suitable radionuclide can be used to visualise the spleen. This is particularly useful for detection of spleenuncli, postsplenectomy. The blood is added to acid citrate dextrose (ACD)* which is a non-penetrating medium, and centrifuged. The cells are washed, also with ACD, to remove plasma and the packed cells are then equilibrated with pertechnetate, in a minimum volume of saline, in an incubator. Stannous ion, in ACD, is then added to bind the technetium, and the cells shaken in a cold water bath. The cells are now washed twice with saline to remove uncomplexed technetium, and finally are heated at a controlled temperature until converted into aspherocytes. Since the labelled cells are now reinjected, it is important to use aseptic technique throughout (Eckelman *et al* 1971).

Bone imaging

Delineation of bone is dependent upon the ability to prepare a radiopharmaceutical with an affinity for calcified tissue. Exchange of the calcium in the bone crystal with calcium-47 is not a practicable proposition and strontium-85 and strontium-87 m proved useful substitutes. Fluorine-18 as fluoride ion gives excellent bone to tissue ratios quite quickly but the use of multimillicurie quantities of a radionuclide with a half-life of 110 minutes requires the user to be sited fairly near to the cyclotron.

At present phosphates and phosphonates labelled with technetium-99m are universally used. Of the inorganic compounds many condensed polyphosphates have been used but the simple dimer (i.e. pyrophosphate) is adequate if not superior to the longer polymers (Huberty *et al* 1974). Similarly, although many organic phosphonates have been used the simple methylene diphosphonate appears to be the best (Subramanian *et al* 1975). It is interesting to compare the structures:

Pyrophosphoric acid   Methylene diphosphonic acid

In each case the reductant is tin(II) and care has to be taken to prevent oxidation and hydrolysis (see above, chelates).

* Sodium dihydrogen phosphate 0.015 g, trisodium citrate 3 g, dextrose 0.2 g, water to 100 ml.

Other preparations

Many organic compounds are capable of acting as ligands and forming complexes or chelates with reduced technetium-99m. The excretion pattern is generally unchanged and the radioactive content enables the organ through which the material is eliminated to be visualised.

Thus labelled mercaptosuccinic acid provides one of the best renal imaging agents (Enlander *et al* 1974). Gluconate, glucoheptonate and penicillamine–acetazolamide complexes have also been used (Boyd *et al* 1973; Halpern *et al* 1972).

Sodium phytate (^{99m}Tc) which forms a colloid *in vivo* had a vogue for liver and spleen imaging (Subramanian *et al* 1973). Tetracycline (^{99m}Tc) (Dewanjee *et al* 1974) and D-penicillamine (^{99m}Tc) (Tubis *et al* 1972) have been used as cholescintigraphic agents and pyridoxylidene glutamate (^{99m}Tc) (Baker *et al* 1975) is an excellent hepatobiliary agent, though it passes from the liver rather quickly. All these are quite easily prepared and commercial kits are also available for some.

Other short-lived radionuclides are used but unless they can be obtained from a generator are difficult to obtain in sufficient quantities. One of the most promising is iodine-123 which can be used to label iodohippuric acid by fusion (Elias *et al* 1973) for renal studies and rose-bengal (Serafini *et al* 1975) for hepatobiliary studies.

MEASUREMENT OF RADIOACTIVITY

The number of atoms per unit mass of a pure radionuclide is given by N/M, where N is Avogadro's number and M is the atomic mass.

Since the curie is defined as 3.7×10^{10} transformations per second and λ can be expressed as:

$$\lambda = \frac{\log_e 0.5}{t_{\frac{1}{2}}}$$

where $t_{\frac{1}{2}}$ is the half-life in seconds, then the maximum specific activity S_{max} of 1 gram of a pure radionuclide is

$$S_{max} = \frac{6.02 \times 10^{23}}{\text{at. wt.}} \times \frac{\lambda}{3.7 \times 10^{10}} \, \text{Ci/g}$$

which reduces to $\dfrac{1.123 \times 10^{13}}{\text{at. wt.} \times t_{\frac{1}{2}}} \, \text{Ci/g}$

The radioactive concentration of a solution states the radioactivity in terms of unit volume, usually per millilitre.

Though the classical methods of detecting radioactivity, through the ionisation of gases and the production of scintillations in responsive materials remain unchanged, the associated electronic means of amplification and measurement have, for obvious reasons, become highly sophisticated.

Ionisation of gases

Ion chambers

When beta or gamma radiation enters a gas, some of the atoms are split into electrons and residual positive ions. If a potential difference is induced between two electrodes placed in the gas, recombination is prevented, since the electrons are then collected by the anode and constitute a current, which can be amplified and measured. With moderate voltages, the current arising from a single beta particle is very small and sensitivity to gamma radiation is even less, so the instrument is used for measuring activities in the range of $10\,\mu Ci$ to 1 Ci. At these activities a great many transformations will be occurring simultaneously. The standard reference chamber in this country is the AERE Type 1383A air chamber, but pressure chambers are available filled with argon at 2020 kPa, having enhanced characteristics in respect of sensitivity, volume and geometry. Ion chambers are connected to an electrometer amplifier with picoammeter. Compact instruments are usually termed calibrators. By setting an isotope factor, related to the energy of the emitter, a read-out is given in millicuries. It also gives the concentration in millicuries per millilitre should that information be required.

The magnitude of such ionisation currents is small but, provided the extra high tension (EHT) is stabilised, is proportional to the level and intensity of the radiation.

Geiger–Muller counters

If the applied voltage is greatly increased, the electrons are accelerated and acquire sufficient energy to cause ionisation of further gas atoms in their path. This is a multiplication effect as exemplified by the well-known Geiger–Muller (GM) tube. To prevent this cascade process from continuing indefinitely a quenching agent, usually a halogen, is included in the tube. This is ionised by the positive ions and when the halogen ions reach the cathode the pulse collapses. No current flows until another pulse is initiated by another beta particle entering the gas. GM tubes are virtually 100% responsive to beta radiation but have a low efficiency (less than 1%) as detectors of gamma rays. The advantage of GM tubes lies in the fact that within a certain voltage range (the plateau) the count rate is largely independent of the EHT, which means that it is not necessary for it to be stabilised. GM tubes are largely used as contamination monitors. A glass or aluminium GM tube will admit gamma photons, but windows of either very thin aluminium or mica must be inserted to allow the entry of beta particles, and the thinner the window the greater is its fragility. For low-energy beta-counting, windowless tubes, which require a continuous flow of gas, are generally used. Helium/isobutane and argon/ isobutane mixtures are available for such purposes.

Radiochromatogram scanners

The principle of these instruments is continuously to detect changes in radio-activity which has been deposited on paper, or thin-layer supports, and distributed by development of the chromatogram with a suitable solvent system. Electrophoretograms are similarly treated. Windowless gas flow tubes are used in these instruments and collimation effected with adjustable slits. The ionisation currents are amplified and fed through a ratemeter to operate the servo mechanism of a pen recorder. An integrating recorder which integrates the counts in each peak is a great advantage. Otherwise, especially for accurate assay of impurity levels, it will be necessary to isolate and count the individual peaks in a well counter.

Scintillation counting

When beta or gamma radiation is dissipated within a phosphor, light is produced, which is proportional in amount to the energy absorbed.

Well counters

For gamma radiation the detector is usually a single crystal of sodium iodide, activated with a small proportion of thallium. The crystal is cylindrical with a blind hole on the axis and is encased in aluminium except for the bottom, which usually is in contact with an integral photomultiplier system. Although the pulse emerging from the anode is proportional to the energy, the efficiency is related to the size of crystal used. With the sample inserted in the hole, almost all the gamma photons will traverse the detector but, unless the crystal is very large, many will escape without interaction. Associated with the well crystal is an amplifier and a scaler/timer (or else a ratemeter), and generally, the instrument contains a discriminator circuit which rejects pulses below the limit to which it is set. When combined with a pulse height analyser, which accepts only those pulses within a further limit, a voltage channel results, often termed a window. Provided the energies are sufficiently separated, one radionuclide can then be counted in the presence of another. When so used, the instrument functions as a single-channel gammaspectrometer, but for accurate work, multichannel analysers are used in conjunction with an analogue/digital converter and teletype. Such instruments may have from 100 to more than 1000 channels and the price is commensurate with the facilities provided. Solid state semiconductors, such as lithium-drifted germanium detectors, have greatly improved resolution and can be used with multichannel analysers, but they require cryostats and are expensive. Well counters must, of course, be sufficiently shielded.

Liquid scintillation counting

To avoid the problems of self absorption, especially with low-energy emitters such as carbon-14 and hydrogen-3, the sample can be intimately mixed with a liquid organic phosphor. Such methods are used in pharmacy for investigating the metabolism of isotopically labelled drugs, or the affinity of labelled drugs for specific tissue receptors, but have no particular place in radiopharmacy as such.

Calibration

At hospital level, radiopharmaceuticals are assayed for activity by measurement in an ion-chamber, which has been calibrated with a standardised solution of the radionuclide concerned. The long-term stability of most instruments is reasonably good, but it is advisable, after lengthy periods of use, to repeat the calibration. It should be noted that the radiopharmaceuticals included in the BP (1973) are subject usually to limits of $\pm 10\%$ for radionuclidic content, which may seem excessive, but this variation is dependent upon the degree of accuracy with which the ion-chamber used for measurement can be standardised.

The response of well chambers is examined with the aid of similar standards, but since the position of gamma peaks is important, it is customary to conduct such checks frequently, even daily. For short-lived radionuclides this is not practicable since such standardised solutions are only available from time to time and they are expensive. Therefore recourse is made to mock standards which simulate the energy of the principal gamma photon of the short-lived radionuclide, but have extended half-lives. Examples are the use of cobalt-57 in lieu of technetium-99m, barium-133 for iodine-131 and caesium-137 for molybdenum-99. For indium-113m an equilibrium mixture of tin-113 and the daughter may be used. Naturally the gamma-ray spectra of multienergetic emitters will not correspond with those of such mock standards but approximations can sometimes be achieved by a combination of selected radionuclides.

LABORATORY FACILITIES AND DESIGN

In order to specify the conditions required before the manufacture of radio-pharmaceuticals can be undertaken, it is necessary to consider the dual nature of such preparations. By definition, they are, firstly, radioactive and thus subject to the relevant sections regarding safety, disposal and laboratory design which are contained in the *Code of Practice for the Protection of Persons against Ionizing Radiations arising from Medical Use* (DHSS 1972). Secondly, they are medicines within the meaning of the Medicines Act 1968, which entails compliance with the recommendations of the *Guide to Good Pharmaceutical Manufacturing Practice, Appendix I (revised)*.

It must be emphasised that these two publications are complementary and, in general, premises which comply with 'clean area' and 'aseptic area' requirements will also meet 'radiation standards'. The converse, however, is far from true and laboratories designed solely to meet radiation hazards are rarely acceptable for pharmaceutical purposes. The majority of radiopharmaceuticals are administered parenterally and for sterile product manufacture the premises must have the approval of the Medicines Inspectorate. To provide the standards required for sterile product manufacture, in every case where radiopharmaceuticals are prepared, would be inordinately expensive. Ordinarily such facilities will be required only at Regional Centres for Nuclear Medicine but, if the circumstances warrant, may sometimes have to be provided at Area level. At District and Hospital levels some restriction must be imposed on the methods of preparation so that they may be undertaken under less rigorous conditions. This may be done by resorting to 'closed procedures'. In effect this entails having all the reagents prepared, standardised and sterilised in advance. Such 'kits' may be prepared in an approved sterile products unit or purchased. Preferably, the reagents should be packed in single-use containers, but if a bactericide is not detrimental, multi-use containers may be employed. The basic 'kit presentations' are so devised that simple addition of a sterile solution of the radioactive reagent (the primary reagent) produces a labelled compound which is pharmaceutically acceptable. Other kits require the sequential addition of reagents other than the primary reagent, and may include a heating stage or a filtration stage via an integral filter. The primary requirement is that addition or withdrawal is made to or from a sealed container under conditions of pharmaceutical cleanliness. This may only be done in a room or part of a room which is used exclusively for this purpose and which complies with the appropriate recommendations concerning the handling of radioactive materials. It must be understood that if such relatively simple premises are 'improved', the nature of the work being undertaken cannot be upgraded in any way, unless the 'improvement' is to full clean-area and/or aseptic-area requirement. There are no half-measures (see Chapter 5).

Unidirectional-flow work stations

A laminar-flow cabinet, which provides a small-scale clean-room facility, cannot ever be used for handling unsealed sources because the exhausted air, which is discharged through the front opening, may contain radioactive particles and so contaminate the laboratory environment. The conventional design must be modified by fitting an extraction unit in the base and then balancing the input and output so that a neutral zone is created at the front opening; neither is unfiltered air drawn into the cabinet nor is any internal air discharged into the laboratory. A low-speed anemometer and ventilation smoke tubes are essential to ensure correct performance. Some recirculatory systems are self balancing and have the further advantage of a partial intake through a front grille which gives a greater assurance of containment of radioactive contamination within the system. The usual pharmaceutical conditions with regard to continuous operation and/or washing down with a suitable disinfectant are applied in the usual manner.

Fume cupboards

Fume cupboards are always specified as an essential feature of any laboratory handling radioactive material. They must have flush interior surfaces which are easily cleaned and be supplied with an efficient exhaust system which must discharge into a safe area. The regulations must be studied carefully, for compliance is essential. It should be noted that under no circumstances can a fume cupboard be placed in the same room as a balanced-flow work station, unless a system of interlocking switches is employed to prevent simultaneous operation.

Drains

Wash basins and even waste disposal must often be provided in 'clean areas' and even in 'aseptic areas' when radioactive materials are being used. Considerable thought must be given to the design of waste fittings, preferably excluding water-seal types. They must be readily cleaned, even sterilised, and never connected to any other part of the hospital system if a blockage could result in radioactive waste being diverted into other sinks and wash basins elsewhere.

These notes are for general guidance only and whereas pharmaceutical safety is a pharmaceutical prerogative the advice of the Radiological Protection Advisor and/or the Radiation Safety Officer must always be sought in matters pertaining to radiation safety. No conflict of interest need arise.

REFERENCES

BAKER R. J., BELLEN J. C. & RONAL P. M. (1975) *Journal of Nuclear Medicine* **16,** 720.

BENJAMIN P. P. (1969) *International Journal of Applied Radiation and Isotopes* **20,** 187.

BOYD R. E., ROBSON J., HUNT F. C., SORBY P. J., MURRAY I. P. C. & McKAY W. J. (1973) *British Journal of Radiology* **46,** 604.

BROOKMAN V. A. & WILLIAMS C. M. (1970) *Journal of Nuclear Medicine* **11,** 733.

CASTRONOVO F. & CALLAHAN R. J. (1972) *Journal of Nuclear Medicine* **13,** 823.

CISCATO V. A., NICOLINI J. O. & PALCOS M. C. (1969) *International Journal of Applied Radiation and Isotopes* **20,** 115.

COHEN M. B. (1970) *Journal of Nuclear Medicine* **11,** 767.

COLOMBETTI L. G., GOODWIN D. A. & HERMANSON R. (1969) *Journal of Nuclear Medicine* **10,** 597.

COTTON F. A. & WILKINSON G. (1972) *Advanced Inorganic Chemistry*, p. 430. Wiley, New York.

CRAGIN M. D., WEBBER M. M., VICTERY W. K. & PINTAURO O. (1969) *Journal of Nuclear Medicine* **10,** 621.

DAVIS M. A., JONES A. G. & TRINDADE H. (1974) *Journal of Nuclear Medicine* **15,** 923.

DEWANJEE M. K., FLIEGEL C., TROVES S. & DAVIS M. S. (1974) *Journal of Nuclear Medicine* **15,** 176.

DUNSON G. L., THRALL J. H., STEVENSON J. S. & PINSKY S. M. (1973) *Radiology* **109,** 387.

ECKELMAN W., RICHARDS P., ATKINS H. L., HAUSER W. & KLAPPER J. F. (1971) *Journal of Nuclear Medicine* **12,** 310.

ELIAS H., ARNOLD C. H. & KLOSS G. (1973) *International Journal of Applied Radiation and Isotopes* **24,** 463.

ENLANDER D., WEBER P. M. & DOS REMEDIOS L. V. (1974) *Journal of Nuclear Medicine* **15,** 743.

GARZON O. L., PALCOS M. C. & RADICELLA R. (1965) *International Journal of Radiation and Isotopes* **16,** 613.

HALPERN S., TURBIS M., ENDOW J., WALSH C., KUNSA J. & ZWICKER B. (1972) *Journal of Nuclear Medicine* **15,** 34.

HANEY T. A., ASCANIO I., GIGLIOTTI J. A., GUSMANO E. A. & BRUNO G. A. (1971) *Journal of Nuclear Medicine* **12,** 64.

HARPER P. V., LATHROP K. A. & RICHARDS P. (1964) *Journal of Nuclear Medicine* **5,** 382.

HILL T., WELCH M. J., ADATEPE M. & POTCHEN E. J. (1970) *Journal of Nuclear Medicine* **11,** 28.

HUBERTY J. P., HATTNER R. S. & POWELL M. R. (1974) *Journal of Nuclear Medicine* **15,** 124.

JOHNSON A. E. & GOLLAN F. (1970) *Journal of Nuclear Medicine* **11,** 564.

LIN M. S. & WINCHELL H. S. (1972) *Journal of Nuclear Medicine* **13,** 58.

LIN M. S., WINCHELL H. S. & SHIPLEY B. A. (1971) *Journal of Nuclear Medicine* **12,** 204.

LIN T. H., KHENTIGAN A. & WINCHELL H. S. (1974) *Journal of Nuclear Medicine* **15,** 34.

MURRAY I. P. C. (1972) *Symposium on Medical Radioisotope Scintigraphy*. SM-164/164. IAEA, Vienna.

SERAFINI A. N., SMOAK W. M., HUPF H. B., BEAVER J. E., HOLDER J. & GILSON A. J. (1975) *Journal of Nuclear Medicine* **16,** 629.

STAUM M. M. (1972) *Journal of Nuclear Medicine* **13,** 386.

STERN H. S., ZOLLE I. & McAFEE J. G. (1965) *International Journal of Applied Radiation and Isotopes* **16,** 283.

STERN H. S., McAFEE J. G. & SUBRAMANIAN G. (1966) *Journal of Nuclear Medicine* **7,** 665.

SUBRAMANIAN G. & McAFEE J. G. (1971) *Radiology* **99,** 192.

SUBRAMANIAN G., McAFEE J. G., BLAIR R. J., KALLFELZ F. A. & THOMAS F. D. (1976) *Journal of Nuclear Medicine* **16,** 744.

SUBRAMANIAN G., McAFEE J. G., MEHTER A., BLAIR R. J. & THOMAS F. D. (1973) *Journal of Nuclear Medicine* **14,** 459.

SZYMENDERA J., ZOLTOWSKI T., RADWAN M. & KAMINSKI J. (1971) *Journal of Nuclear Medicine* **12,** 212.

TUBIS M., KRISHNAMURTHY G. T., ENDOW J. S. & BLAHD W. H. (1972) *Journal of Nuclear Medicine* **13,** 652.

ZOLLE I., RHODES B. A. & WAGNER H. N. (1970) *International Journal of Applied Radiation and Isotopes* **21,** 155.

FURTHER READING

BRITISH INSTITUTE OF RADIOLOGY (1975) *Guidelines for the Preparation of Radiopharmaceuticals in Hospitals*. Special report 11. British Institute of Radiology, London.

DEPARTMENT OF HEALTH AND SOCIAL SECURITY (1972) *Code of Practice for the Protection of Persons against Ionising Radiations arising from Medical and Dental Use*. HMSO, London.

INTERNATIONAL ATOMIC ENERGY AGENCY (1970) *Analytical Control of Radiopharmaceuticals*. STI/PUB/253. IAEA, Vienna.

INTERNATIONAL ATOMIC ENERGY AGENCY (1971) *Radiopharmaceuticals from Generator-produced Radionuclides*. STI/PUB/294. IAEA, Vienna.

INTERNATIONAL ATOMIC ENERGY AGENCY (1973) *Radiopharmaceuticals and Labelled Compounds*. STI/PUB/344. IAEA, Vienna.

SUBRAMANIAN G., RHODES B. A., COOPER L. & SODD L. (eds.) (1975) *Radiopharmaceuticals*. Society of Nuclear Medicine, New York.

WILSON B. J. (ed.) (1966) *The Radiochemical Manual* Radiochemical Centre, Amersham.

8

Drug analysis and quality control

I. COUPER & N. DRIVER

The quality of a product has been defined as its 'fitness for a purpose' (Caplen 1972). 'Quality control' could be defined as any process, or series of processes, which guarantee the fitness of a product for a given purpose.

Unfortunately, the popular concept of quality control is somewhat narrow in outlook, in that the term tends to be associated with those analytical procedures which are applied during production and to the final product to ensure its reliability. This is not an acceptable idea since the term 'quality control' should extend from the birth of the drug or preparation to the moment it is handed to the patient. In hospitals, this is more apposite since the hospital pharmacist may have greater control over the medical product than does his industrial colleague. Thus, if one takes hospital quality control to its logical conclusion, it must be said that every pharmacist who checks measurements and calculations of a technician's manufactured product, who tests the acceptability of appearance of a cream or suspension, who is concerned with correctness and neatness of labelling is practising 'quality control'. Further, in a hospital environment, the ward level pharmacist who screens patients' drug records for incompatibilities and overdoses is controlling the quality of patient care and therapy.

This concept of 'quality control' is very much wider than that which was formerly used. The term 'quality control' is in fact not a suitable title to describe all the processes involved in hospital pharmacy, and therefore a different terminology, such as 'quality assurance', should be adopted, with 'quality control' confined to those analytical procedures etc. involved in production control and final product analysis. These terms are defined in the *Guide to Good Pharmaceutical Manufacturing Practice* ('Orange Guide'; DHSS 1977) and for the remainder of this chapter, the terms 'quality control' and 'quality controller' will be used in the contexts laid down in the 'Orange Guide'.

DUTIES AND RESPONSIBILITIES OF THE QUALITY CONTROL LABORATORY

The duties of the quality control department are many and varied and will be discussed in detail later. The quality controller has however only one responsibility; that is to ensure, as far as possible, that every product issued from the hospital pharmacy has attained a satisfactory standard of fitness, and will keep that standard until used, for the purpose for which it was intended.

While many quality control techniques require sophisticated equipment and skilled personnel, a large number of assays for active ingredients may be carried out using simple titrimetric methods. Thus while Regional and Area analytical facilities will be necessary, many items manufactured in smaller hospital pharmacies may be subjected to a final product control using simple,

Table 8.1   Availability of analytical facilities in quality control laboratories

Type of laboratory	Facilities available	Comments
Regional	Gas–liquid chromatography Ultraviolet/Visible and infra-red spectrophotometry Atomic absorption spectrophotometry Particle counting and identifying apparatus	This advanced type of equipment should be *in addition* to the routine facilities mentioned below. Instruments should be of research grade where possible.
Area	Particle counting apparatus Ultraviolet/visible spectrophotometry Polarimetry Refractometry pH Meters	Equipment for routine counting of particulate contamination of parenteral fluids should be available for Area Sterile Fluids Laboratories. Analyses which cannot be handled at this level should be referred to the Regional Services. Area Labs. should handle quality control for all hospitals in each Area.
Hospital	Titration equipment pH Meter	Hospital laboratories should handle simple routine tests on their own manufactured products, passing on more complicated samples to Area or Regional level.

efficient titrimetric techniques which require very little space and only the most basic laboratory glassware and reagents.

In the smaller hospitals, materials which cannot be assayed by those simple methods should be passed on to Area or Regional laboratories for analysis. This 'tiered' system was envisaged in the Noel Hall Report (DHSS 1970). Some examples of facilities which should be available in different types of hospital are shown in Table 8.1.

It cannot be overemphasised that lack of analytical facilities does not mean lack of quality control. In pharmacies where no formal quality control service is available, it is the responsibility of the pharmacist in charge to ensure that the medicines in his department are of adequate standards, either by referring samples to other laboratories for testing or by good supervision of his own production procedures.

EQUIPMENT AND TACTICS

Equipping a laboratory

It is often thought that the chief considerations in equipping a laboratory are the important analytical instruments. Whilst these major instruments merit considerable attention, the more mundane pieces of furniture are also essential, since little work can be performed without these basics.

The first of these is obviously the room and services. The more fortunate quality controller will be able to plan a new building, but more often the choice will fall upon what space is available. In this case, every effort must be made to obtain as much space as possible since it will often be found that what is thought to be adequate now may prove to be very cramped quarters in future to the detriment of the work. If possible, the room should have north-facing windows, and plenty of natural light. It should also contain some area which can be darkened, or partially so. The provision of electric sockets cannot be overdone, and ideally, one sink unit should be supplied per operator. A fume cupboard is necessary, and also some secure storage for the noxious chemicals such as bromine and acetic anhydride. It is required that all volatile solvents (i.e. those having a flashpoint below 32°C), should be stored in fire-resistant secure cabinets.

Lastly in the basics are the reagents, and whilst these will be obtained as required, a comprehensive range should be obtained at the start. Reference to the pharmacopoeial appendices will give indications of what is required. For volumetric solutions, the concentrated solutions available in ampoules cover most needs, and save time in standardisation which can be better utilised in analysis. They also allow small quantities to be prepared as required.

Secondly the 'nuts and bolts' of analytical chemistry must be chosen and a comprehensive range of glassware and small items obtained. It is also essential that volumetric glassware should be of class A standard as required by the pharmacopoeias. Since dilution of samples forms a large part of the work, the smaller pipettes (1ml and 0.5 ml) should be of the 'blow out' variety. Frequently, reaction and distillation apparatus is required, and for these assays, ground-glass joint apparatus should be available with sufficient adaptors and connectors to enable assembly of all likely outfits.

Replacement of broken glassware is becoming increasingly expensive: for obvious safety reasons the use of cracked or chipped glassware cannot be allowed. In some cases, if an item is expensive to replace, it may be 'salvaged' by an experienced glassblower, whose skills are also useful for production of 'one-off' pieces of equipment to a user's specification.

Choosing an instrument

The range of equipment available can be obtained by studying the advertisements in journals such as *Chemistry in Britain, Manufacturing Chemist* and *Laboratory Practice,* and also by attending exhibitions such as those organised by the Royal Institute of Chemistry. A review of the available equipment with the following points in mind may be of assistance in making the final choice.

Accuracy

Since price always increases with sophistication, it is uneconomic to purchase an instrument which has specifications within 'research' limits when only routine estimations are to be carried out. Routine instruments, which are less expensive, usually have a lesser degree of accuracy, but are completely acceptable for normal laboratory work and may be easier for technicians to operate. Specifications regarding accuracy are given in manufacturers' literature, and most companies market a range of 'routine' instruments for laboratory work.

If the user also wishes to carry out research, an instrument with a higher degree of accuracy should be considered. It may be desirable, if a large amount of research work is to be done in a Regional Laboratory, to choose and keep instruments specifically for this purpose.

Versatility

The wide range of products manufactured in a pharmaceutical department make it essential that an instrument should be able to cope with various adaptations which may be required.

Ease of operation

It must be borne in mind that most technical staff in hospital pharmacy have, as yet, very little training in the use of analytical equipment. Therefore simplicity of operation should be a key factor in the choice of an instrument. The appropriate sections on operation in instrument handbooks should be studied where possible. Some manufacturers are now designing their instruments so that the smallest number of controls are needed, or alternatively, those controls which are not in constant use are under a covering plate to prevent inadvertent or unauthorised adjustments.

Efficiency of repairs

For equipment in regular use, efficient repair of breakdowns is essential. It is important therefore to consider whether a service engineer for a particular company is near at hand to deal with emergencies. The physics department of many large hopsitals are also able to assist.

Cost

The factor of price should be considered only in relation to the other factors mentioned. Most instruments of similar specification are competitively priced. When one is costing an instrument, one should include accessories, for example recorders or printers, which may be required.

Compatibility of accessories

The increasing trend towards automation in analysis has led to the development of aids, such as recorders and printers, which can be fitted to instruments to give a written record of results. Electronic recorders are particularly useful accessories giving a visual presentation of the result obtained. If, however, it is desired to choose or use a recorder not recommended or sold by the instrument manufacturers, care should be taken to ensurethat it is compatible (e.g. does the output in millivolts match that of the recorder?). Dedicated recorders are often very desirable since they are made to follow closely the instrument, and the chart paper is printed so as to conform to the calibration of the instrument. This is very desirable in ultraviolet (UV) spectra, and essential in infrared (IR) spectra. If an instrument will accept any one of a variety of accessories, then one such accessory may be purchased which is compatible with a number of pieces of equipment, thus saving on the cost of unique accessories.

The value of an accessory must be carefully assessed since it is easy to find that the accessory has only limited value. For example, a fluorimetric attachment to a UV spectrophotometer is useless for nearly everything except quinine, since in most instruments, there is insufficient energy to give enough sensitivity.

Most companies will arrange for a demonstration of their equipment on request, and the potential buyer is strongly advised to examine a number of instruments in this way. Ideally, one should keep the instrument for a few days, testing it in situations which might routinely arise. It is useful to obtain the views of other users of the instrument. Many companies will supply names of laboratories where their equipment is in routine use.

Once a particular instrument has been chosen, there are certain practical considerations which must be made, such as installation and safety factors. The site for a particular piece of equipment must be chosen with care, taking into account such factors as mechanical stability, sensitivity to 'noise' and draughts and effects of atmospheric pollution. An instrument such as an analytical balance which is affected by mechanical vibrations must be set on a bench designed to absorb shock produced by normal mechanical movement, and if possible protected from draughts in a position away from the main 'traffic course' of the laboratory. Ideally, instruments should be housed in an area of the laboratory which is partitioned off from the main working areas: samples should be prepared outside and taken into the 'instrument area' for testing. Reagents should be removed as soon as possible to minimise the risk of damage to instruments due to spillage of possibly corrosive materials. If such a system is not feasible, then instruments should be placed on benches separated from the routine work bench and staff should be encouraged to carry out all dilutions etc. at the work bench, transporting samples to and from the instruments as necessary. Electronic particle counters are sensitive to electrical 'noise' and if the laboratory is in the vicinity of machine shops, X-ray machines or any large concentration of electrical equipment, an electrical interference filter should be fitted to screen off background 'noise' which would affect results. Such particle counters may also be 'earthed' by fitting a metal cage round the sampling chamber to further cut down interference. This also serves to protect the sample from contamination by atmospheric dust.

If gas cylinders are required, for example hydrogen, nitrogen, acetylene or nitrous oxide for gas chromatographs or atomic absorption equipment, fire regulations require the cylinders to be in separate outhouses and the gases piped to the instruments. Needle valves in the pipeline close to the instrument are desirable for control purposes. Suitable extraction facilities are required to vent exhaust fumes produced with atomic absorption and fluorescence spectrophotometers. The instrument manufacturer and hospital specialists such as engineers and electricians should be consulted on the design of such additional requirements to conform to the necessary safety regulations.

Maintenance and monitoring of reliability

Service contracts can be arranged with most firms for regular yearly or twice-yearly checks on equipment. It is advisable to ensure that such servicing is carried out, since a great deal of expense on repairs may thus be saved.

These comprehensive checks, carried out by experts on the electronics of each instrument, are however no substitute for regular laboratory monitoring of instrument performance. Most instrument handbooks list various tests which may be carried out to challenge the reliability of results. Weekly or monthly procedures should be laid down in instruction manuals for laboratory staff.

Some examples of routine laboratory checks are given below.

pH Meters. Weekly calibration of electrodes with standard buffer solutions; visual examination of electrodes for cracks.

Spectrophotometers. Challenging of calibration curves with standards; checking wavelength with a holmium oxide filter and absorption response to potassium-dichromate solutions recommended in handbooks.

Particle counters. Weekly calibration of threshold counts with standard latex or spore suspensions; visual checks of orifice for blockage or damage.

The above are tests which should be applied to instruments in use in the quality control laboratory. It is also the duty of the quality controller to monitor the reliability of other equipment used for production, for example stills, autoclaves and laminar flow cabinets.

Fault finding

All operators of instruments should be capable of locating and correcting simple faults. Most instrument manuals contain sections on fault finding, and provided the instructions are followed carefully there is no reason why a number of minor repairs should not be effected without the need to call in a service engineer. When incorrect results are being obtained, or it appears that the instrument is not functioning correctly, it is useful to have available some solution or filter whose characteristics are known to test for malfunction. For example, a holmium oxide filter will check the wavelength scan, the photometric accuracy and the performance of the recorder for a spectrophotometer. Similarly, a mixture of hydrocarbons C_9 to C_{12} can be used to check a gas–liquid chromatogram.

Having found that the instrument is functioning correctly, then contamination of standards or reagents should be looked for. For example, when unusual spectrophotometer traces are obtained, the cleanliness of the cells should first be ensured, then the reference standards checked for purity.

Development of standards and limits for starting materials and final products

It is generally agreed that all raw materials should be tested before being released for use in manufacturing processes. Monographs for raw materials usually contain a number of standards, and while ideally each test specified should be carried out, shortage of staff may not allow for this, and a compromise may be necessary. One should remember that the 'raw materials' purchased by a pharmacy are *ideally* the 'finished products' of reputable manufacturers.

While one may assume a certain degree of quality of product, an identification test at least for major constituents of the product is essential. The number of other tests carried out by the quality controller will depend on the degree of confidence he has in a particular supplier, but a reasonable recommendation is that an identification test be carried out on every container of each batch, together with at least two other qualitative and/or quantitative tests to be performed on a representative sample of each batch. At set intervals, once again dependent on the confidence in the manufacturer, all the appropriate monograph tests on a particular product will be undertaken. It is possible that different gradings for raw materials may be used, for example there may be a sodium chloride for parenteral use, for internal use and for external use. Specification sheets and labels must state clearly the appropriate grade of raw materials.

A committee consisting of the Regional Pharmaceutical Officer, the quality control pharmacists in the region and representatives from a School of Pharmacy should be formed to decide on standards regarding assays, raw materials, limits and sampling procedures. Specification sheets for each raw material should be produced based on the decisions of this committee and every batch of raw material tested accordingly. Items brought into the pharmacy stores should be 'quarantined' until tested by the quality control department. A label of distinctive colour, carrying the date of issue and a batch number corresponding to the specification test number, should be attached to each container after testing, without which no material may be used for manufacture.

Since it is the responsibility of the quality control department to monitor storage conditions, certain tests for adequate storage should be adopted. Tests for insect contamination and foreign organic matter may be employed; tests for absence of degradation products may be useful indicators of efficient storage conditions.

When a raw material is particularly unstable, an assay for major constituent (and for degradation products) should be performed immediately before the material is used in manufacture; sodium iodide and phenol are two typical examples.

It is of interest to note that the pack size purchased is of some importance. Degradation occurs at a much greater rate in opened packs. If only a small quantity of material is to be used at any one time, it may be more economical to purchase a smaller pack size, especially with unstable materials, rather than discard the remainder of a large pack which has fallen below its specifications when next required for manufacturing purposes.

In hospitals where research is carried out by medical staff, non-official preparations are often requested. In many cases the raw materials themselves are non-official products. Standards and assay methods must be laid down, once again in agreement with all quality controllers in the region. The following factors should be taken into consideration:

1. Use of end product (i.e. whether it is for parenteral, oral or topical administration).

2. Toxicity of material. This will affect the percentage variation from the labelled amount which will be allowed.

3. Stability. This will affect the shelf-life of the product and influence the decision on the expiry date required.

4. Toxicity of possible degradation products. This will affect the shelf-life of the final products.

5. Toxicity of adulterants. This will influence the decision on which qualitative and quantitative tests should be performed.

The term 'starting materials' should be understood to include containers and closures of all types (i.e. glass, plastic, rubber or metal) and these should be subject to similar specifications as other raw materials. Products which are purchased in bulk and broken down into smaller pack sizes must also be controlled, since these are, in a sense, 'starting materials'. This is particularly true in the case of tablet prepacking which is often carried out on a large scale at Area level. Tablet prepacks should be subjected at least to identification tests for active ingredients. Specifications and policy must be decided for control of prepacked items in a similar manner to other starting materials.

Other items which should be the responsibility of the quality controller are containers used for mixing and preparation of products, weights and measuring vessels, detergents used in cleaning, and labels and labelling equipment. All these items should conform to certain accepted standards.

ROUTINE PROCEDURES

Analytical techniques

The function of an analyst in the hospital environment is likely to be concerned with: identification procedures; assay procedures of sterile and non-sterile preparations; suitability of raw materials; complaints regarding all of these; surgical dressings. Thus the analyst should have a full knowledge of all analytical methods commonly in use so that the above quoted procedures may be accommodated. In addition, the senior quality controller should always be aware of newer techniques being brought into use. A thorough reading of current literature is essential, and also some index system of applications reported which could have a bearing on pharmaceutical analysis. The quality control department should build up a library not only of British and foreign pharmacopoeias but also of textbooks on analysis, monographs on instrumental techniques, and instrument, labware and chemicals catalogues. Subscriptions should be taken for appropriate journals on an Area basis, and the journals should be circulated to all quality controllers within the Area.

The following is a review of important techniques and instruments currently in use.

The balance

As the balance is the starting point and the ultimate reference in an analytical laboratory, it should be carefully chosen and properly sited. The tendency today is to require reference standards, and these must be weighed out in small amounts as the amount supplied is limited; often only 100 mg or less. Thus a five-decimal-place balance is desirable if reasonable accuracy is to be attained.

Spectrophotometry

Spectrophotometry, one of the most widely used of all analytical techniques, has many pharmaceutical applications which may interest the quality controller (Hummel & Kaufman 1972).

Ultraviolet/visible spectrophotometry

This is the technique of greatest use in analysis. It is above all the instrument of choice for many applications and it is the instrument for quantitative assay. To this end, the greatest proportion of the allocated funds should be given to the purchase of a suitable instrument. Since very many substances can only be conveniently assayed by this technique, the precision and accuracy should be as great as is consistent with the price.

   The earlier instruments were single beam, calibrated linearly in transmission. We are concerned solely with *absorbance*; transmission is only a means to this end. An instrument, preferably a double-beam system, calibrated linearly in absorbance, and with scale expansion should be chosen. The newest instruments have digital read-out, and this is a considerable advance, and a great convenience. If possible, a recorder should accompany the instrument, and be of the dedicated variety so that standard scans of the spectrum can be obtained. This means that it is possible to obtain an identification of many solutions at the same time as the assay. To this end, a library of spectra of those substances commonly used should be compiled under standard conditions in acid, alkaline and alcoholic solution.

   For many substances, simple dilution in water or dilute acid, and measurement at a maximum in the region 200–360 nm is all that is required. Calculation using $E_{1\,cm}^{1\%}$ values yields the desired result. If there is no absorbance in this region, or it is of a low value, then it is often possible that reaction with some other compound will yield a coloured solution with a maximum absorbance in the 360–700 nm region. Again, calculation using $E_{1\,cm}^{1\%}$ value gives the desired result (Beckett & Stenlake 1976).

   Sometimes, two or more compounds are present together, and if the absorbance peaks are well separated, then the two compounds can be assayed together, and the results calculated using simultaneous equations. The estimation of nicotinamide and pyridoxine in Strong Thiamine Compound Tablets is an example of this technique.

The advantages of ultraviolet/visible spectrophotometry are that it is quick, accurate, highly specific and easy to perform. Adulteration of samples or incorrect compounds can be detected if the spectrum is scanned, unexpected peaks or shifts of wavelength being obtained. The method is very versatile, being applicable to gases, volatile liquids, microquantities and turbid solutions, and can be adapted for flow through use or to receive fractions directly from a fraction collector.

Examples of some substances which may be analysed by this method in the ultraviolet region are atropine (Fig. 8.1), ephedrine, physostigmine, chlorhexidine (Fig. 8.2), cocaine, chloramphenicol, lignocaine and cyanocobalamin, and in the visible region morphine, folic acid and adrenaline.

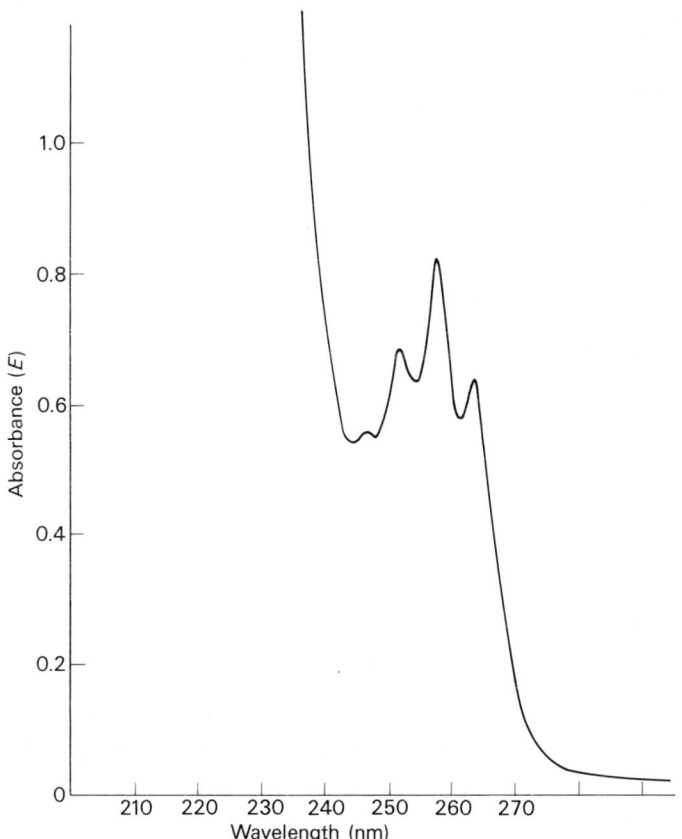

Fig. 8.1   The ultraviolet spectrum of atropine sulphate from Atropine Eyedrops. The reference (blank) solution is 0.02% benzalkonium chloride solution, the preservative used in the preparation of the eyedrops; λmax: 258 nm.

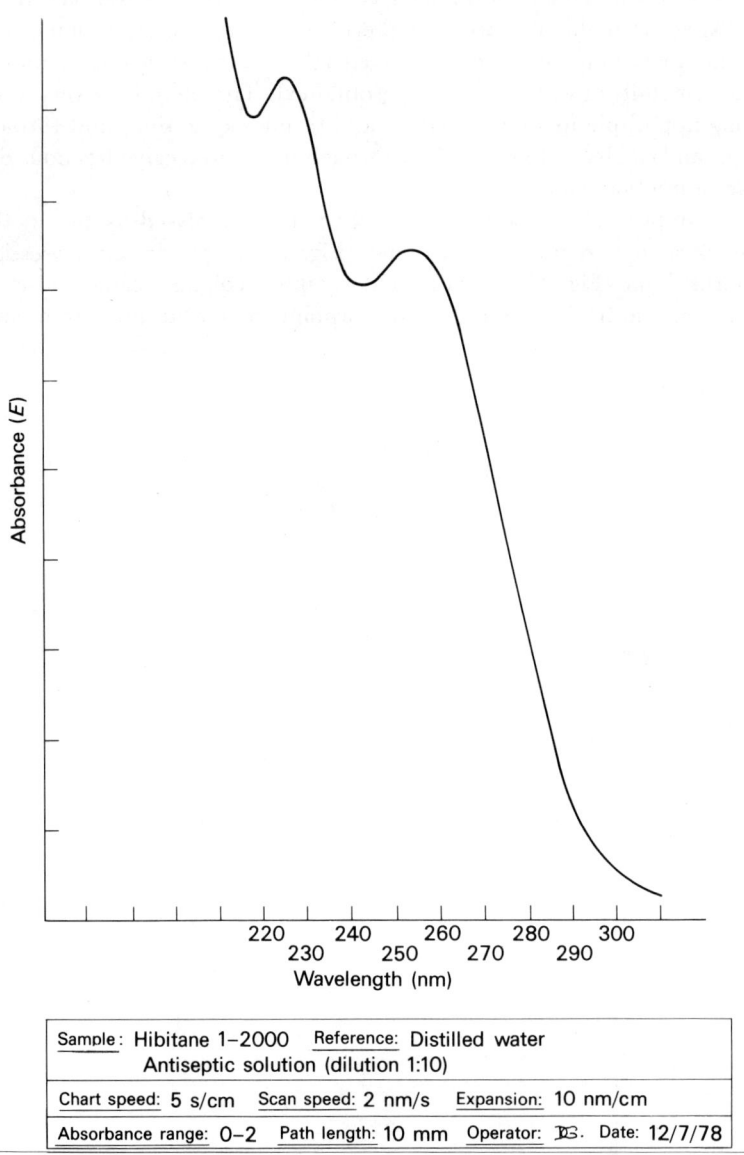

Fig. 8.2   A recorded trace of the ultraviolet spectrum of a sample of chlorhexidine gluconate (Hibitane) solution.

Infra-red spectrophotometry

This is above all the method for the identification of compounds. In hospital pharmacy, the concern is mainly with confirming identity, not establishing it. A library of spectra of the compounds of interest should be compiled, and thought given to the preparation of the sample. There is no universal method of sample preparation. The potassium bromide disc has the advantage that no bands are present in the 4000–650 cm^{-1} range, but has the disadvantage that a hydraulic press is needed, and that isomorphous changes may occur. The mull technique is quick and easy to use, and if two spectra are run, one in liquid paraffin and one in hexachlorobutadiene, then the whole spectrum is covered. Liquid samples, solid samples, pastes, ointments, creams and gases can also be examined. In some cases it may be necessary to use an attenuated total reflectance (ATR) unit.

Absorption/emission spectrophotometry

The simple flame emission photometer, which is a filter instrument, suffices for the majority of samples which have either sodium or potassium present. This is a simple instrument for routine work which is what is required for a unit producing intravenous products. The disadvantage of the instrument is that large dilutions are required. Instruments are available which automatically dilute the sample presented, and give a direct digital read-out of concentration if the instrument has been previously calibrated. This type of instrument has the capacity for a very large workload.

Just as the ultraviolet/visible spectrophotometer was developed from simple colorimeters, so has the atomic absorption spectrophotometer developed from the flame photometer, and in a like manner it is a very accurate and sensitive instrument. Practically all metallic elements can be determined, provided one has the necessary hollow cathode lamps, but the halides and other inorganic anions cannot. This limits its usefulness in the application for measuring trace elements in raw materials. Special care must be taken, in the preparation of standards, to avoid contamination by trace quantities of elements such as lead and sodium; due to the extreme sensitivity of the technique, false results may be obtained caused by contamination of standards by lead or sodium leached from containers. The atomic absorption spectrophotometer is a very expensive instrument, the cost being greater than that of an ultraviolet spectrophotometer. Its cost can only be justified where specialised work is undertaken.

The instrument usually requires an air – acetylene flame for ignition of the samples, and extraction ducts are necessary if poisonous elements (e.g. mercury) are being determined. If the flammable gases are used, then an instrument with safety gas controls should be chosen.

Fluorescence spectrophotometry

The main applications of this technique in pharmacy are for quinine and quinine-like preparations, vitamins and digoxin. For all except digoxin, a filter instrument is adequate, but if dissolution studies of digoxin are undertaken, then a spectrofluorimeter is essential.

Titrimetry

The importance of this classical method of analysis must not be underestimated. Titrimetric analysis is a highly adaptive technique which finds wide use in pharmacopoeias. There are pharmaceutical applications for almost all of the many forms of titrations, from the simplest acid–base determination to more complex non-aqueous or 'redox' analyses. Garratt (1964) and Beckett and Stenlake (1976) quote many pharmaceutical analyses in which titration is used. In the Royal Infirmary, Glasgow, about 50% of all assays performed utilise titration in some form, either wholly or as part of the final analytical techniques. Where numerous repetitive titrations are involved, automated titrating equipment may be used. This equipment can be used either semiautomatically or fully automatically. In the semiautomatic mode the normal method of manual titration can be utilised together with the advantage of the accuracy of the piston burette, and if sufficient number of burette and reservoir units are available then time is saved by not having to fill and empty burettes. The amount of titrant added is displayed digitally by the instrument. The fully automatic mode is useful where difficulties in normal titration occur such as obscured end points, small inflexions as during titration of poly basic acids. The mode used can be either one which gives the normal 'S' curve or the first derivative curve. The apparatus can be set for either fast or slow titration, and the rate of addition can be slowed as the end point is approached. It is also possible to stop the titration at any particular point. A full written record is obtained by means of the recorder.

Since titration involves measurement of chemical reactions, and many compounds tend to react in a similar manner, this lack of specificity of the technique means that titration results should only be relied on where one is certain that there can be no interference from similarly reacting compounds in the sample, or where steps are taken to correct for such interference.

Individual variations in the ability of operators to recognise colour changes at end points tend to be a disadvantage of titrimetric analysis. Inexperienced operators should be supervised carefully to ensure that they are obtaining reproducible results.

Chromatography

Chromatography is a technique for separating mixtures of compounds, and finds wide pharmaceutical application in both quantitative and qualitative analysis.

Gas–liquid chromatography (GLC)

Gas–liquid chromatography provides the means whereby mixtures of compounds can be separated, identified, and quantitatively analysed. Various detectors are in use (e.g. katharometer, flame ionisation and electron capture), but for pharmaceutical use the flame ionisation detector is the most widely used. A dual flame ionisation temperature programmed instrument with a suitable recorder should be chosen. An integrator is an advantage. The retention time is a characteristic of the compound under standard conditions, but for positive identification two or more columns should be used. The peak height or area is proportional to the concentration of the compound, but as the injection cannot be reproducibly repeated, the use of an internal standard is common practice.

The method, while requiring a sound knowledge of the technique, is invaluable in the estimation of many compounds. In most cases, direct injection of a simple extraction suffices. It is specific and effects a considerable reduction in time for many assays. For example, camphor or methyl salicylate can be quickly estimated in ointments or liniments. Chloroform can be reliably estimated in aqueous solution to very low levels, which is certainly not the case for colorimetric methods. Ethanol, in galenicals, can be determined in a Poropak Q column, and other alcohols and hydroxy compounds, such as glycerol, may be determined in a similar manner.

A silicone gum SE30 column is a useful general-purpose column. Purified forms of silicone, the OV series, are useful for more polar substances. Greenwood and Guppy (1974) have shown that a silicone OV17 column can be used for aqueous solutions of salts of nitrogenous bases. Thus procaine, amethocaine, lignocaine, belladonna alkaloids, antihistamines and morphine and pethidine can be determined by injection as their salts in aqueous solution.

Steroids and barbiturates may also be determined by GLC. As the determination of steroids requires the use of glass columns, it is suggested that the laboratory has suitable glass columns available.

High-pressure liquid chromatography (HPLC)

The apparatus consists of an injector, column and detector and the moving phase flows through the column under high pressure usually at room temperature.

Injection of the sample into the system can be by syringe as in GLC but the use of a sampling valve overcomes difficulties which arise from the high pressures in the system (up to 5000 lb/in², 400 bar).

The column is normally shorter than in GLC because of the greater separating efficiency of the packing materials which have been developed. The packing materials consist of small porous particles of size 30 μm or less.

Detection of the sample can be by spectrophotometry, refractive index or flame ionisation, but the more usual is the spectrophotometric. The spectro-photometric technique requires a very stable spectrophotometer capable of measuring reliably below 0.01 A on small volume cells (about 8 µl). The earlier models were designed for working at a fixed wavelength (250 nm) but there are considerable advantages in having variable wavelength. Sugars for example are detected at 190 nm, steroids at 220 nm, cyanocobalamin at 360 nm.

The separation in the column is by partition or adsorption. Partition chro-matography is either normal or reverse phase. Separation by adsorption is on the recently developed column of controlled diameter silica gel or alumina particles.

Elution is by means of the moving phase. This moving phase is critical to the separation and usually consists of a mixture of organic solvents. The particular mixture used will depend on the type of materials to be separated. Where methods have to be developed or a mixture of two or more components has to be separated, it is often necessary to vary the compositions of the moving phase; this is termed gradient analysis. Gradient analysis is achieved by the use of two supply systems (usually pulseless pumps) and varying the ratios of the mixture components by electronic control of the pumps.

Column chromatography

This method of separation usually finds application in qualitative analysis. It may be useful to adopt this technique, prior to further quantitative investiga-tion, for separation of mixtures of closely related compounds. A variation in the column chromatographic technique is the substitution of an ion-exchange resin for the normal column adsorbent. This enables compounds, which may be weakly basic or acidic, to be converted via the ion-exchange column to more easily analysed compounds. The assay for sodium perchlorate (Analar Standards 1967) can be adopted for analysis of sodium perchlorate injections. Sodium and potassium phosphate solutions and sodium sulphate solutions may be assayed by this method, being eluted from the column and determined as phosphoric or sulphuric acids respectively.

Thin-layer chromatography (TLC)

Numerous articles have been published on the use of TLC, both qualitative and quantitative, in analysis of countless types of products. It is certainly the most useful qualitative method: it is rapid, versatile, accurate and requires only inexpensive equipment. Since very small quantities of sample are required for analysis, the method is ideal for identification of unknown substances and Clarke (1969) quotes TLC systems for identification of large numbers of drugs.

Quantitative TLC has been suggested for the analysis of many pharma-ceutical preparations, but the method requires a skilled operator constantly engaged in the work, so that the number of variables which may interfere with accuracy and reproducibility is reduced.

While it is unlikely that quantitative TLC will find use as a routine tool in hospital analysis, a semiquantitative method of determination based on measurement of sizes of spots may be useful in certain instances where the concentration of a compound is questioned. Since concentration is directly proportional to size of spot obtained with a given system, an indication of concentration may be given by running the compound under test with standards of known concentration and comparing the sizes of the spots obtained after development of the plate.

As a qualitative method for identification of unknowns, for screening samples for adulteration, for detecting the presence of impurities or degradation products, the technique is invaluable. Almost any substance may be subjected to TLC, by varying solvent systems or plate coatings.

Paper chromatography

This technique has little value in routine hospital work; it has the same uses as TLC but is much slower in operation. It has a use as an aid for teaching or demonstration purposes.

Other instruments

The major instruments have already been discussed but there remain other smaller instruments which are required.

Polarimeter

This is essential where dextrose, laevulose and fructose preparations are being tested. The deficiency of the older instruments is the visual judgement of the balance point by the operator, and this makes the method somewhat tedious. There is now a polarimeter in the lower price bracket which uses an electronic balance method. The polarimeter is perhaps the best instrument to distinguish between quinine and quinidine, quinine being laevorotatory and quinidine being dextrorotatory.

Refractometer

The refractometer is used for the measurement of refractive index of essential and fixed oils. Provided a calibration curve has been made, the refractometer can determine glycerol/water and sorbitol/water mixtures.

Microscope

The microscope has many uses, the main ones being the identification of structures, but it is also used for the measurement of particle size (e.g. corticosteroid suspensions).

Disintegration and dissolution apparatus

These may be necessary where tests on tablets or capsules are to be performed. The disintegration test is official for both coated and uncoated tablets and capsules. The *British Pharmacopoeia Addendum* (1977) describes a dissolution test which is to be applied to one product, digoxin tablets. The technique used is the rotating basket system similar to that described in the *United States Pharmacopoeia*. This technique can be applied to most tablet and capsule formulations and can be made automatic if the liquor from the apparatus is pumped by a peristaltic pump through a flow cell in a spectrophotometer set to record at a fixed wavelength.

Adaptations or alterations in official methods

While one must recognise the necessity to use official assay methods where possible, there are many cases where procedures set down in the pharmacopoeias are not suitable for the final products submitted for analysis to the quality controller. Development of analytical methods for pharmaceutical preparations is dealt with in Chapter 9.

Incorrect results

Some comments on the procedure to be adopted when results are obtained which do not fall within the set limits may be appropriate. The position can be divided into three classes.

1.   Incorrect assay procedure.
2.   Operator error.
3.   The sample is incorrect.

Any one, or all of these conditions may be present and a deductive method must be applied to eliminate where possible.

It is first necessary to establish that the correct assay method has been used, and that it is known to be reliable and accurate. In the cases where the assay method is used for the first time this may not be known, and the possibility of an unreliable assay method may have to be considered. Secondly, the reliability of the operator must be questioned, and whether other similar samples have been assayed at the same time. For example, if three samples of normal saline have been examined, and only one is wrong, then the possibility is that it is a production error. However, if two are only just within the limits, and the third just outside, it could possibly be an operator error. If it is considered that the operator is at fault, then the operator should be carefully taken through all the stages, checking that each has been correctly performed. The quality of the reagents used should be checked, remembering that certain reagents such as sodium nitrite solution need to be freshly prepared. If this does not yield the clue to the fault, then repeating the method with a known correct preparation could yield useful information on operator and instrument performance.

Sampling and interpretation of results

Sample size

Official recommendations for sample sizes for sterility testing (*European Pharmacopoeia* 1971) may be taken as useful guidelines for sampling for quantitative analysis. However, from a purely practical point of view one must consider the time involved in testing the recommended number of samples, and the cost in 'wastage' of final containers which are utilised for analysis. From a typical autoclave load of 250 containers, the recommended number for analysis is ten. If duplicate tests are carried out on each container to ensure accuracy of results, then for each batch of material, 20 separate procedures are to be performed. In addition to the containers removed for quantitative analysis, another ten will be required for sterility testing, five for particle counting. Samples for pyrogen testing may also be required, therefore at least 25 of the 250 containers, or 10% of the batch, is 'lost' in the testing procedure.

Conversely, for small batches of ampoules, the recommended sample size may not give sufficient material to perform adequate assays. For example, from a batch of 30 × 2 ml containers, the sample size is stated as 10% or four whichever is greater. In this case four ampoules would be chosen, but 8 ml of material may not be sufficient to carry out the necessary analyses.

The quality controller must ensure that adequate samples are taken to perform the necessary tests and give a representative picture of the total batch, without constituting a 'waste' of final product.

Sampling procedures

Ideally, samples should be chosen at random from any point in a batch. For a given autoclave load, this would entail choice of samples by random numbers or by numbering each bottle, writing the numbers on slips of paper, and drawing the required number of slips 'from a hat'. This is an extremely time-consuming process, and in busy hospital quality control departments a compromise may be necessary. We have found that when sampling for quantitative analysis from batches of sterile products, it is possible to choose effectively random samples by taking test bottles from those which have failed visual inspection for particles to which every container of sterilised material is subjected. These 'rejects' are almost certainly distributed at random throughout the autoclave load. This method has two advantages, the first being that since 'reject' material is used, there is no 'wastage' of bottles which may be passed into stock. The second is that this method can be suggested to other hospitals where material is to be sent to another department for analysis. The Guide to Good Pharmaceutical Manufacturing Practice (DHSS 1977) recommends that quality control staff should be involved in choosing samples for analysis to avoid any possible bias on the part of the production team, but where no quality controller is on the premises, the above sampling technique can be suggested to the production team who are choosing samples, and will result in a representative sample being examined.

Truly random sampling will give an overall picture of the *average* contents of ingredients in a batch. However, consider a case where a production fault has resulted in inadequate mixing of the batch. One would expect a higher concentration of ingredient at the bottom of the mixing vessel and a lower concentration at the top. Therefore the first container filled (from the top of the vessel) would on analysis be weaker than the last containers, filled from the bottom of the vessel. A randomly chosen sample of containers may or may not be chosen from the bottles in the centre of the filling process where the concentration of ingredient may fall within the required limits and the production fault could be missed. If containers were chosen from the beginning, middle and end of the process, the variation in concentration would be detected and the fault could be remedied. This 'stratified' method of sampling has been suggested by Caplen (1972) to give a more representative picture of the whole batch than truly random sampling. The stratified procedure recommended in the 'Orange Guide' for sterility testing, where samples from each level of the autoclave load are taken, should be used when examining dextrose or laevulose solutions for breakdown products (5-hydroxymethylfurfural) where slight changes in sterilising temperatures will result in different concentrations of breakdown products.

Borderline decisions

When results of an analysis indicate that the content of a sample falls on, or just outside, the stated lower or upper concentration limits, it is the duty of the quality controller to decide whether or not the material may be released, or must be discarded. Before making this decision, a number of points could be considered:

1.   The demand for the product. If the product is required urgently, it may not be possible to prepare another batch in time to meet the demand.

2.   Toxicity or potency of material. It is necessary to judge whether the variation in the amount present would constitute a hazard to the recipient or user of the product.

3.   Operator error. Certain analysts, particularly if inexperienced, when using titrimetric techniques tend to read either 'high' or 'low' because of individual variations in recognition of the indicator colours at the end point. Examination of past records of the operator's performance may show whether the result obtained is a true high or low reading, or a reflection of such personal variation.

4. Cost. The cost of the product, in terms of man hours spent in preparation, starting materials, containers and labels must be weighed against any hazards involved in use of a product whose content of ingredient is slightly outside accepted values. For instance, one might ask if the cost to the Health Service of the loss of a batch of Dextrose 5% Injection which was found to be 4.6% w/v Dextrose was justified when the difference in calorific value of the final product administered to the patient was calculated.

It may be possible as an emergency measure to 'salvage' small batches of material whose contents fall outside stated limits by relabelling the containers with the actual concentration found on analysis.

Spot checks

In larger pharmacies where a considerable variety of products is manufactured, it may not be possible for every item to receive an analytical test on a routine basis. While this is the ultimate ideal of the quality control department, we must realise that initially staff and equipment shortages will mean that a decision will have to be taken on which items receive final analysis and which do not.

It is good practice for the quality control department to carry out 'spot checks' on material not routinely analyzed. Spot checks are useful for a number of reasons.

1. To ensure that items not regularly analysed attain adequate standards.
2. To monitor purity of 'contract' non-proprietary products.
3. To check on standards of drug companies' products.
4. As an aid to monitoring storage conditions in laboratories and wards.
5. To check on manufacturing techniques of staff.

Analysis for particulate contamination

The occurrence and hazards of particulate contamination of parenteral fluids are well documented. Garvan and Gunner (1971) and Groves (1973a and b) have listed types of contaminants which may be found in parenteral solutions.

Instrumental techniques

Large-volume parenteral fluids must now conform to a standard for the number of particles of a given size (BP 1973). There are a number of instrumental methods which may be used to analyse particulate contamination.

Some of the most common techniques are listed below, together with practical advantages and disadvantages encountered with each method.

Measurement of changes in electrical resistance

The principle of this technique is that particles suspended in an electrolyte solution are passed through an aperture between two electrodes. Each particle displaces its own volume of electrolyte when passing through the aperture, and thus causes a small change of resistance between the electrodes. Changes in resistance may be detected and displayed on an oscilloscope and digital representation of numbers of particles counted may be obtained.

Advantages

1. The instruments are relatively cheap and readily available.
2. A variety of thresholds may be set from 1 micron upwards for measurement of particles above given sizes.
3. A good library of reference is available.
4. The large number of such instruments in use throughout the country may facilitate the setting-up of collaborative studies into particle counting techniques and manufacturing standards.

Disadvantages

1. The sampling orifice tube, being glass, is easily broken and is expensive to replace.
2. Regular calibration of the instrument with standard particles of known dimensions is recommended; this procedure is complicated and time consuming but is necessary as a routine check on performance and when new orifice tubes are installed.
3. Instrument performance is affected by interference from heavy electrical equipment in the vicinity necessitating the fitting of an electrical filter: mechanical vibration and draughts may also be the cause of variations in readings.
4. The solution being tested must be capable of carrying an electric current, or must be rendered polar by addition of a filtered electrolyte solution; the dilution procedure must be carried out with care to avoid introduction of extrinsic particulate contamination.
5. Particles are counted but not identified.
6. Aggregates of particles may be counted as one single particle: air bubbles will displace electrolyte and are thus counted as particles.
7. The test is destructive in that samples must be removed from their containers for testing.

Light scattering techniques

This technique utilises a laser beam which oscillates as it passes through the sample. The beam of light is deflected by particles entering its path. Each deflection is detected and counted and the particle count displayed digitally (Groves 1974).

Advantages

1. The analysis is non-destructive of sample, since the whole container is presented to the counter without being opened.
2. Very slight interference from electrical equipment is experienced.
3. The operation is extremely quick and simple to perform.
4. The sample is placed on an illuminated table which enables visual checking and counting procedures to be carried out simultaneously.
5. The sample does not require to be polar.
6. There are no easily breakable components.
7. Volumes of 1 ml are counted with each operation.

Disadvantages

1. Particles are counted but not identified.
2. Aggregates of particles will be counted as one single particle, air bubbles will be counted as particles.
3. The instrument is expensive.
4. Results are read from a three-figure display, thus the instrument is of limited value where high levels of contamination (>1000 particles/ml) are involved.
5. Flaws in the walls of the containers will cause errors in readings.

Microscopic methods

The technique, in its simplest form, involves filtering of the contents of the sample bottle through a membrane filter, which is usually gridded to facilitate counting, drying of the filter in ultraclean conditions and examination of the filter with a microscope using incident light. A further refinement may be adopted by 'clearing' the filter, that is collapsing the membrane structure using an organic solvent, thus leaving only the contaminants which may be examined with transmitted light. The apparatus required for this technique is fairly inexpensive. This method has been described in great detail for analysis of particulate contamination (Millipore Corporation 1967).

Advantages

1. The apparatus required is inexpensive.

2. The whole bottle is sampled and not just a portion as with the other techniques.

3. Particles are both identified and counted.

4. The filter can be kept as a permanent record.

Disadvantages

1. Great care must be taken in preparing samples to prevent extraneous contamination.

2. The procedure must be standardised to give meaningful results.

3. The method is more time consuming than those mentioned above.

More sophisticated microscopic techniques involving scanning microscopes with television cameras and computers are now available for particulate analysis. These instruments have been developed mainly for powder technologists and metallurgists, but can be adapted for use by the pharmaceutical analyst, and indeed some pharmaceutical manufacturing companies are utilising this technique. The sample is treated basically in the same manner as for 'manual' microscopic examination. The filter is fitted to a microscope stage and the membrane is scanned by a television camera which displays an image of the field being scanned. Different features of the contaminants may be selected by means of a discriminating unit, and a computer and printout facility is used to count particles and present results of particle size, area, or any other feature required. For identifying a source of particulate contamination, a microscopic method is required. While the sophisticated computer systems could find many uses in research departments and are of great interests, the 'manual' microscopic technique provides an acceptable method of identification of particles. This method can be used for troubleshooting to locate sources of contamination, both in parenteral fluids and in production environments (Millipore Corporation 1970).

There is a need for multicentre studies to standardise methods of sampling and to compare performances of different types of instrument.

It must be emphasised that, no matter how sophisticated or accurate is the method of analysis of contamination, there can be no substitute for adequate control of the production process or for good manufacturing technique.

Sterility and pyrogen testing

Sterility and pyrogen testing are fields in which, until recently, the pharmacist has played little part, being content to allow the bacteriologist to perform sterility tests, and to send samples for pyrogen testing to other laboratories.

One disadvantage of the sterility testing method in use in most laboratories is that only samples of each bottle and not whole contents are incubated. The

European Pharmacopoeia recommends a membrane filtration technique which involves sampling of the whole container. The technique involves drawing the cóntents of the sample bottle through a membrane filter and incubating the filter in a suitable medium. The operation is carried out under strict aseptic conditions. The procedure requires great care in operation to eliminate environmental contamination and must be carried out by well-trained, conscientious staff. The method gives more meaningful results than those obtained with the 'sampling' technique.

A final 'sterility test' can only be carried out on a limited number of containers chosen at random. The problem is, as with choosing samples for particulate analysis, to choose a number which will give a representative picture of the batch and at the same time is economical in terms of loss of final product. It must be understood that final sterility testing should only be considered as an adjunct to total production control. Other indicators of sterility must also be used, for example chemical or biological indicators placed in bottles in each autoclave load and electronic recorders for temperature control incorporated into sterilisation cycles.

None of those controls can guarantee sterility of the whole batch, but can only give information on the efficiency of the manufacturing process. Once again, as with all types of quality control, there is no substitute for good manufacturing practice.

The official pyrogen test which is carried out using rabbits is extremely expensive and has the disadvantage that in many cases the nature of the product being tested is such that the material itself produces a pyrogenic reaction *in vivo*.

Other types of *in vitro* pyrogen testing have been suggested. These cannot be considered as alternatives to the official method but may prove useful as inline controls and for testing starting materials.

Benfante and Labarre (1969) suggested a method for pyrogen testing of parenteral products based on culturing of Millipore filters. Cooper *et al* (1972) showed that a cell lysate prepared from amoebocytes of *Limulus polyphemus* (the horseshoe crab) is a sensitive and rapid test for the presence of bacterial endotoxin. The sample is treated with the reagent and incubated at 37°C for about 1 hour. The presence of a firm gel after incubation indicates the presence of an endotoxin. However, this technique is not always reliable and may give false results.

From a practical point of view, it must be borne in mind that if sterility and pyrogen testing procedures are to be carried out by the hospital quality control department, a separate laboratory area will be required for this purpose, with facilities for incubation of samples and subsequent destruction of any organisms.

STAFF AND STAFF TRAINING

Staffing requirements

From a review by Furber *et al* (1974), it would appear that inefficient use is being made of resources in quality control laboratories to ensure that hospital departments operate to the standards required by the *Guide to Good Pharmaceutical Manufacturing Practice* (DHSS 1977).

Adequate numbers of specially trained staff are necessary for the efficient operation of a quality control department.

The head of the quality control department should be fully conversant with all methods of pharmaceutical analysis, and should strive to keep up to date with new developments in this field. While a further degree, or special training, in analytical methods is useful, it is not essential. There are many advantages in having a pharmacist, as opposed to an analyst, as the head of the department, since the pharmacist's catholic training in the fields of pharmaceutical manufacture, engineering, microbiology and chemistry will enable him to understand production problems involved in other units within the pharmacy. The quality controller should have the ability not only to carry out his own research but also to direct the work of other members of staff. An ability to supervise and train staff is essential, as is the art of communicating with other workers in the service.

Technicians employed in a quality control department should ideally have a special training in analytical methods and be familiar with operation of instruments, possibly to ONC or HNC level. Pharmacy technicians who show an interest in analytical duties should be accommodated provided they receive suitable training.

Preregistration students have a special place in the quality control department. Their recent training enables them to operate instruments without further supervision and their enthusiasm and knowledge may be utilised in the performance of short projects of interest to the department.

Education

All staff employed in quality control, no matter at what level, will require further education. A training policy should be laid down by the quality controllers and education pharmacists.

Graduate and preregistration pharmacists may require only refresher courses and some practical experience, while technicians, according to their level of knowledge, may require more in-depth education. Pharmacy technicians' study courses at present offer only basic teaching in analysis and it may be necessary, if pharmacy technicians are to be employed in the quality control department, to present a course of lectures on basic chemistry, instrumentation and analytical techniques. The quality controller must therefore be aware of teaching aids which are available to enable him to instruct staff at all levels.

All staff must be made aware of their individual responsibilities to their colleagues and employers and/or employees under the recommendations of the Health and Safety at Work etc. Act 1974.

All pharmacists and preregistration students should be given the opportunity to work in a quality control department, if only for a limited time. A rota system could be employed to allow all staff an equal opportunity in this field. Individual research by staff should be encouraged, provided their work is useful to the department. Regular staff meetings and in-service training programmes should be instigated. All personnel should be encouraged to report on their own research and make suggestions about improvements in working techniques.

Instruction Manuals

Written instructions on use of instruments, analytical techniques and safety precautions are essential for the efficient operation of any department. The quality controller should ensure that standard techniques are used in all laboratories under his control and should prepare instruction manuals in collaboration with other quality control staff.

One of the obvious disadvantages of official monographs is that no reasons are given for any procedure which is carried out during an assay. This is surely a dangerous practice, since staff learn to follow the instructions by rote without any real understanding of the functions involved. The provision of instruction manuals with explanation of each step of a procedure will prove an invaluable aid in the training of staff. Essential information on safety precautions for use of dangerous chemicals and expensive instruments could be included, and a short section on theory of analytical techniques would provide the basis for a useful handbook which would allow staff to carry out simple quality control procedures without the need for constant supervision.

SPECIAL DUTIES

Troubleshooting

An efficient quality control department will soon become the logical recipient of 'problems' which arise in other parts of the pharmacy and in hospital departments. Many different types of problem may be encountered, and the quality controller should be prepared to deal with them as well as his resources permit. If their complexity puts them outside his scope, he should be aware of other establishments where such work may be handled.

Some examples of the types of problem which may be encountered are discussed:

Identification

The identification of unknown tablets has become easier with the increase in popularity of coded tablets; nevertheless there are still cases where the analyst is presented with an unmarked white tablet for identification. If there are no clues as to the identity and only a limited amount of sample is available normal qualitative tests are of little value and the investigator must turn to more advanced techniques, for example ultraviolet or infra-red spectroscopy, or chromatography. A procedure manual for handling unknown materials should be developed and a library of UV and IR spectra obtained from unknown tablets and capsules compiled for future reference.

Formulation

The task of formulating new dosage forms or non-official preparations which are requested by clinicians falls to the pharmacist. The quality controller should be involved not only in the final stages in analysis of the product, but throughout its development, giving advice on matters which may affect stability and quality of the formulation. It is possible with fairly simple inexpensive equipment to carry out 'accelerated storage' studies to provide useful data on shelf-life and storage conditions.

Analysis

Apart from routine analyses and development problems discussed earlier, there may be cases where analysis of a sample is requested if concentration of ingredient is in doubt or an adverse reaction is suspected. It may be that another quality control department requires some further testing of, or a 'second opinion' on, a product. Staff must be trained to handle such one-off analyses confidently and efficiently.

Manufacturing and production

The locating of faults in a manufacturing process, and advising on manufacturing techniques are possible duties for the quality controller. He may also be required to test equipment to be used in manufacture and advise on its suitability.

Investigation of suspect material

It can happen that pharmaceutical products are returned to the pharmacy, suspected of having adverse effects on patients.

The investigation of such suspect material is a form of trouble-shooting which deserves special mention, since it affords an excellent opportunity for a collaborative effort between the pharmacist and other hospital staff.

An Adverse Reaction Policy would be of great assistance in the control of reactions to intravenous fluids and in detection of incompatibilities. Such a policy document could provide advice for nursing and medical staff on what steps to take if a product is suspected of causing a reaction, and could name members of staff, for example the bacteriologist, quality controller and ward pharmacist, who should be notified in this event. Suspect material can be tested for bacteriological contamination (if an i.v. fluid is involved, tests should also be carried out on administration sets, needles etc.); samples should be sent for analysis to the quality control department, and the results of the tests relayed by the information pharmacist to the appropriate parties. This should provide a rapid feedback of information to medical and nursing staff and product manufacturers.

FUTURE OF QUALITY CONTROL

Pharmacokinetics and bioavailability studies carried out by analytical pharmacists will enable the quality control department to contribute to the production of more stable, efficient and safe hospital-manufactured medicines.

As pharmacists move further into the clinical field, the quality controller must become concerned not only with the quality of medicines administered to patients, but also with the total quality of care received by patients during hospitalisation. Thus the quality control pharmacist has a part to play in the role of monitoring of blood levels of drugs, in collaboration with his colleagues of the biochemistry and toxicology teams.

REFERENCES

ANALAR STANDARDS (1967) *Analar Standards for Laboratory Chemicals.* 6th edn, p. 510. Analar Standards, London.
BECKETT A. H. & STENLAKE J. B. (1976) *Practical Pharmaceutical Chemistry.* Part I, 3rd edn, pp. 99–134. Athlone Press, London.
BENFARTE P. & LABARNE J. (1969) *Drug Intelligence and Clinical Pharmacy* **3,** 286.
CAPLEN R. H. (1972) *A Practical Approach to Quality Control.* Business Books, London.
CLARKE E. G. C. (1969) *Isolation and Identification of Drugs in Pharmaceuticals, Body Fluids and Post-Mortem Material.* Pharmaceutical Press, London.
COLES J. & TREDREE R. L. (1972) *Pharmaceutical Journal* **209,** 194.
COOPER J. S., HOCHSTEIN H. O. & SELIGMAN E. B. (1972) *Bulletin of the Parenteral Drug Association* **26** (4), 153.
DEPARTMENT OF HEALTH AND SOCIAL SECURITY (1970) *Report of the Working Party on the Hospital Pharmaceutical Service.* The Noel Hall Report. HMSO, London.

DEPARTMENT OF HEALTH AND SOCIAL SECURITY (1977) *Guide to Good Pharmaceutical Manufacturing Practice*. HMSO, London.

EUROPEAN PHARMACEUTICAL SOCIETY (1971) *European Pharmacopoeia*. Council of Europe, Maisonneuve, S.A. France.

FURBER T. H., STEANE M. A. & BOOTH T. G. (1974) *Journal of Hospital Pharmacy* **32** (6), 104.

GARRATT D. C. (1968) *The Quantitative Analysis of Drugs*, 3rd edn. Chapman & Hall, London.

GARVAN J. M. & GUNNER B. W. (1971) *British Journal of Clinical Practice* **25,** 119.

GREENWOOD N. D. & GUPPY I. W. (1974) *The Analyst* **99,** 313.

GROVES M. J. (1973a) *Pharmaceutical Journal* **210,** 185.

GROVES M. J. (1973b) *Parenteral Products. The Preparation and Quality Control of Products for Injection*. Heinemann, London.

GROVES M. J. (1974) *Pharmaceutical Journal* **213,** 581.

HUMMEL R. & KAUFMAN D. (1972) *Analytical Chemistry* **44,** 535R.

FURTHER READING

BETHRIDGE D. & HULLAM H. E. (1972) *Modern Analytical Methods*. Chemical Society, London.

CHATTEN L. G. (ed.) (1969) *Pharmaceutical Chemistry*. Vols. 1 and 2. Marcel Dekker, New York.

COOPER M. S. (1972) *Quality Control in the Pharmaceutical Industry*. Vol. 1. Academic Press, New York.

PATTISON J. B. (1973) *A programmed introduction to gas–liquid chromatography*. Heyen, London.

WILLARD L., MERRITT L. & DEAN L. (1965) *Instrumental Methods of Analysis*. Van Nostrand, London.

WILLIAMS D. H. & FLEMING J. (1973) *Spectroscopic Methods in Organic Chemistry*. McGraw-Hill, New York.

Reference books

HASKMI H. (1973) *Assay of Vitamins in Pharmaceutical Preparations*. John Wright, Bristol.

The Merck Index. 8th edn. Merck, Rahway, New Jersey.

WEAST R. C. (1977) *Handbook of Chemistry and Physics*. 57th edn. CRC Press, Cleveland, Ohio.

9

Development of analytical methods

A. L. GLENN

GLOSSARY

The present author has coined several special terms and has also employed certain other terms which, although well used in the literature, may not be understood by all readers.

Baseline method (or correction). A spectrophotometric assay which minimises the effect of irrelevant absorption by means of a calculation involving $E(1 \text{ cm})$ at three or more wavelengths (BPC 1973; Donbrow 1967).

Compensation method. A spectrophotometric assay which minimises the effect of irrelevant absorption by including, in the reference cell, a suitable concentration of the compound (X) undergoing assay. A balance point occurs when reference and sample cells contain the same concentration of X, in which case the observed spectrum is entirely due to irrelevant absorption and shows none of the features of compound X (Beaven *et al* 1961).

Feasible method. A rough and ready process which seems to work (see p. 242).

One-off assay. An assay which meets the short-term need of a special investigation and may never be used again.

Primary optimisation. See p. 257.

Proven method. A well-designed and thoroughly tested process (see p. 270).

Relative molarity. The molarity of a constituent, divided by the molarity of the major constituent in the preparation.

Relative parts/10^6. Parts per million of a constituent, divided by the parts per million of the major constituent in the preparation.

Secondary optimisation. See p. 270.

Working method. A well-designed process which can be used with reasonable confidence (see p. 257).

ΔE Method. A spectrophotometric assay which minimises the effect of irrelevant absorption by use of a difference (ΔE) between two forms of the compound undergoing assay (BPC 1973, p. 663; Donbrow 1967).

INTRODUCTION

This chapter is aimed at the recent graduate, who has emerged from an academic course with a fair knowledge of analytical techniques but with no experience of applications. An ability to modify official methods and to develop new assays and tests is of obvious importance to hospital pharmacists who are concerned with the control of quality. Such concern often refers to preparations which are just a little different from their official equivalents but, even with official preparations, there may be good local reasons for replacing an official method by an alternative method of 'equivalent accuracy'. In these circumstances, a recent graduate may suffer a mildly traumatic experience, on discovering that pharmaceutical analysis is no longer just a matter of following the official monograph (or class schedule) but often requires some original thought, coupled with an ability to reach decisions and generally stand on one's own scientific feet. What was once a bore, may then become a fascinating occupation!

In designing an assay or test for a pharmaceutical preparation, we take the relevant sections of an academic course and cement them together with a few general principles and a large measure of common sense. Among the relevant sections the following can be included:

1. The theory, scope and limitations of analytical techniques in common use.
2. Practical experience of analysis.
3. Relationships between 'analytical' properties (e.g. spectra) and molecular structure.
4. Practical knowledge of pharmaceutical preparations, as may be acquired from practical pharmaceutics.
5. Statistics, which is the true foundation of quality control.

To such knowledge, we must add a general background, which includes the whole of pharmaceutical chemistry and large parts of pharmaceutics and pharmacognosy. All such knowledge is, of course, assumed in this chapter, which is mainly concerned with a few general principles and a measure of common sense, so necessary to a correct orientation of the relevant knowledge.

The following discussion refers to the design of a manual assay of the nominal constituents of a preparation. Although, with the passage of time, such assays represent a decreasing part of the range of assays and tests, which apply to particular examples, the design of items like tests of identity, assays of toxic impurities and estimates of biological availability is amenable to the same general principles. The same does not however apply to the automated assays, which are rapidly gaining ground in the pharmaceutical industry and which demand a substantially different approach to the problem of design. Nevertheless, even after allowing for the rapid changes which currently affect hospital pharmacy, the manual assay seems likely to dominate the scene for some years to come.

Available facilities

The design of an assay is often affected to a marked extent by local facilities. In the absence of a good level of knowledge and experience on the part of both analysts and technicians there is much to be said for the simplicity of 'classical wet methods' while, in the matter of equipment, no hospital laboratory can hope to provide the large range of techniques mentioned in Table 9.1, which affords a broad overview of the techniques of pharmaceutical analysis.

When choosing a technique, we need to consider a number of characteristics such as cost, specificity, precision and sensitivity, indicated by the codes (C4, D1, P2, S3) in Table 9.1 and given as a very rough guide (there are many exceptions).

Table 9.1 Techniques which are relevant to pharmaceutical analysis

Titration (with indicator) [C1, D1, P3, S1]
Potentiometric titration [C2, D2, P3, S1]
Gravimetric analysis [C1, D1, P3, S1]
Solvent extraction [C1, D1, P2, S1]
Melting point, specific gravity etc. [C1, D1, S1]
Optical rotation [C2, D1, P2, S1]
Refractive index [C2, D1, P3, S1]
Absorptiometry (visible) [C2, D1, P2, S2]
Turbidimetry [C2, D1, P2, S3]
Visible spectrophotometry [C2, D2, P3, S2]
UV spectrophotometry [C3, D2, P3, S2]
Nephelometry [C2, D1, P2, S3]
Spectrofluorimetry [C3, D3, P2, S3]
Emission spectrography [C3, D3, P1, S3]
Flame photometry [C2, D2, P2, S2]
Atomic absorption spectrophotometry [C3, D3, P2, S2]
Infra-red spectrophotometry [C3, D3, P1, S1]
Laser raman spectrophotometry [C4, D3, P2, S1]
NMR spectroscopy (^{1}H and ^{13}C) [C4, D3, P2, S1]
Optical rotatory dispersion [C4, D2, P2, S1]

Table 9.1—contd   Techniques which are relevant to pharmaceutical analysis

Circular dichroism [C3, D1, P2, S1]
X-ray fluorescence [C4, D2, P3, S2]
Photoelectron spectroscopy [C4, D3, S3]
Mass spectrometry [C4, D3, P1, S3]
Gas chromatography/mass spectrometry [C4, D3, S3]
Gas chromatography [C3, D2, P1, S2]
High pressure liquid chromatography [C3, S2, P2, S2]
Column chromatography [C1, D1, S1]
Thin-layer chromatography [C1, D1, S2]
Paper chromatography [C1, D1, S2]
Paper electrophoresis [C2, D1, S2]
Conductimetry [C2, D1, P2, S1]
Coulometry [C3, D1, P3, S3]
DC polarography [C2, D2, P2, S2]
Amperometric titration [C1, D1, P2, S1]
AC polarography [C3, D2, P2, S2]
Cathode-ray polarography [C3, D2, P1, S3]
Pulse polarography [C4, D2, P2, S3]
Membrane electrodes (including glass) [C2, D1, P1, S2]
Thermometric titration [C2, D1, P2, S1]
Thermogravimetry [C3, D1]
Differential thermal analysis (DTA) [C3, D2, P1, S1]
Differential scanning calorimetry (DSC) [C4, D2, P1, S1]
Radioisotope dilution [C3, D2, P2, S2]
Radioimmunoassay [C3, D3, P1, S3]
Neutron activation analysis [C4, D3, P1, S3]

Although comprehensive, the above list is by no means exhaustive. A number of techniques (e.g. X-ray fluorescence) are of great value in providing answers to a limited number of problems which defy the more conventional techniques (e.g. UV spectrophotometry). In order to provide a rough impression of cost, specificity, precision and sensitivity, comments on each technique are coded as follows:

C1, trivial cost (e.g. titration with indicator)
C2, low cost (e.g. pH meter)
C3, medium cost (e.g. UV/visible spectrophotometer)
C4, high cost (e.g. gas chromatography/mass spectrometry)
D1, low specificity (e.g. titration with indicator)
D2, medium specificity (e.g. UV/visible spectrophotometry)
D3, high specificity (e.g. infrared spectrophotometry)
P1, low precision in the measurement of concentration* (e.g. infra-red spectrophotometry)
P2, medium precision in the measurement of concentration* (e.g. polarography)
P3, high precision in the measurement of concentration* (e.g. UV/visible spectrophotometry)
S1, low sensitivity (e.g. infra-red spectrophotometry)
S2, medium sensitivity (e.g. UV/visible spectrophotometry)
S3, high sensitivity (e.g. spectrofluorimetry)

* In a few cases (e.g. differential thermal analysis), 'concentration' refers to the concentration of an element or compound in a solid sample.

Specificity

Although Aspirin Tablets, which contain 10% more aspirin than the upper BP limit, are unlikely to harm a patient, an accidental substitution of strychnine (for aspirin) is certain to kill. Hence, of the various characteristics of an assay (or test) for a given compound, specificity is by far the most important.

If we regard specificity as an ability to distinguish one given compound for all other compounds, we are immediately concerned with distributions of the kind shown in Figs. 9.1 and 9.2. Thus, in Fig. 9.1, we show the distribution of λmax, obtained when a large number of drugs and related substances are measured in acid solution. Bearing in mind that:

1. Sixty-eight per cent of the compounds show absorption peaks between 245 nm and 285 nm;
2. Only a small proportion show peaks above 350 nm;

It is not too difficult to see that a measurement of λmax in acid solution is rather more efficient in identifying a drug with a peak of 360 nm than in identifying a drug with a peak at 260 nm. In other words, the specificity of the test, 'λmax in acid solution' is strongly influenced by the *value* of λmax.

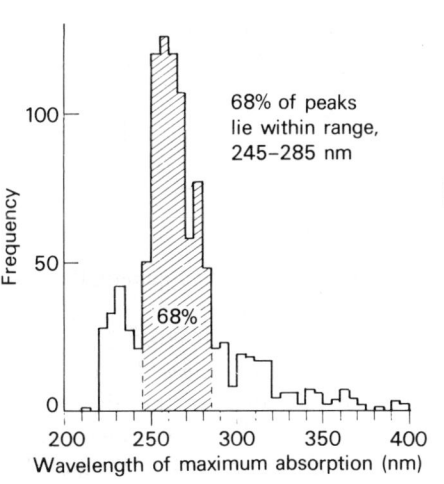

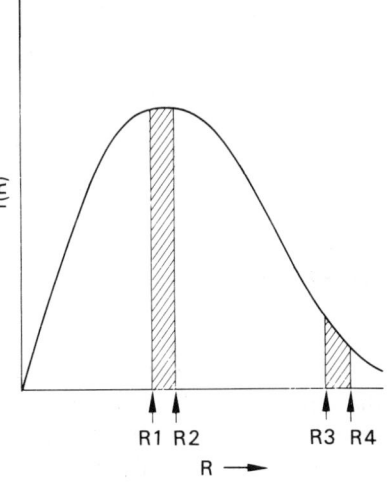

Fig. 9.1 Distribution of λmax among compounds which absorb in the UV (under acid conditions) and are listed by Clark (1969, 1975).

Fig. 9.2 Possible distribution of results (R) for a given quantitative test of identity. f(R) is the frequency of results whose values fall between R and R + δR.

The above discussion is further developed by Fig. 9.2, which shows the distribution of results (R), which might emerge if a given quantitative test of identity (e.g. melting point) were applied to all compounds, known and unknown. All quantitative tests are subject to error and, at the end of a test, all we can ever claim is that the true result lies somewhere between lower and upper limits, for example, R1 and R2 in Fig. 9.2. Hence, in performing the test, we have identified a *group* of compounds, which possess values of *R* between R1 and R2, and only on very rare occasions will the 'group' contain just one compound. Moreover, the probability that the test will give a result between R1 and R2 may be calculated from a ratio of areas, namely, the shaded area (between R1 and R2) divided by the area beneath the whole curve. On this basis, the probability of a result between R3 and R4 is a good deal less than the probability of a result between R1 and R2—thereby demonstrating, once again, that the probability of a result is affected by its magnitude.

In the light of the above discussion, *the specificity of a quantitative test for the identity of a given compound is inversely related to the probability that the test will give*

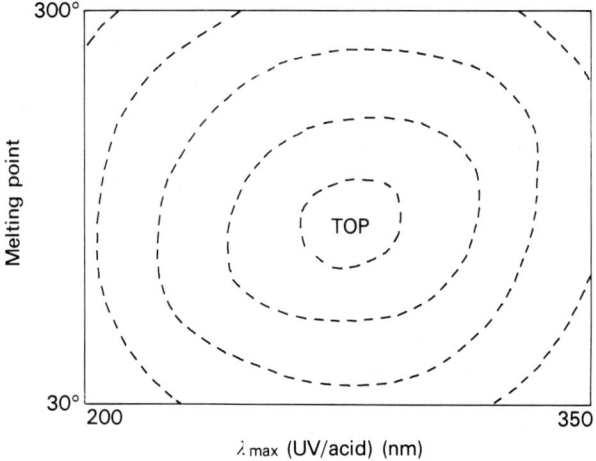

Fig. 9.3 Possible bivariate distribution for a combination of two quantitative tests of identity.

a result within the appropriate limits, when applied to all known compounds (and where the 'appropriate limits', e.g. 250–252 nm, are decided by the given compound). The specificity of such a test is also affected by its accuracy, which determines the interval between the lower and upper limits (e.g. R1 and R2) in Fig. 9.2. The more accurate the test, the smaller the interval and, hence, the probability that the test will 'give a result within the appropriate limits, when applied to all known compounds'.

If we combine two quantitative tests of identity, the frequencies of the various combinations of results are represented by a bivariate distribution (Fig. 9.3) in place of the univariate distributions of Figs. 9.1 and 9.2. Moreover, in Fig. 9.3, we use contour lines to represent the (three-dimensional) bivariate distribution in just the same way as we represent a hill on an ordinary contour map, the heights in Fig. 9.3 being proportional to the frequencies of various combinations of results. The top of the hill corresponds with a melting point of about 165° and a λmax of about 270 nm, which combination of results would occur more frequently than any other combination, if the two tests were applied to all compounds, known and unknown.

The specificity of a combination of two quantitative tests of identity usually exceeds the specificity of either individual test alone and, in most cases, the combination causes a large increase. In the bivariate distribution (Fig. 9.3), the coordinates of particular combinations of results extend over an area of the diagram while, in the relevant univariate distributions, the coordinates of individual results are confined to a line, namely, the abscissa scale in each case. Hence, by combining two tests, we increase the space available for coordinates and, thereby, decrease the probability of a clash between any two combinations of results.

Combinations of three or more quantitative tests of identity are associated with multivariate distributions (which cannot be represented in a space of three dimensions) and also with greater specificity, as one might expect. Combinations of tests are also subject to the same rules in regard to accuracy and values of results, as apply to individual tests. The specificity of a combination of tests is enhanced by:

1. An increase in the accuracy of the tests.
2. A decrease in the frequency of the combination of results.

For example, the specificity is smaller for those (frequent) combinations, which contribute to the top of the hill in Fig. 9.3, than for those (less frequent) combinations which contribute to the 'low-lying regions'.

Having dealt with quantitative tests of identity, we now consider the specificity of assays in terms of a simple example, which shows that a measurement of concentration may be rather non-specific—even though it involves a method (e.g. UV spectrophotometry) which is reasonably specific when used as a quantitative test of identity. In a nutshell: whenever we assay compound X in a pharmaceutical preparation, there is a remote possibility that we may obtain a reasonable result, even though the preparation contains some other compound (Y) in place of X. Thus, 2% of compound Y might give the same result as 1% of compound X and, thereby, obscure a serious mistake in manufacture. Moreover, as may be seen from Fig. 9.4, the process, 'measure $E(1 \text{ cm})$ at 250 nm' has a much lower specificity than the process, 'check that a maximum occurs at 250 nm', even though the same technique is involved in the two processes. If, as in Fig. 9.4, the assay is subject to limits of 90–110% of the nominal concentration, there are many other absorbing compounds which, at suitable concentrations, would give a result within the required limits. Such compounds are, in fact, far more numerous than those which exhibit maxima in the vicinity of 250 nm.

Bearing in mind that 90% of all drugs absorb in the range, 200–300 nm, a UV spectrophotometric assay is almost certainly less specific than a titration with alkali to a phenolphthalein end point—unless it is also accompanied by the observation of a maximum within specified limits (this being a stronger requirement than the rather vague, 'at a maximum at about *x* nm', found in the official compendia). The same does not, however, apply to assays which measure less common properties, such as fluorescence or polarographic reduction. For example, a spectrofluorimetric assay is fairly specific, even in the absence of an observation of maxima.

Despite important omissions, the above discussion should clarify the meaning of 'specificity', used elsewhere in the chapter. It also emphasises the fact

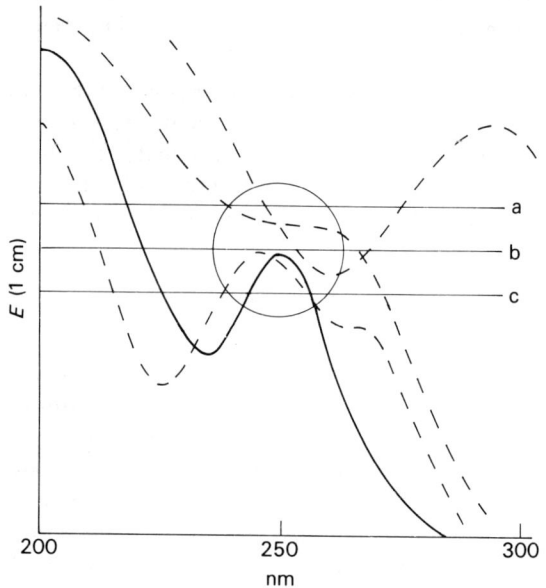

Fig. 9.4   When combined with official limits (90–110%), the process, 'measure $E(1 \text{ cm})$ at 250 nm' will, not only accept the right drug (solid line) at the right concentration, but will also accept a very large number of wrong drugs (broken lines) at other concentrations. (a) upper limit (110% nominal); (b) nominal concentration; (c) lower limit (90% nominal).

that, in a given situation, the specificity depends upon a collection of methods and standards (as occur in an official monograph), rather than upon individual tests and assays. The specificity will, therefore, suffer if a given test of identity is excluded from the collection or, otherwise, ignored at the time of execution. In this context, however, we are using 'test of identity' in a rather broad sense and would include any assay or test (e.g. weight per ml) which may help to distinguish the relevant compound from all other compounds. Although important in their own right, assays and tests which refer to impurities within the relevant compound, rarely contribute to the specificity of a collection of methods and standards.

Table 9.2 Lack of specificity of official monographs, revealed by a sample of hydrocortisone acetate

	BP (1958)	USP XVI	Sample
Specific rotation	+157–167°	+158–165°	+159.1°
Loss on drying	≯1%	≯1%	0.02%
Sulphated ash	≯0.1%	'Negligible'	0.02%
Melting point	About 220°	216–222°	218.4°
Assay (UV)	96–104%	nil	101.3%
Related foreign steroids	nil	'Complied'	
Tetrazolium assay	nil	nil	90.5%

The number of assays and tests, which we include in a given collection, is always limited by economics and, by adding a further test, we sometimes receive a shock, as in the case of a sample (Table 9.2) which passed all assays and tests in two pharmacopoeial monographs but gave a very low result (90.5%) when subjected to an additional assay using tetrazolium blue.

Of those assays and tests, which contribute a measure of specificity, a minority refer to entire molecules while the majority refer to parts of molecules. For example, in Fig. 9.5, various parts of the chloramphenicol molecule are encircled and keyed to the relevant tests, thereby emphasising that some tests (melting point, IR spectrum and mass spectrum) refer to the whole molecule, while others refer to parts of molecules, such as the '*p*-nitrobenzyl' part, which determines the UV spectrum. Hence, when considering the specificity of a test, the analyst should always identify that part of the molecule, which generates the result, and then assess the therapeutic relevance of the part in question.

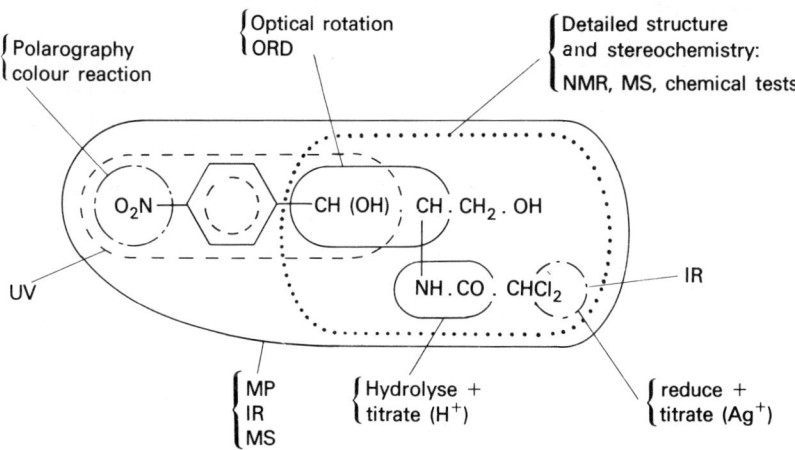

Fig. 9.5 Most assays and tests refer to a given part of a molecule (chloramphenicol in this example), while a minority refer to the whole molecule.

Separation of constituents

All assays involve an estimate of the quantity of material, contained in a given quantity of sample, but not all assays involve a separation. Moreover, an estimate of quantity may either be non-specific (e.g. the weight of a precipitate) or specific to some degree (e.g. the $E(1\ cm)$ at a given wavelength) and, on this basis, we can recognise three classes of assay:

1. A specific method for estimating quantity without separation (e.g. the assay of chloramphenicol in Chloramphenicol Eyedrops BPC).
2. A separation followed by a non-specific method for estimating quantity (e.g. the assay of quinine dihydrochloride in Quinine Dihydrochloride Injection BP).
3. A separation followed by a specific method for estimating quantity (e.g. the assay of vitamin A in cod-liver oil).

Of those separations which are most relevant to pharmaceutical analysis, we may comment as follows:

Solvent extraction

Still the most common form of separation, although frequently laborious and a major source of error in some assays. Nevertheless, by virtue of good correlations between partition coefficients and ratios of solubilities, the design of a solvent extraction is often predictable from the armchair and so there is much to be said for a solvent extraction in the case of a 'one-off' assay, which demands some form of separation.

GLC and HPLC

Both methods combine a process of separation with an estimate of quantity, which is often low in specificity (e.g. estimates of quantity provided by a flame ionisation detector (but see p. 261). Moreover, the separation, itself, may be less specific than some analysts appear to think.

GLC and HPLC are compact and 'fully instrumental' techniques which demand less analytical ability than other techniques of chromatography. Nevertheless, in common with the latter, the design of an assay, involving GLC or HPLC, is difficult to predict from the armchair and usually demands a considerable amount of 'suck it and see' in regard to solvent system, stationary phase, flow rate, temperature, etc.

Other chromatographic techniques

Column chromatography (e.g. on alumina or alginic acid) constitutes the main technique in this category, other techniques like quantitative TLC and paper chromatography affording a much lower standard of precision in most cases.

In providing what amounts to a further test of identity (e.g. 'the compound is more soluble in chloroform, than in water at pH 4'), a process of separation will always contribute to the specificity of an assay.

Methods for estimating quantity, unlike separations, are either predictable with high probability (e.g. titrations) or are well documented (e.g. IR) and so the design of a working method may entail rather more experimental work, if a separation is included. Moreover, with the exception of GLC and HPLC, a separation not only increases the labour of assay, but also demands a high standard of analytical ability. In these circumstances, separations are best included as necessities, rather than 'optional extras'.

STAGES IN THE DESIGN OF AN ASSAY OR TEST

While each assay (or analytical test) poses its own peculiar problems in the matter of design, there is much to be said for the general scheme, given in Fig. 9.6. Cogitation forms a major part of the entire process and is important in all stages, including a clear statement of the problem, which should occur at the outset. How far we proceed with the scheme in Fig. 9.6 depends on circumstances.

In Fig. 9.6, the design of an assay is divided into three stages, of which stage 1 combines a good deal of thought with a certain amount of 'quick and dirty' experimental work and leads to a feasible method or, in other words, a rough and ready process which seems to work. Whenever we are involved in 'troubleshooting', we are usually concerned with major errors, in which case, we rarely proceed beyond stage 1 in the case of any 'one-off' assay which we need to develop.

In Stage 2, we develop the feasible method into a working method, largely on the basis of refined experimental work, guided by a set of theoretical principles which are grouped under the heading, primary optimisation (see p. 257). A working method is a well-designed process which can be used with reasonable confidence.

If the assay is to receive frequent use by several analysts and by several laboratories over a long period of time, we ought to proceed with stage 3 and subject our working method to a process of secondary optimisation (see p. 270), thereby arriving at a proven method or, in other words, a well-designed and thoroughly tested process.

Specification of the method requires careful thought at the end of stages 2 and 3 since, apart from the specification, there is no other channel of communication between designer and analyst. By means of a good specification, the analyst becomes aware of all essential features of the designer's superior knowledge of the process.

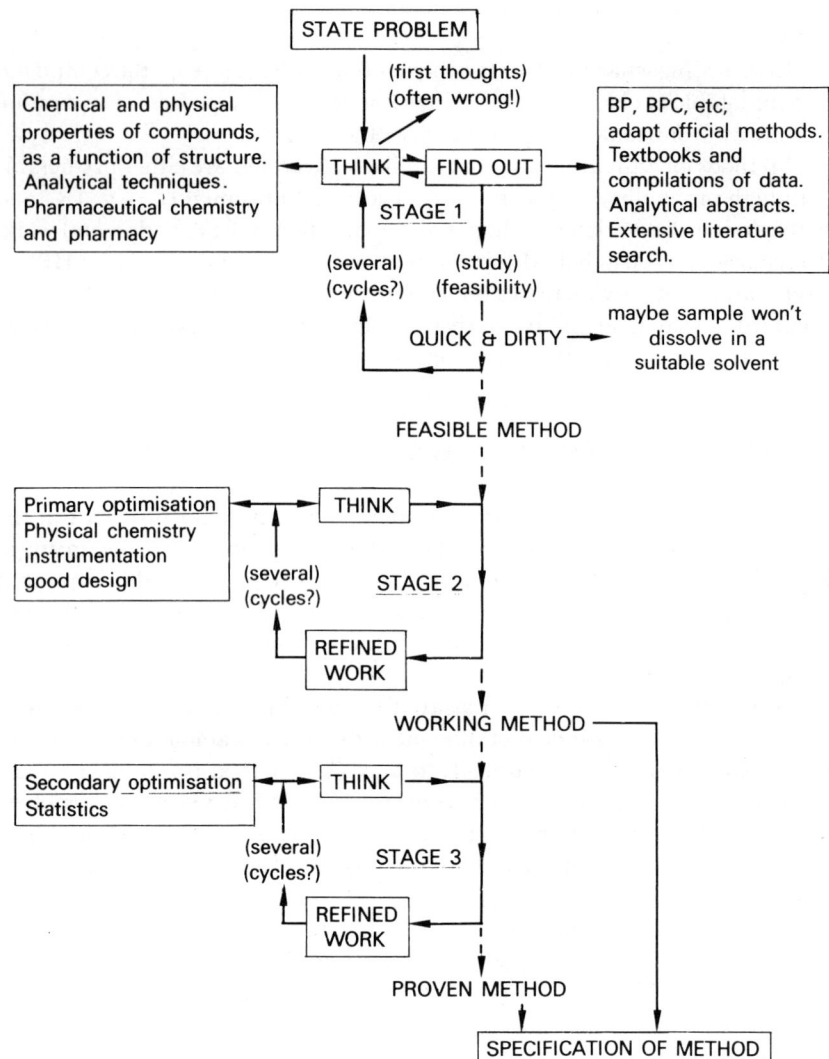

Fig. 9.6   Stages in the development of an assay or test.

In Fig. 9.6, 'quick and dirty' refers to those qualitative and semiquantitative experiments which afford a quick indication of feasibility and which often anticipate a repetition under refined conditions, involving good standards of analytical technique. Although there is a place for quick and dirty work in all stages of development, the greatest need arises in stage 1, which sometimes demands a rapid assessment of several ideas, spawned from the armchair.

Sound judgements concerning the roles of quick and dirty, and refined work are rather important if the design is to proceed with a minimum of frustration. Although refined work is usually wasteful in establishing the feasibility of a process, a quick and dirty approach may be so quick and so dirty that misleading results emerge, thereby discrediting a genuinely good idea or, otherwise, frustrating later refined work.

The rest of the chapter is mainly concerned with the development of feasible and working methods.

Statement of problem

When listing the constituents, which we intend to control, we must often restrict our attention to the active constituent(s) and, thereby, ignore the rest of the preparation. We may also take note of any special requirements in regard to limits of content, bearing in mind that the standard deviation of assay must not exceed a small fraction (e.g. one-tenth) of the difference between upper and lower limits.

For an assay to exert an effective control over manufacture, the errors of assay must always be less than the errors of manufacture. But, such errors are rarely known at the time of stating the problem and, in these circumstances, one can only rely upon primary optimisation (see p. 257) as a means of decreasing the errors of assay as far as possible.

In the absence of a special requirement, limits of content are best fixed in the light of experience of the first ten batches, two replicate assays being performed on each batch. In a subsequent analysis of variance, one can then estimate the variances, Va and Vm, where Va denotes the variance of assay and Vm denotes the variance of manufacture. On this basis, one can establish the following limits of content:

$$\text{lower limit} \approx c_n - 3.25s \text{ and upper limit} \approx c_n + 3.25s$$

where c_n is the nominal (i.e. midrange) concentration, 3.25 is student's t for 9 degrees of freedom and $P=0.01$ and

$$s = \sqrt{Va + Vm}$$

Having chosen t at the level of probability, $P=0.01$, the above limits are likely to fail about 1% of all batches, which are manufactured with the same amount of care as the first ten batches (used to establish the limits). Although the above limits will, therefore, fail a small proportion of good batches, wider limits would accept a larger proportion of batches which have not received the usual amount of care during manufacture.

In establishing limits, which are relevant to good manufacture, we must obviously ensure that the same condition applies to all batches which affect the calculation of s.

First thoughts on a feasible method

In developing a feasible method (see p. 239), cogitation, references to the literature and quick and dirty experimental work need to proceed, hand in hand, from the very outset of stage 1. Nature is apt to thumb her nose at the products of the armchair and the sooner we get down to the bench, the sooner we shall detect those unforeseen snags which can jeopardise the most promising of ideas. Although IR may have seemed 'the very thing' as we sat in our arm-chair, we may be due for a nasty jolt on discovering that our sample is too insoluble in any of the usual solvents to provide a suitably intense peak, when run at an acceptable pathlength.

Our approach to the literature is coloured by two considerations. In the first place, properties like spectra, pK, optical rotation, solubility, etc. are often more accessible by direct observation than by reference to a library. Samples of the compounds to be assayed are part of the birthright of a pharmaceutical analyst and, when we need the spectrum of a compound, the library is often an inefficient source of information by comparison with our own spectrophoto-meter, which can produce a spectrum in a few minutes under the conditions which relate to our own investigation and which may not apply to any of the spectra, we may eventually cull from the library. Such rapid acquisitions are, of course, assisted by the abridged information contained in well known laboratory handbooks and we must not forget that with some techniques (e.g. atomic absorption), the heuristic approach may prove both inefficient and misleading.

With regard to the second consideration, the design of a satisfactory assay is unlikely to cause a hospital pharmacist to breach the frontiers of analytical chemistry and, in these circumstances, the official compendia (which contain the fruits of a great deal of analytical development) are a valuable source of information. Assays of the BP, BPC and USP are therefore of considerable interest in stage 1 of the development and, after stating the problem, we shall immediately wish to know how the official handbooks cope with related prob-lems.

For further information, we may turn to general analytical textbooks, com-pilations of data and then to analytical abstracts, which usually constitute a rapid source of information by comparison with the, more comprehensive, chemical abstracts. For the latest information we shall need to scan the latest journals (*Journal of Pharmacy and Pharmacology, The Analyst, Anal. Chim. Acta, Analytical Chemistry, Journal of Pharmaceutical Sciences*).

With regard to cogitation, we can say that knowledge in the head is alto-gether more useful than knowledge in the library and, to that end, we shall need to pluck the fruits of our undergraduate courses (see p. 230), in which respect, the following items are extremely relevant:

1.   Analytical methods (both classical and instrumental) together with their scope and limitations.

2. Chemical and physical properties of elements and compounds together with the relationship between properties and molecular structure.

When designing an assay for formulation, it is a good plan to convert all concentrations to molarities (macromolecules excepted) or parts 10^6, where relevant. The molarities of minor constituents should be supplemented by relative molarities, which facilitate comparisons with the molarity of a given major constituent. It is also advisable to list the elements present (other than C, H and O) and to write down the structures of organic constituents.

A list of standard questions, on the following lines may be useful.

Major or minor constituent?

Assays of major constituents are apt to require less sensitive methods than assays of minor constituents, while the assay of a minor constituent is usually affected by, apparently inert, major constituents, which may change the properties (e.g. solubility, UV spectrum, etc.) of the minor constituents, or increase the blank result of a number of methods.

Need for a process of separation?

A decision, 'to separate or not to separate' (see p. 238) exerts a major effect upon the design of an assay.

Importance of specificity?

The need for a 'specific assay' (see p. 233) is often greater in the case of an active constituent than in the case of a formulation additive. Moreover, the need for a specific assay may diminish if the assay is combined with a test for identity.

Nature of preparation?

If the preparation is a solid (e.g. capsules containing a powder), is it soluble in one or more common solvents? If the preparation is a semisolid, is it miscible with one or more common solvents? If the preparation is a liquid, is it aqueous or non-aqueous? If the preparation is a non-aqueous liquid, is it miscible with one or more common solvents?

Presence of additives?

The preparation may contain additives (e.g. bactericides in the case of injections, issued in multidose containers) not mentioned in the formula or liable to change throughout a sequence of batches, prepared over a period of time.

Choice of method?

You have no option but to choose a technique, which is available to you and, apart from considerations (e.g. specificity) mentioned elsewhere, you also need simplicity, reliability, speed and cheapness.

Availability of sample?

The sample may be:

1.   Plentiful and cheap.
2.   Plentiful but expensive.
3.   Restricted, because it comes from a small, one-off batch.
4.   Restricted with 'legal overtones', because a patient suffered ill effects. In these circumstances, we may reject a method (e.g. titration) merely because it consumes too much sample.

A sample which is 'restricted with legal overtones' demands a considerable amount of experience, and sometimes access to less available methods, like mass spectrometry. This kind of sample must be carefully protected from contamination and only subjected to those tests, which are very likely to succeed, each test being validated in a previous trial on other material (usually a good batch of the same preparation). By validating each test, we avoid the unnecessary wastage of a crucial sample in tests which fail, on account of faulty reagents, analytical ignorance or a lack of success in scaling down a conventional test (with the object of conserving sample). Complete consumption of the sample in one or more inept tests is a 'mortal sin' and, at the end of our work, sufficient sample should remain for subsequent investigation by another laboratory.

How many samples per week and for how many years?

The effort we expend in developing a working method, or in transforming a working method into a proven method (see p. 270), will naturally depend upon the frequency of assay.

First thoughts on feasible methods for a number of preparations

Several examples will now be used to illustrate those thoughts, which are specific to the problem, in contrast to the more general thoughts, listed on p. 242. It must, however, be emphasised that first thoughts are often misleading and that some of the 'genuine first thoughts', listed below, have already failed at the bench.

Although the following preparations are official, we approach them as new problems and largely ignore the official compendia (which would normally receive our very careful attention at the start of any real problem). Moreover, in the first example, we check through the list of techniques (see p. 231) item by item.

Lignocaine injection

Table 9.3   Constituents of Lignocaine Injection

Constituent	Quantity	Molarity
Lignocaine Hydrochloride	2 g	0.07
Water for Injection	100 ml	

Among the list of techniques (see p. 231), there are a considerable number of possibilities:

1.   *Titrimetry?*

    a.   *Estimate Cl⁻ with AgNO₃?*

Volhard's method would be possible, although the easier Mohr's method is contraindicated by low pH. Potentiometric titration using a silver electrode would be quicker than Volhard's method, although silver electrodes are known for quixotic behaviour. Nevertheless, Cl^- is a non-active moiety and, hence, a rather unspecific indication of the lignocaine content. NaCl may also be present to adjust the isotonicity, in which case, $[Cl^-]$ will exceed the concentration of lignocaine.

    b.   *Extract the base and titrate with sulphuric acid?*

An assay, which refers to the tertiary aliphatic amino group, is not very specific. On making alkaline and extracting with ether, phenolic bactericides should stay in the aqueous phase and should not, therefore, interfere with the assay; the same applies to NaCl, if present.

By using a back titration, there is no need to extract the base as a solid. The assay is tedious, although used in the BP.

2.   *Gravimetry?*

    a.   *Estimate Cl⁻ as AgCl?*

Uneconomic and subject to the criticisms in **1a**.

    b.   *Extract the base and weigh the residue?*

A tedious and non-specific method, although NaCl and phenolic bactericides should not interfere. By contributing further information as to identity, a melting point on the base would increase the specificity but, in this case, the melting point might be rather low.

3.   *Solvent extraction?*

Already covered in **1** and **2**.

4.   *Optical rotation?*

There is no asymmetric centre.

5.   *Refractive index?*

As a measure of concentration, refractive index is both insensitive and non-specific and, in this case, contraindicated by the low molarity and possibility of interference from bactericides.

6.   *Absorptiometry (visible)?*

Lignocaine is colourless but might form a suitable colour if we hydrolysed the amide linkage and then diazotised and coupled the resultant primary aromatic amine with *N*-(1-naphthyl)ethylenediamine.

7.   *Spectrophotometry (visible)?*

Comments in **6** are also relevant here together with the observation that spectrophotometry is inherently superior to absorptiometry in the matter of specificity.

8.   *Spectrophotometry (UV)?*

By characterising the arylamido group, UV spectrophotometry would be fairly specific and would also provide a quick, precise and direct measurement of the concentration of lignocaine. Moreover, in the presence of a phenolic bactericide, we might combine UV spectrophotometry with the separation mentioned in **1b** although the assay would then be tedious and, in the hands of inexpert analysts, less reliable than the method suggested in **1b**.

9.   *Spectrofluorimetry?*

This molecule is not expected to fluoresce!

10.   *Flame photometry or atomic absorption spectrophotometry?*

No suitable elements are present (apart from Na which may have been added as NaCl).

11. *Spectrophotometry (IR)?*

IR spectrophotometry is rarely suitable for aqueous samples. We might, however, extract the base which could then be dried, weighed and subsequently identified by comparing the IR spectrum (of a thin film) with that of an authentic specimen of the free base. Such combination of an assay of low specificity with a highly specific test of identity might be used in a 'one-off' investigation, if we suspected a serious mistake in manufacture or were interested in the hydrolysis of the amide link. UV spectrophotometry could also be used in a similar way, particularly in the absence of a bactericide.

12. *Spectrophotometry (laser raman)?*

Irrelevant at the present time, although highly specific assay for drugs in aqueous solutions may have emerged from this technique by 1984.

13. *Nuclear magnetic resonance?*

Unsuitable for aqueous samples and it would, therefore, be necessary to transfer the base to D_2O by a modification of **1b**. NMR is often inferior to IR in the matter of specificity.

14. *Optical rotatory dispersion?*

There is no asymmetric centre.

15. *Photoelectron spectroscopy, mass spectrometry or GLC/mass spectrometry?*

Unsuitable for aqueous samples and none of these techniques would show much advantage over IR spectrophotometry in the kind of 'one-off' investigation, mentioned in **11**.

16. *Gas chromatography?*

A gas chromatograph, equipped with flame ionisation detectors, is not very suitable for an aqueous sample, which contains a small molarity of the volatile substance. We would, however, extract the base with chloroform and inject the extract, in which case, phenolic bactericides should not interfere and the assay would be fairly specific. (A successful assay, involving direct injection of the diluted sample, verifies an earlier comment that first thoughts are sometimes misleading!)

17. *High pressure liquid chromatography?*

The aliphatic amino group augers well for an efficient separation on an ion exchange column, while the aromatic chromophore would be 'seen' by a UV detector. There should be no difficulty in separating the lignocaine peak from a peak due to a phenolic bactericide.

18.   *Chromatography (other than GLC and HPLC)?*

Qualitative information on decomposition products might emerge from paper chromatography, thin-layer chromatography or paper electrophoresis.

19.   *Conductimetry?*

Use of conductimetric titration to estimate [Cl⁻] is subject to the objections, mentioned in **1a**.

20.   *Polarography (DC, CR or pulse)?*

A direct polarographic assay is not feasible, in the absence of an 'electroactive' group, although, if the amino group were to form a complex with Cu^{++}, an indirect assay might succeed.

21.   *Potentiometry using membrane electrodes?*

Only two membrane electrodes (i.e. those reversible to H^+ and Cl^-) are relevant to the present problem. The glass electrode would serve the needs of a potentiometric titration in **1b**, while a chloride (membrane) electrode would afford a direct indication of [Cl⁻]—but see criticisms in **1a**.

22.   *Thermal methods?*

Of the thermal methods given on p. 232, only thermometric titration could further the present problem and, to that end, a 'thermal end-point' might facilitate a direct titration with alkali (not, otherwise, possible by indicator or potentiometric end point). Nevertheless, in view of the small molarity, the result of a thermometric titration would not be very precise and, because it referred to the amino group, the assay would not be very specific.

Checking through a list, on the lines of the above discussion, is a useful exercise for a beginner and will help to stimulate the first thoughts, which are so necessary to the development of a feasible method. In the present case, there are many ways of obtaining a result, which is proportional to the concentration of Lignocaine Hydrochloride, and a number of techniques which are relevant to the 'one-off' investigations, required in troubleshooting. There is, of course, no point in using a sledge hammer to crack a walnut and techniques, like GLC/MS, will scarcely enter the thoughts of a more experienced analyst, when developing a method for the control of an injection solution. At the same time, however, a good analyst will always be aware of these more specialised techniques and of their possible relevance to problems which may eventually arise.

Conclusion

In the absence of a bactericide, there is much to be said for an assay involving UV spectrophotometry, which technique is available in most hospital control laboratories. By combining a determination of $E(1 \text{ cm})$ with an individual determination of λmax, the process would be fairly specific.

In the presence of a bactericide, UV spectrophotometry might still succeed on the basis of:

1. A 'two-substance analysis' preceded, if necessary, by partial extraction of the bactericide.
2. A quantitative separation of lignocaine by column chromatography.

Assay of bactericide (if present)

Table 9.4 lists the bactericides which may accompany Lignocaine.

Table 9.4

Bactericide	% w/v	Molarity
Phenol	0.5	0.053
Cresol	0.3	0.028
Chlorocresol	0.1 (a mixture)	0.007
Methyl paraben	0.2	0.013
Phenylmercuric nitrate	0.001	0.00003

As a matter of convenience, we would hope to assay the bactericide by the same technique as used for lignocaine and, in this respect, there are good prospects for UV spectrophotometry in the assay of all four phenolic bactericides, listed above. Although used in smaller molarities than lignocaine, the phenols may well contribute a large share of the total absorption at longer wavelengths, in view of the greater intensity of the phenol chromophore (by comparison with the amido-dimethyl-benzene chromophore of lignocaine) in the same part of the spectrum. Moreover, if a simple UV assay were to prove unsatisfactory, the ΔE-method might succeed in distinguishing a phenolic bactericide from lignocaine.

On grounds of low molarity, coupled with the low intensity of the benzene chromophore, phenylmercuric nitrate is not amenable to a UV spectrophotometric assay, its absorption being swamped by that due to lignocaine (and, by the same token, a UV assay of lignocaine would not be affected by phenylmercuric nitrate). Hence, if it were necessary to assay phenylmercuric nitrate in Lignocaine Injection, we would consider some other technique, such as polarography or atomic absorption spectrophotometry.

In divulging his first thoughts on the remaining four examples, the author omits many of the ideas, which may occur to a reader who checks through the list on p. 231. It is then possible to concentrate on those ideas which offer the greatest promise.

Chloramphenicol eye-drops

Table 9.5 Constituents of Chloramphenicol Eyedrops

Constituent	Quantity (g)	Molarity	Relative molarity
Boric acid	1.5	0.243	1.00
Chloramphenicol	0.5	0.015	0.062
Borax	0.3	0.008	0.033
Phenylmercuric nitrate	0.002	0.00003	0.00012
Purified water	to 100 ml		

Although the major constituent (boric acid) is unlikely to affect the first two proposed methods, it may well affect such calibration curves, as we may eventually establish.

Assay of chloramphenicol

On account of large differences in molarity and chromophoric intensity, the absorption of phenylmercuric nitrate (or acetate) will be swamped by the absorption of chloramphenicol and, since no other absorbing compounds are present, the chloramphenicol could be assayed by UV spectrophotometry.

Assay of phenylmercuric nitrate

UV spectrophotometry and polarography are both contraindicated, the response of phenylmercuric nitrate being swamped by the chloramphenicol response in both cases and, in these circumstances, we may resort to atomic absorption spectrophotometry.

Assay of boric acid and borax

Following the well-known method for mixtures of boric acid and borax, we could titrate (to methyl red) with sulphuric acid and then add glycerol, before titrating (to phenolphthalein) with sodium hydroxide, which process might well succeed in the presence of chloramphenicol and phenylmercuric nitrate (or acetate). On the other hand, the efficiency of a borax buffer is more easily assessed by an estimate of buffering power, on the following lines:

1. Measure the pH.
2. Add x ml of sodium hydroxide 0.5 N aq. to y ml of the eyedrops and remeasure the pH, both pH values being subject to narrow limits (e.g. correct pH ± 0.05).

By adopting the second alternative, we would save a significant amount of analytical labour but might run the risk of overlooking a mistake in manufacture, which increased the boric acid/borax concentrations by a factor of 10, while maintaining the correct ratio. A rogue sample might then pass our test and generate a complaint from the ward.

Intraperitoneal Dialysis Solution (Acetate)

Table 9.6 Constituents of Intraperitoneal Dialysis Solution (Acetate)

Constituents	Quantity (g)	Parts/10^6	Relative parts/10^6
Sodium chloride	5.56	2190 Na	1.00
Sodium acetate	4.76	805 Na	0.37
Calcium chloride	0.328	60 Ca	0.027
Magnesium chloride	0.152	18 Mg	0.0082
Sodium metabisulphite	0.15	36 Na (0.0008 molar)	0.016
Dextrose	17.0	1.7% w/v	
Water	to 1000 ml		

The presence of two major constituents (NaCl and NaAc) may tend to undermine our first thoughts about the minor constituents; for example, the assays of Ca and Mg may prove difficult in face of a large excess of Na. In these circumstances, the following thoughts are more tentative than usual.

Dextrose

Optical rotation (after mutarotation, catalysed by NH_4OH).

Sodium, Calcium, Magnesium

Atomic absorption spectrophotometry (using Na and Ca/Mg lamps) should afford quick assays of high specificity, while membrane electrodes (Na, Ca and Mg) could be used for the 'in-process' control of individual solutions of salts, before mixing.

Metabisulphite

Add excess iodine and titrate with sodium thiosulphate.

Chloride

A chloride (membrane) electrode might give results of sufficient accuracy but, if not, use Volhard's method.

Acetate

Potentiometric titration (with sulphuric acid 0.5 N aq.)

Methyl Salicylate Ointment

Table 9.7   Constituents of Methyl Salicylate Ointment

Constituent	Quantity (g)
Methyl salicylate	500 (0.0033 mol/g)
White Beeswax	250
Hydrous wool fat	250

Beeswax and wool fat are of little interest and only modest precision is required in the assay of methyl salicylate by one of the following methods:

UV spectrophotometry

Beeswax and wool fat are not very soluble in alcohol, in which case, we could melt the ointment in warm alcohol and hope to extract 99% of the methyl salicylate, which could then be assayed by UV spectrophotometry. Irrelevant absorption from the ointment base is unlikely to cause a serious error but, if it did, we could resort to a baseline correction.

IR spectrophotometry

Take up in chloroform and, if the solution is cloudy (on account of moisture from the hydrous wool fat), clarify with anhydrous sodium sulphate and so protect the rock salt windows. Place in a sample cell and apply the compensation method; methyl salicylate bands disappear when the concentration of methyl salicylate in the reference cell is equal to that in the sample cell.

   IR measurements on a thin film of ointment would afford a quick assessment of homogeneity, by using a ratio between the extinction of a prominent band in the spectrum of methyl salicylate and the extinction of a prominent band in the spectrum of the ointment base.

Gas chromatography

Take up in chloroform; add a known amount of standard (e.g. benzyl alcohol or methyl benzoate) and inject onto a suitable column; evaluate areas and refer to a calibration curve. The choice of a suitable standard, stationary phase and oven temperature may entail rather more experimental work that is required to develop the two methods above.

Dimethicone Cream

Table 9.8   Constituents of Dimethicone Cream

Constituent	Quantity (g)
Water	444
Liquid paraffin	400 (40% w/w)
Dimethicone 350	100 (10% w/w)
Cetostearyl alcohol	50 (0.0195 molar)
Cetrimide	5 (0.015 molar)
Chlorocresol	1 (0.007 molar)

Three points are immediately apparent:

1.   The two major constituents are insoluble in water and, hence, unlikely to affect the assays of the minor constituents.
2.   Liquid paraffin, Dimethicone and cetostearyl alcohol are characterless substances, which may be difficult to separate and will fail to respond to most of the techniques on p. 231.
3.   No assay can proceed until the emulsion has been cracked. On referring to official monographs, we find that all three oily constituents are soluble in ether, in which case, our first thoughts are as follows:

Separation of oily constituents from water-soluble constituents

In this kind of problem, a satisfactory process for cracking the emulsion is prerequisite to first thoughts on methods of assay and should, therefore, be settled by a quick and dirty evaluation at the very outset! The emulsion may crack under the influence of heat and by the addition of chemical reagents (solvents, strong acid, strong alkali and neutral salts). Nevertheless, by adding a large quantity of reagent, we may complicate the rest of the assay with an unwanted major constituent (e.g. sodium sulphate).

After cracking the emulsion, we would hope to retain the cetrimide and chlorocresol in the aqueous phase (after addition of alkali), while separating the oily constituents by extraction with ether.

Chlorocresol

Assay by UV spectrophotometry, making use of ΔE or baseline methods, in the event of a substantial irrelevant absorption.

Cetrimide

As an indication of the cetrimide concentration, a bromide assay would probably fail on account of low molarity and possible contamination with chloride, which would give high results. We may, therefore, prefer a titration with sodium lauryl sulphate (see official compendia).

Liquid paraffin, dimethicone and cetostearyl alcohol

An IR spectrum of the well-dried mixture of oily constituents should reveal:

1. An O-H band (about $3600\,cm^{-1}$) from cetostearyl alcohol.
2. A C-H band (about $3000\,cm^{-1}$) from liquid paraffin and cetostearyl alcohol.
3. An Si-O band (about $1250\,cm^{-1}$) from dimethicone, in which case, we could proceed as follows:

1. Determine the % w/w of oily constituents in a sample of the emulsion.
2. Use the compensation method to compare the mixture of oily constituents with a reference mixture, accurately prepared from the same batches of material, as were used to manufacture the cream. With a thin film of the extract in the sample cell and a thin film of the reference mixture in a micrometer (reference) cell, we would adjust the micrometer so as to minimise the number and intensities of the peaks in the difference spectrum. We would then compare the latter with a standard set of difference spectra, obtained from accurately prepared mixtures, which represented the maximum deviations, acceptable from good manufacture.

Tricks and dodges

Having tackled the above examples in terms of 'vertical' thought (e.g. 'the compound does not fluoresce and so we cannot use spectrofluorimetry'), we now emphasise the value of 'horizontal' thought in terms of a number of 'tricks and dodges', which may speed the development of a feasible method.

1. *A weak acid can sometimes be strengthened* by complexing (Fig. 9.7a) or by solvent extraction (Fig. 9.7b).
2. *A strong acid can be further strengthened* by complexing with a non-aqueous solvent.

$$HClO_4 + CH_3.COOH \rightleftharpoons ClO_4^- + CH_3.COOH_2^+$$
$$\text{(a stronger acid)}$$

3. By means of indirect determinations, we can extend the range of a technique to include compounds, which would not otherwise produce a response:

a. By quantitative liberation of a suitable reagent; for example, we can assay copper sulphate by titration with thiosulphate, even in the absence

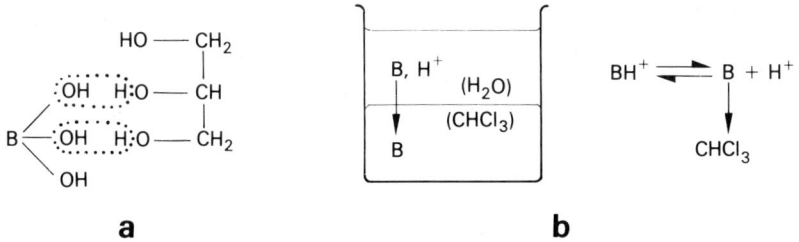

a   **b**

Fig. 9.7 (a) Addition of glycerol converts boric acid (pKa 9.14) to a stronger acid (glycerylboric acid, pKa 5.2); (b) a layer of chloroform extracts some of the base from the cation acid (BH^+) of a base (B), thereby liberating H^+ and causing an apparent increase in the strength of BH^+.

of a direct reaction between the two compounds (iodine acting as intermediate).

$$2CuSO_4 + 4KI \rightarrow Cu_2I_2 + I_2 + 2K_2SO_4$$

titrate with thiosulphate

b. By quantitative precipitation. For example, 'soluble aluminium' can be made insoluble and, hence, amenable to gravimetry.

$$Al_2(SO_4)_3 + 6H(\text{oxinate}) \rightarrow 2Al(\text{oxinate})_3 + 3H_2SO_4$$
(soluble)   (insoluble)

c. By quantitative solubilisation. For example, a 'non-electroactive' aminoacid can be assayed by polarography (by solubilising an insoluble cupric compound into a form which is reducible at the dropping mercury electrode).

$$Cu_2(OH)PO_4 + 4CH_3.CH.COOH \rightarrow$$
(insoluble) $\qquad\qquad |$
$$\qquad\qquad\qquad NH_2$$

$$2(CH_3.CH.COO)_2Cu + H_2O + H_3PO_4$$
$\quad | $
$\quad NH_2$

(soluble and reducible at the
dropping mercury electrode)

d. By quantitative development of colour (i.e. chromogenic reaction). We can assay a colourless compound by absorptionmetry or spectrophotometry. To produce a colour, the compound is either coupled to some other compound, which is already coloured (e.g. methylene blue in the assay of imipramine), or subjected to an extension of its chromophore (as in diazotising a primary aromatic amine and coupling to *N*-(1-naphthyl)ethylenediamine). Chromogenic reactions, which are used in quantitative analysis, have usually emerged from certain well-known colour tests of qualitative analysis and, in the absence of a chromogenic reagent which is already known to be suitable for quantitative analysis, we can only resort to a colour reaction of unknown suitability in that respect.

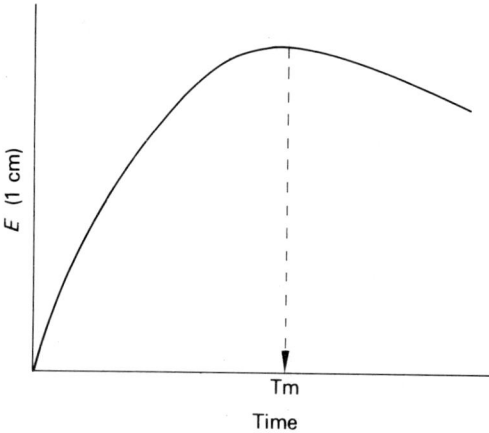

Fig. 9.8　Change of *E* (1 cm) with time in a typical chromogenic reaction. It is important to measure *E*(1 cm) at a definite time (Tm) after addition of reagent.

The chemistry of a chromogenic reaction is usually complicated and obscure. Stable colours are extremely rare (Fig. 9.8) and so *E*(1 cm) must be measured at the correct time, while some colours are extremely sensitive to small variations in temperature and in the composition of reagents.

e.　By quantitative modification of a compound's absorption spectrum (equivalent to a small change in 'colour', as in the Δ*E* method), we can sometimes distinguish the compound from other constituents of the mixture.

f.　By quantitative development of fluorescence. For example, by the action of concentrated sulphuric acid on some steroids. Fluorogenic reactions resemble the chromogenic variety in being complicated, obscure, unstable and sensitive to variations in reagents and temperature.

4.　Use of enzymes. For example, amylase will dissolve small quantities of starch, which would otherwise require filtration; enzyme electrodes enable a pH meter to determine an increasing number of organic compounds.

5.　Instrumental tricks. For example, the compensation method.

Primary optimisation

At the end of stage 1 (see p. 239), we arrive at a feasible method, which may achieve the status of a working method after 'primary optimisation' in stage 2. Primary optimisation involves a number of decisions, taken in the armchair, and a number of decisions, based upon refined laboratory work. These decisions may include such items as weight of sample, solvent, dilution factor, mode of dilution, pH, mode of extraction, requirements for complete extraction, time of heating, wavelength, pathlength, stationary phase, oven temperature, etc.

Physicochemical aspects

1. Avoid unstable conditions of assay. By varying a certain parameter (e.g. temperature), we may find a corresponding variation in the result of an assay (Fig. 9.9) and, in these circumstances, it is important to avoid those values of the parameter, which correspond with a slope in the graph; otherwise, small

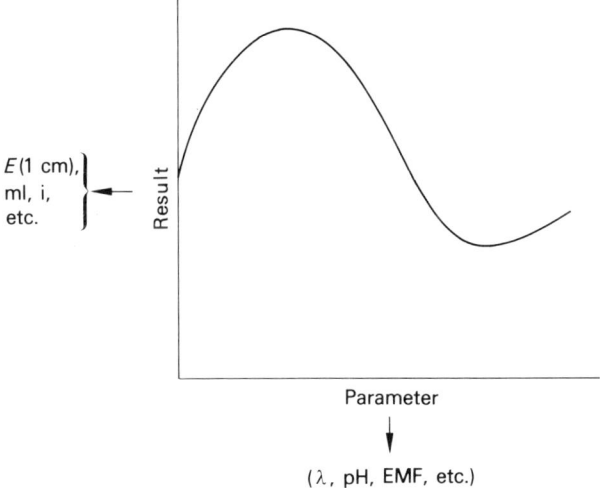

Fig. 9.9 Effect of parameters (e.g. λ, pH, EMF) upon the result of an assay. In choosing stable conditions for an assay, we must avoid those values of a parameter which correspond with a slope in the graph of result vs. parameter.

variations (in the parameter) will affect the result and lead to error. Hence, in developing a working method, we need to plot graphs (result vs. parameter) for all those parameters, which are likely to affect the result. For example, the graphs in Fig. 9.10 relate to an assay, in which the result is affected by wavelength, pH and time.

Fig. 9.10 refers to a compound which possesses a 'pH-sensitive auxochrome' and, hence, an absorption curve which shifts with pH. The compound also decomposes at the extremes of pH and, therefore, denies our use of one of these extremes as a means of stabilising the absorption curve. Moreover, if we decide to work at pH 5 and measure $E(1 \text{ cm})$ at λ_2, small errors in pH will produce large errors in $E(1 \text{ cm})$, in which case, we shall need to add a precise quantity of an accurately prepared buffer and, in these circumstances, we may well prefer to measure $E(1 \text{ cm})$ at the isosbestic point (λ_1) and to run the gauntlet of a gentle slope in the absorption curve and the consequent need for a careful setting of the wavelength. In this example, two of the parameters

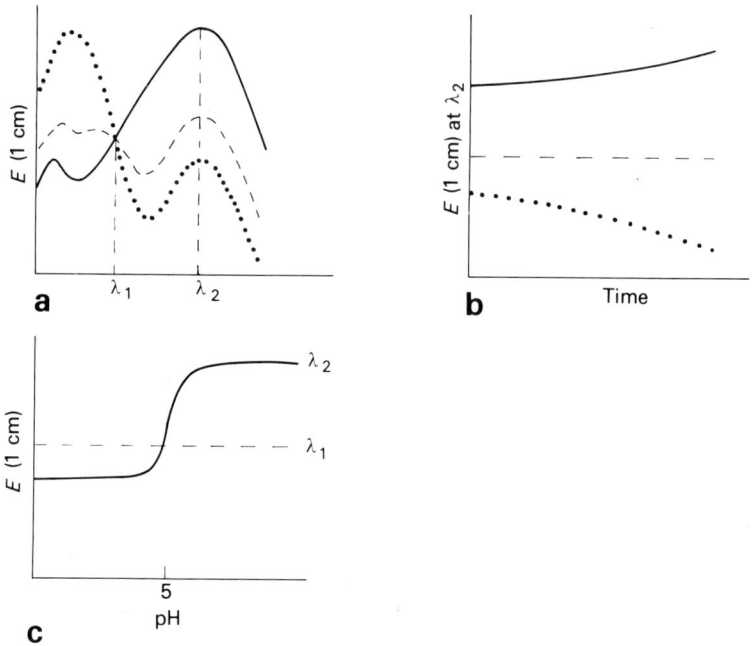

Fig. 9.10   Typical graphs of result vs. assay parameter. In (a) and (b) dotted line is pH 2, broken line is pH 5 and solid line is pH 11.

(i.e. pH and time) are in conflict while, in regard to the third parameter (wavelength), we are lucky to find a gentle slope at λ_1.

Although a certain parameter may affect the result of an assay, neither a maximum nor a minimum may occur on the graph (result vs. parameter) and we must then find conditions which minimise the slope. For example, in DC polarography, the limiting current is usually associated with a slope in the polarogram and, if the slope depends upon some parameter (e.g. pH in Fig. 9.11), we can sometimes find a value, which minimises the slope.

2. When assaying a minor constituent, allow for the influence of a major constituent. The assay of a minor constituent is often complicated by the presence of one or more major constituents, which may:

    a. Swamp the response of the minor constituent; the terms, 'major' and 'minor' referring to response, in this case. Thus, in some injections, the absorption of an active constituent (e.g. lignocaine) is swamped by the absorption of a bactericide (e.g. methyl paraben) and, on such occasions, we must either change to a different technique or remove the major constituent by means of a separation (which need not, necessarily, reach completion).

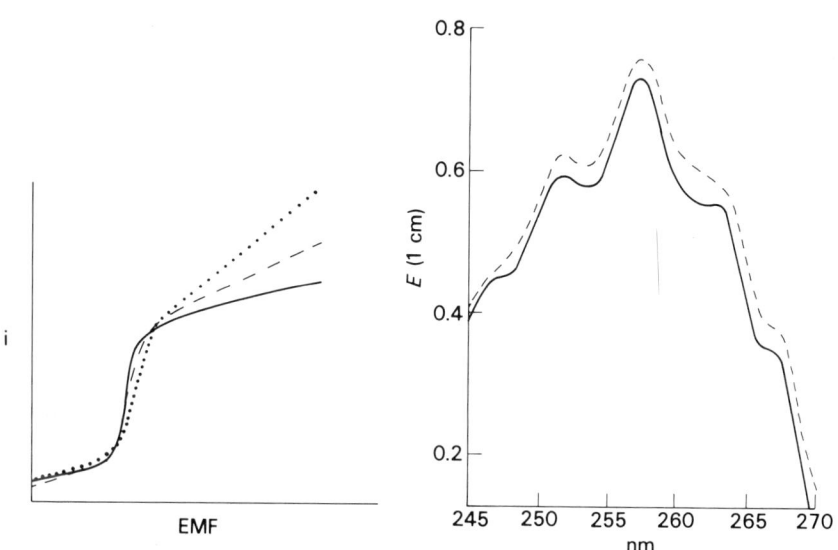

Fig. 9.11 (left) Effect of pH on the polarogram of chloramphenicol in citrate-phosphate buffer; the limiting current is associated with a minimum slope at pH 8. Dotted line, pH 4; broken line, pH 6; solid line, pH 8.
Fig. 9.12 (right) Effect of sodium chloride upon the absorption spectrum of benzyl alcohol. Solid line, spectra in water; broken line, in NaCl 3.8 M aq.

    b. Contribute impurities which affect the result. For example, sucrose in syrups contributes a substantial irrelevant absorption below 250 nm. Moreover, in making the necessary correction, we must remember that a blank determination may prove unsatisfactory on account of differences between batches of the major constituent, or even between different samples of one batch. In correcting for irrelevant absorption, a blank determination is often inferior to a baseline correction.
    c. Shift the calibration curve. For example, $E(1\%, 1\ cm)$ of an aromatic compound is affected by a large concentration of electrolyte (Fig. 9.12).

Moreover, in allowing for such an effect, we can only recalibrate in the presence of the major constituent(s) (at the concentration(s) specified in the preparation) and, to that end, an ordinary calibration curve is superior to the method of standard addition (see p. 268).

3. Minimise the effects of impurities. For example, in UV spectrophotometry, the use of a short pathlength (e.g. 1 mm) will reduce the effect of absorbing impurities in solvents while, by using a longer wavelength, we can often reduce the effects of absorbing impurities in both solvent and sample.

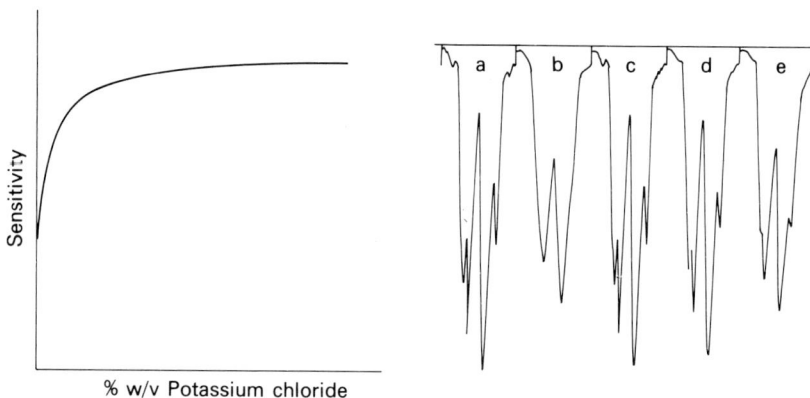

% w/v Potassium chloride

Fig. 9.13   (left) Effect of potassium on the assay of strontium, using a C_2H_2/N_2O flame. By filling the flame with electrons, the atoms of an alkali metal suppress the ionisation of strontium and, thereby, increase the sensitivity of assay. Traces of alkali metals, therefore, lead to variations in sensitivity, and hence to variable results, in which circumstances, the effect is carried to a limit by adding a large excess of the salt of an alkali metal.

Fig. 9.14   (right) Effect of resolution, gain and scan speed upon the spectrum of polystyrene (2700–$3300 cm^{-1}$). Resolution: normal throughout (apart from spectrum b, obtained at low resolution). Gain: normal throughout (apart from spectra d and e, obtained at low gain). Scan speed: low throughout (apart from spectra c and e, scanned at high speed).

In coping with impurities which lead to variable results (but not to a catastrophic fall in sensitivity), we can sometimes remove the variations by adding a large concentration of the offending impurities; in other words, 'if you can't beat them, join them'. Thus, in polarography, the limiting current is greatly affected by small concentrations of non-electroactive electrolytes and, by adding a large excess of supporting (i.e. non-electroactive) electrolyte, we carry the effect to a limit at which the limiting current is unaffected by further contamination with the same impurities. The same device is also used in atomic absorption spectrophotometry whenever the result is affected by traces of 'more easily ionisable' elements, like sodium and potassium. For example, when strontium is assayed in the nitrous oxide/acetylene flame (Fig. 9.13), we add a large excess of potassium chloride in order to remove the variations which would, otherwise, result from traces of sodium and potassium.

Instrumental aspects

Some knowledge of instrument physics is essential to the correct adjustment of instrumental parameters, this being an important part of primary optimisation. For example, the shapes of IR absorption peaks are strongly influenced by such instrumental parameters as gain, resolution and scan speed (Fig. 9.14). Within limits, most instruments can be stretched to meet unusual requirements.

The nature and adjustment of instrumentation may exert a marked effect upon the specificity of an assay. In general, the greater the resolution, the greater the specificity although, by increasing the resolution, we tend to lose precision and, hence, accuracy. Moreover, as the example in Fig. 9.14 will have shown, the resolution is an important parameter in IR spectrophotometry and, although we can vary the resolution of any one instrument, there is also a large difference between the resolutions obtainable from the various commercial instruments—so much so, that the spectrum, which emerges from a cheap IR spectrophotometer, is often a grossly distorted version of the spectrum which emerges from an expensive, research type, instrument. (Much, however, depends upon the sample examined and, in this respect, a cheap IR spectrophotometer is adequate for most pharmaceutical analysis.)

Similar comments apply to the specificities of GLC and HPLC, which are markedly affected by the choice and adjustment of several parameters. Moreover, in both techniques, the specificity is strongly affected by the choice of detector. Thus, for GLC, we can obtain detectors, which will only respond to those compounds which contain one particular element (e.g. P,N,S,F,Cl), and such detectors afford a large gain in specificity, by comparison with the specificity obtainable from the conventional, but virtually non-specific, flame ionisation detector.

Sensitivity is the one parameter common to all instruments and is defined as follows:

$$\text{sensitivity} = \frac{\delta \text{ (response)}}{\delta \text{ (concentration)}}$$

or, in other words, the slope of the calibration curve at any point. Sensitivity depends upon instrumental parameters such as wavelength, applied voltage, burner height, etc. For example, in UV spectrophotometry, a change from 10 mm to 1 mm pathlength will reduce the sensitivity by a factor of 10, while the very opposite occurs on changing from 10 mm to 100 mm. The sensitivity is also affected by the setting of an electrical 'sensitivity control' in most instruments.

Of the various parameters, which require adjustment, scanning speed (where relevant) and sensitivity are easily understood. It is rather obvious that, if a spectrum is scanned too fast, the trace will be distorted while, if the sensitivity is set too high, the pen (or meter needle) will be driven off the scale on any instrument. Nevertheless, most sensitivity controls involve a source of error which may fox a beginner who expects that, with a given sample, he will exactly double the reading by switching from 'X1' to 'X2'. Thus, in most instruments, the sensitivity control is composed of resistances, which may vary by $\pm 1\%$ of the true value, and in these circumstances, significant discrepancies between actual and nominal sensitivities are the rule, rather than the exception. Unless, we are sure that such discrepancies are negligible by comparison with the other errors of assay, we should obtain all results (involved in calibration and measurement) at one given sensitivity.

Although an assay can never be too specific, it may be too sensitive, as will inevitably occur when assaying a major constituent by means of a rather specific, but highly sensitive technique, like spectrofluorimetry and, unless we take steps to desensitise the technique, the sample will require excessive dilution. Moreover, in the case of spectrofluorimetry, the use of a markedly off-peak wavelength of excitation will afford a substantial drop in sensitivity, while preserving a linear relationship between fluorescence and concentration.

In order to further one's knowledge of instrumentation and keep abreast of the latest developments, it is a good idea to join the relevant 'national groups', which deal with particular branches of instrumental analysis, information on any of these groups being obtainable from the appropriate manufacturer. Some of these groups are affiliated to The Chemical Society, while others are accessible through the columns of *European Spectroscopy News*.

Minimisation of random error by good design

Analytical measurements are associated with two kinds of error, namely, 'random error' and 'bias or systematic error'. Random errors fluctuate in sign between replicates and arise from a lack of precision on the part of operator and equipment, while errors due to bias possess a definite sign, which does not fluctuate between replicates, and reflects one or more permanent deficiencies in apparatus and/or method. For example, when using a particular set of volumetric apparatus to replicate the assay of a given sample, the spread of results is assigned to random error, while any difference between the mean result' and the true result is assigned to bias and attributed to defects in apparatus and/or method. Thus, our 25 ml pipette may actually deliver 24.97 ml, on average, and the assay may tend to overestimate the true result by 0.62%.

In developing a working method, we can take reasonable account of random error but can do very little about bias. While random error is amenable to commonsense, bias is a quixotic error which is difficult to predict and is, necessarily, ignored in the present discussion. Any bias, associated with equipment, is best taken into account at the time an assay is performed and may involve the use of a reference standard together with a decision to keep some item(s) of equipment (e.g. a UV spectrophotometer) constant throughout the comparison of sample with reference standard.

In pharmaceutical analysis, relative errors are often more important than absolute errors and, in most assays, there is one source of error which overshadows all other sources and mainly determines the total error. Furthermore, if it were possible to identify the practical operation, which generated the largest error, we would focus our attention on the design of that one operation and ignore all other sources of error, until such time as we had reduced the largest error to something less than the 'next contender' in the hierarchy of errors.

Although a shrewd guess will sometimes identify the operation, which generates the largest error, the issue is often obscure and can only be settled by a suitable statistical approach at the stage of secondary optimisation. Hence, in developing a working method, it is advisable to adopt a 'blunderbuss approach' and design the assay in such a way that we minimise *all* sources of error, thereby attending to the largest source of error at some point in a design, which needs to take account of the following items:

Preparation of solutions

At our earliest opportunity in the development of a working method, we need to design a good scheme for preparing solutions; in other words, a scheme which avoids:

1. Imprecise steps (e.g. weighing 10 mg on a macrobalance, use of a 1 ml bulb pipette, etc.).
2. An unnecessary number of steps.
3. An inadequate quantity of solution at any stage (thus, 25 ml of solution is not enough to rinse and fill a 25 ml pipette!).
4. Wastage of expensive solvents.
5. Final readings which fall outside the optimum range of measurement.

In designing the scheme, we need to consider each step in turn and specify the conditions (e.g weight of sample) in such a way that no step is likely to generate a relative error in excess of 0.3%. For example, a weighing is subject to a more or less constant *absolute error* (x) and, if the weight of sample is less than $333x$, the relative error will exceed 0.3%. In the case of a macrobalance (i.e. a 'four place' balance), the weighings are subject to absolute errors of about 0.2 mg and so a '10 mg weighing' is apt to incur a relative error of

$$\frac{0.2}{10} \times 100 = 2\%$$

while a '100 mg weighing' is subject to a relative error of 0.2%. Hence, if we are to limit the relative error in accordance with the above target (0.3%), the weight of sample must not be less than 70 mg.

Deliveries from a burette are also subject to an absolute error ($\pm$0.03 ml, in the case of a 50 ml burette) and require the same approach as in weighing, while the very opposite applies to devices, like bulb pipettes and volumetric flasks, which are concerned with the measurement of fixed volumes and are so designed as to make the *relative error* (typically $\pm$0.05 to $\pm$0.2%) substantially independent of volume. To this end, the smaller pipettes and volumetric flasks are equipped with stems of smaller diameter than those employed for the larger vessels and, in these circumstances, a given displacement between meniscus and calibration mark generates much the same relative error throughout a considerable range of pipettes and flasks. Nevertheless, for reasons of mechanical strength and convenience, the smallest mumbers of a given class (e.g. a 3 ml volumetric flask) are apt to depart from the general rule and give rise to relative errors which are unusually large.

With such thoughts in mind, we now consider an example, namely, a scheme for preparing solutions for the assay of Zinc Sulphate Eyedrops by atomic absorption spectrophotometry. Moreover, to implement the calibration recommended on p. 267, we need the following four solutions:

Solution A. Diluted sample ($ZnSO_4,7H_2O$).
Solution B. Standard equivalent to *upper* limit (0.28% w/v).
Solution C. Standard equivalent to *midrange* (0.25% w/v).
Solution D. Standard equivalent to *lower* limit (0.22% w/v).

If the readings are to fall within the optimum range of measurement, the concentrations of all four solutions must fall within the range, 0.5–2.5 µg Zn/ ml, as achieved by the scheme shown in Fig. 9.15.

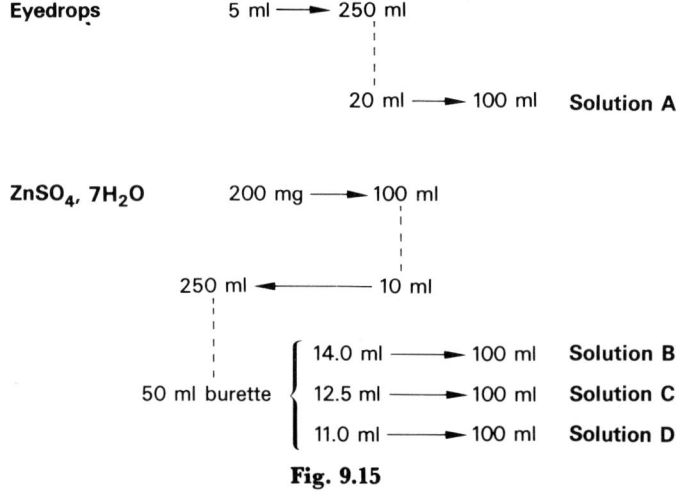

Fig. 9.15

Five ml of eyedrops are diluted to 250 ml and a 20 ml aliquot further diluted to 100 ml (solution A); 200 mg of zinc sulphate is dissolved in water and made to 100 ml; a 10 ml aliquot is diluted to 250 ml and the dilution used to fill a 50 ml burette, from which further aliquots (11.0, 12.5 and 14.0 ml) are successively diluted to 100 ml, in preparation of solutions B, C and D.

In designing such a scheme, we must usually exercise a measure of ingenuity and consider a number of possibilities before arriving at a good result. Thus, if the sample needs diluting by a factor of 200, we could use a 5 ml pipette and a litre flask (Table 9.9) when diluting with water, but not when diluting with an expensive solvent, in which case, we might well use an adjustable, high precision, semi-micropipette (set to 125 μl) and a 25 ml flask.

Table 9.9 Dilution factors obtainable from various combinations of pipettes and volumetric flasks

Flask or pipette	25 ml	50 ml	100 ml	250 ml	500 ml	1000 ml
5 ml	5	10	20	50	100	200
10 ml	2.5	5	10	25	50	100
20 ml	1.25	2.5	5	12.5	25	50
25 ml	—	2	4	10	20	40

Pipettes and volumetric flasks are, inevitably, restricted to a small number of sizes (Table 9.9) and so, in achieving the desired concentration, we must often rely upon some more flexible device (balance, burette or adjustable, high precision, semi-micropipette) at some stage in preparing a solution. Nevertheless, by cascading dilutions, pipettes and volumetric flasks are rather more flexible than Table 9.9 might suggest; for example, by cascading two dilutions, each involving a 10 ml pipette and a 25 ml flask, we can dilute by a factor of 6.25 overall.

Size of response

Most scales of measurement (Fig. 9.16) are subject to a more or less constant error, wherever the scale is read (e.g. the scales of a burette and a potentiometer recorder). The relative error is then infinite at the zero end of the scale and a minimum at 'full scale', which means that in many such cases, a well-designed method will produce a reading between 75 and 100% of full scale.

Exceptions arise in those spectrophotometric methods, wherein the concentration of an absorbing compound is proportional to the (negative) logarithm of the response, as opposed to the response (i.e. transmittance) itself. In these circumstances, one can argue from simple theoretical principles that the minimum relative error in concentration will occur at 37% of full scale (Fig. 9.17a).

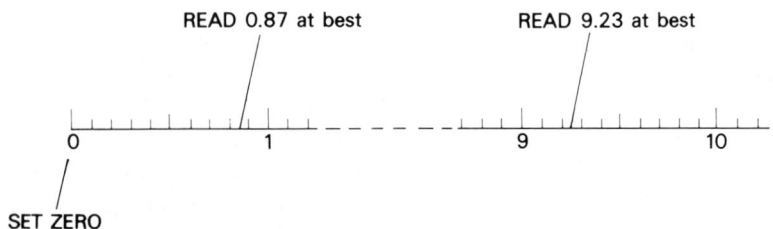

READ 0.87 at best   **READ 9.23 at best**

SET ZERO

Fig. 9.16 Any given measurement involves a relative error which depends upon (a) the absolute errors, entailed in adjusting the zero, in standardising the scale (where necessary) and in taking the reading, and (b) the size of the reading. The absolute errors are often independent of the reading and, in these circumstances, the larger the reading, the smaller the relative error. Hence, in the above example, we expect to read '9.23' with a smaller relative error than '0.87' and, apart from a few exceptions, the same kind of commonsense applies to most scales. The relative error can be further reduced by 'scale expansion' in those cases wherein electronic/mechanical noise is too small to be noticed on the unexpanded scale (otherwise, there is no virtue in scale expansion).

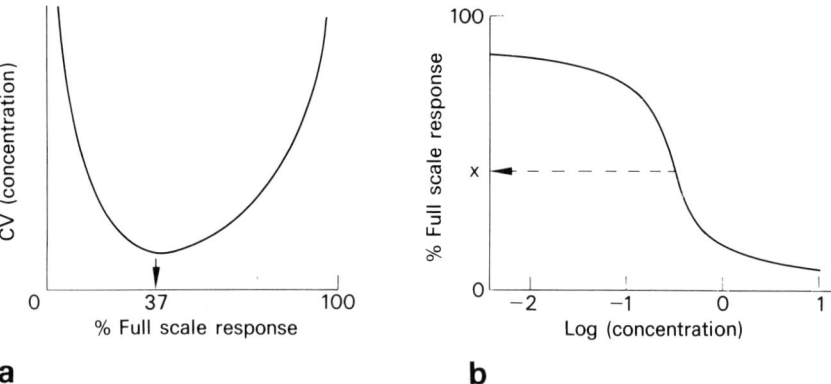

a   **b**

Fig. 9.17 (a) When concentration is proportional to the negative logarithm of the response, the relative error (i.e. coefficient of variation of concentration) is a minimum at 37% of the full scale response (equivalent to an extinction of about 0.43) according to simple theory. (b) In a Ringbom–Ayres plot, we estimate the condition for minimum relative error by noting the response (x) which corresponds with the steepest slope in the graph of % full scale response against log (concentration), thereby exploiting the fact that a given small distance (e.g. 0.1 mm) on any part of a logarithmic scale corresponds with the same relative error in the antilogarithm (i.e. concentration, in this case).

It is also possible to estimate the optimum response from a **Ringbom-Ayres** plot (Fig. 9.17b) and, thereby, allow for such deviations from simple theory, as may occur in practice.

Calibration

While gravimetric assays require no calibration, whatever, and volumetric assays require no more than a standardisation of titrant (against a primary standard), *all* instrumental assays require a calibration curve (i.e. graph of response vs. concentration). Hence, in developing a working method, a calibration curve is often essential and demands attention at an early stage.

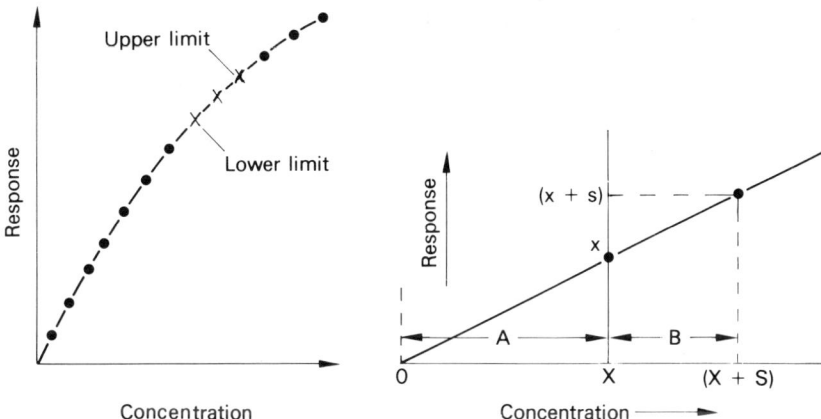

Fig. 9.18 (left) Calibration curve: the points (x), which span the prescribed limits, require frequent revision.

Fig. 9.19 (right) In the method of standard addition, we evaluate a concentration by noting the increase in response which accompanies a known increase in concentration. After measuring a response (x), produced by an unknown concentration (X) of a given compound, we add a known concentration (S) of the same compound before measuring a second response (x+s). The unknown concentration is then obtained by extrapolating a two-point graph to zero response, length 'A' being proportional to concentration X, and length 'B', to concentration S. Moreover, for an accurate extrapolation, B should be large by comparison with A and this requires a large standard addition (S) which will often cause an excessive change in the composition of the sample.

While the quality control of pharmaceutical preparations involves no more than a small segment of the calibration curve (Fig. 9.18), it is always advisable to evaluate the linearity of the entire curve by plotting points for a number of concentrations, equally spaced between zero concentration and a suitable upper limit. Once its overall shape has been established, the relevant segment of curve is easily revised by measuring the latest response at a small number of concentrations, which span the prescribed limits (all other concentrations being irrelevant to the control of quality). Moreover, three points (corresponding with the upper limit, midrange and lower limit) will usually suffice and frequent revision of these three points is superior to a less frequent revision of the entire curve.

Although inferior to a calibration curve, the method of standard addition (Fig. 9.19) is sometimes useful in the quick and dirty calibration which may serve the needs of a one-off investigation. Nevertheless, whatever method we choose, we must always consider the effect of major constituents within the preparation (see p. 259). Thus, if an assay involves only a small dilution of the sample, the major constituent(s) may persist at appreciable concentration(s) in the final dilution to be measured and we may, therefore, anticipate an effect upon the measurement. In these circumstances, a good knowledge of chemistry is a valuable asset but, if we have any doubts in the matter, *all* solutions used in the calibration must contain the major constituent(s) at the *same* concentration(s) throughout, namely those concentration(s) which would occur in the assay of a perfect sample of the preparation. Nevertheless, in those assays involving a large dilution of sample, the concentration(s) of major constituent(s) may drop to negligible values and, on such occasions, simple solutions of the measured compound will constitute a sound basis for calibration.

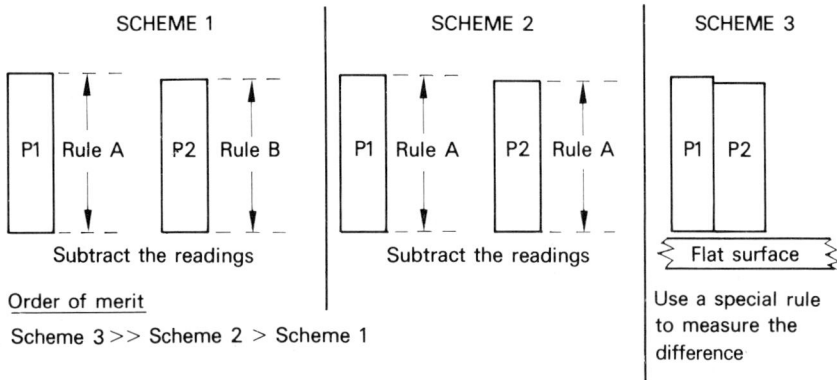

Fig. 9.20   Three schemes for measuring a small difference between the lengths of two planks. Each plank is measured with a different rule in scheme 1, and with the same rule in scheme 2, the observed lengths being subtracted in both schemes. In scheme 3, the two planks are aligned against a flat surface and the difference in length is measured directly, using a rule which is suitable for the measurement of small distances. By using only one measurement taken from a special rule, scheme 3 is more precise than schemes 1 and 2 which each involve two measurements and, in the case of scheme 1, a further possibility that an error will arise from the usual discrepancies between two different rules. Although well understood in all timber yards, the above considerations are not understood by all scientists!

Measurement of small differences

The need to measure a small difference between two chemical systems may sometimes occur, not only in developing a working method, but also in the general course of analysis and, on such occasions, we may be concerned with such problems as:

1. Batch homogeneity.
2. Inertness of a solute to solvent extraction.
3. Detection of absorbing impurities in spectrophotometry. Moreover, in all work of this kind, the results can be downright misleading if we deviate from the principles of good design.

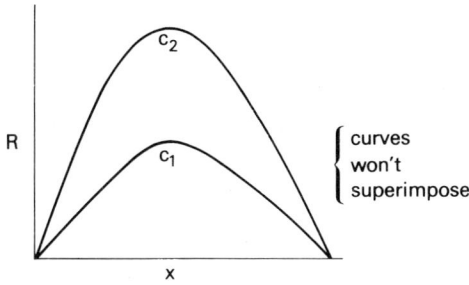

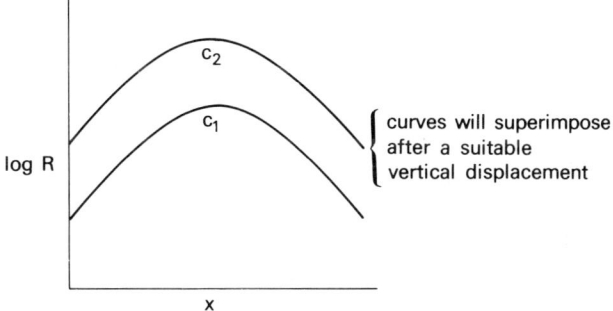

Fig. 9.21 A small difference between the shapes of two curves will only be noticed when the curves are superimposed. Although the curves (R vs. x) for different concentrations (c_1 and c_2) of the same compound won't superimpose (even when the response (R) is proportional to concentration; i.e. $R = Kc$), the related curves (log R vs. x) are superimposible after a suitable displacement of one curve, relative to the other. Hence, by using log R in place of R, we can superimpose the curve of a pure compound upon the curve of a less pure sample of the same compound and note the effect of impurities. The same procedure is also useful in other circumstances (e.g. in the study of solvent effects) and can be used whenever $R = KZ$, where Z is some variable (e.g. concentration) other than x and where K determines the shape of the curve (R vs. x). Thus, $\log R = \log K + \log Z$, where log K varies with x, and therefore determines the shape of the curve, while log Z does not vary with x and cannot affect the shape.

From the example in Fig. 9.20, we must evidently avoid the bias between two measuring devices (e.g. two 50 ml burettes, two spectrophotometers, etc.) and, wherever possible, there is much to be said for differential measurements. For example, the difference in $E(1\ cm)$ between two solutions (X and Y) can be measured directly with solution X in the reference cell and solution Y in the sample cell (analogous to scheme 3 in Fig. 9.20), the observed difference being corrected in accordance with a blank measurement (with Solution X in both cells).

A similar approach may be used to detect small differences between the shapes of experimental curves whenever the response is proportional to concentration. Such differences are sometimes important; for example, small differences in shape between the UV spectrum of a tablet and the spectrum of the active constituent are a sensitive indication that irrelevant absorption from the tablet excipients will cause a positive error in a simple UV assay. Nevertheless, a small difference between the shapes of two curves will only be noticed when the curves are superimposed and, for that purpose, we need to plot the logarithm of the response against the independent variable (e.g. wavelength), as explained in Fig. 9.21.

Secondary optimisation

Secondary optimisation is mainly concerned with the statistical interpretation of refined measurements in stage 3 of the scheme on p. 240 and, therefore, lies beyond the scope of the present chapter. By proceeding with secondary optimisation, we can hope to identify:

1.   The major source of random error.
2.   Sources of bias which have escaped the previous commonsense approach involved in primary optimisation. Nevertheless, such development of a working method into a proven method requires a considerable effort and can only be justified if the method is to receive frequent use by several analysts and by several laboratories over a long period of time.

Specification

In specifying a method, we compose a lucid set of instructions which enable other people to follow our own manipulations in all essential details. An error will occur, if one of the said details is omitted and so, in developing a method, no step is more important than specification; the bias in a method can always be attributed to an omission of some essential detail.

In communicating with the analyst, the specification demands our very best attention. The very lucid instructions, found in the majority of official monographs, are not easy to achieve and even lucid instructions are misunderstood by careless readers. The more detail we give, the longer the specification and the greater the chance that some essential item may be overlooked. We must, therefore, decide what details are important with reference to the knowledge and ability of the analyst(s) who will execute the method. In this respect, the official compendia are rather optimistic and so the need to write our own local specification may even arise with an official method.

The most lucid instructions are written in the imperative tense, using as few words as possible and avoiding long names and difficult sentences. For example, 'prepare a solution by accurately weighing ... and then prepare a second solution by diluting 10 ml of the first solution ...' is inferior to:

Solution A: accurately weigh...
Solution B: take 10 ml of solution A and...

The paragraphs of instructions, so necessary to the conservation of space in official compendia, are rather unsuited to work at the bench and so, when writing a specification for use in our own laboratory, we can achieve a substantial measure of lucidity, merely by breaking our instructions into short easily distinguishable passages:

CHECK that hands are clean and dry.
RULE a baseline on each chromatogram.
CUT out each peak (with great care) and weigh on balance.

CALCULATE $\left(\dfrac{\text{wt. of salicylate peak}}{\text{wt. of benzoate peak}}\right)$ for each solution.

PLOT 'ratio of peak weights' against 'concentration' of methyl salicylate in solutions '1', '2', '3' and '4'.
INTERPOLATE unknown.
CALCULATE the % w/v of methyl salicylate in sample X.

Each instruction commences with a key word (CHECK, RULE, CUT, etc.) which is carefully chosen and enables the analyst to check his progress. Such use of key words, written in capitals, endows each set of instructions with a good deal more character than applies to the, more conventional, use of numbered instructions (the fact that instruction 2 is preceded by instruction 1 and followed by instruction 3 may be classed as 'redundant information' and, unless we need to refer to some prior instruction, there is no point in numbering—but, see later!).

The same approach is even more powerful when writing instructions for complicated equipment and, by labelling each control with a suitable letter, we can avoid the cumbersome phrases in manufacturer's instructions. Provided the controls are labelled in an orderly way, 'Set(A)=2' is more compact and more easily understood than, 'Set the pH/mV mode selector switch to position 2'. Moreover, by invoking some of the well-known tricks of computer programming, it is easy to cope with 'remedial loops' and like situations, which are very difficult to define in more conventional terms. For example, the following excerpt (from instructions for setting up a gas chromatograph) deals with the problem of flame ionisation detectors which may, or may not, light on the first attempt.

> TURN on *hydrogen* by rotating knob clockwise until fine gauge = 50 lbf/in² (but *not* more).
> CHECK that (XC) and (XD) read about *23*.
> (c) SIMULTANEOUSLY turn on *air* (clockwise rotation of knob) and hold (G) depressed *until* 2 loud pops are heard.
> ADJUST air until fine gauge = 40 lbf/in².
> JUMP to step (d) IF cold metal collects mist when placed in effluents from (XP) and (XQ).
> TURN off air until fine gauge = 0.
> RETURN to step (c).
> (d) CHECK that (XG) and (XH) read about *17*.

The result of the first four instructions (TURN, CHECK, SIMULTANEOUSLY and ADJUST) is evaluated by the next instruction (JUMP) and, if both detectors are alight, the analyst jumps to step (d), thereby omitting the next two instructions (TURN and RETURN). On the other hand, if one or both detectors fail(s) to light, the last two instructions (TURN and RETURN) are executed, thereby initiating a fresh attempt to light the detectors. As soon as both detectors are alight, the analyst proceeds with step (d) and, subsequently, with the rest of the instructions.

Given a brief explanation of the objectives and principles behind the above mode of instruction, inexperienced operators can achieve in 30 minutes what would, otherwise, require one or two days on the basis of manufacturers' instructions—which conclusion is amply justified by experience with some 500 undergraduate and graduate operators in London and Manchester.

REFERENCES

BEAVEN G. H., JOHNSON E. A., WILLIS H. A. & MILLER R. G. J. (1961) *Molecular Spectroscopy*. p. 156. Heywood, London.

BECKETT A. H. & STENLAKE J. B. (1968) *Practical Pharmaceutical Chemistry*. Part I, 2nd edn. Athlone Press, London.

CLARKE E. C. G. (1969, 1975) *Isolation and Identification of Drugs*. Vols. 1 and 2. The Pharmaceutical Press, London.

DEAN J. A. (1961) *Chemical Separation Methods*. Von Nostrand, London.

DONBROW M. (1967) *Instrumental Methods in Analytical Chemistry*. Vol. II, Chapter 2. Pitman, London.

FLOREY K. (1972, 1973, 1974) *Analytical Profiles of Drug Substances*. Vols. 1, 2 and 3. Academic Press, London.

KOLTHOFF I. M., ELVING P. J. & SANDELL E. B. (eds.) (1964) *Treatise in Analytical Chemistry*. Interscience, New York.

McFADDEN W. (1973) *Techniques of Combined Gas Chromatography/Mass Spectrometry: Applications in Organic Analysis*. Wiley, London.

STROUTS C. R. N., WILSON H. N. & PARRY-JONES R. T. (1962) *Chemical Analysis*. Vol. II. Clarendon Press, Oxford.

WHITFIELD M. (1971) *Ion Selective Electrodes for the Analysis of Natural Waters*. Australian Marine Sciences Association, Sydney.

III
Patient services

10

Supply of medicines

J. W. BARNETT

The objectives of a medicine distribution system in a hospital, in addition to the obvious supply aspect, include:

1. Minimisation of medication errors to give maximum patient safety.
2. Efficient utilisation of hospital personnel.
3. Minimisation of medicine wastage and abuse.
4. Control of costs.

The supply system is normally triggered by the writing of a prescription and ends with the taking of the medicine by the patient. For outpatients and patients in the community the pharmacist or staff directly supervised by him are responsible for the intervening supply function; for hospital inpatients these responsibilities may be shared to varying degrees according to the system operated, although some suggested future developments have included pharmacists assuming certain responsibilities in the prescribing of drugs and in their administration.

SUPPLY TO OUTPATIENTS

The principal advantages of hospital pharmaceutical departments dispensing medicines to outpatients are:

1. Treatment can be commenced immediately (this may be particularly important for casualty patients).
2. Medicines prescribed may be difficult to obtain or restricted to the hospital service.
3. Medicines may be prescribed as part of a clinical trial.
4. Certain outpatients, particularly at psychiatric hospitals, may fail to obtain their medicines if referred to their GP in order to receive an FP10 form to be dispensed at a general practice pharmacy; this may also apply when a hospital doctor prescribes on form FP10(HP) for presentation at a general practice pharmacy.

5. Patients being discharged from hospital may require sufficient medicines to cover their needs until they can obtain a supply through their general practitioners.

Whether there are financial economies to be made by hospital pharmacists dispensing to outpatients is likely to depend very much on local circumstances, since although the cost of the medicines may be less because of contract arrangements, a pharmacist and/or technician may be grossly underutilised in manning a department which might otherwise be closed.

Method of supply

The method of supply normally follows the pattern of general practice, the patient personally taking the prescription to the hospital pharmacy department to be dispensed by a pharmacist, or technician under his direct supervision. The pharmacist is thus able to confirm that the dosage of medicines is appropriate, that there are no unwanted drug interactions and can give the patient any special directions or warnings regarding his treatment. Rationalisation of prescribed quantities with the cooperation of medical staff and introduction of prepacking systems may save a great deal of time, particularly in psychiatric hospitals (Pritchard 1970). The time interval between a patient's visits to outpatient clinics may be several months. It may thus be necessary to supply very large quantities of medicines on each occasion. A suggestion made by Mattei (1974) in relation to supply of medicines to the chronically ill may have wider application here; the patient is asked to fill in a postcard with his name, address and telephone number at the time the prescription is first dispensed, the pharmacist fills in details of the prescription, and the card is posted to the patient 1 week before his initial issue of medicines is to be exhausted to remind him to collect a further supply.

The bottle label will include the name of the medicine, strength and dosage form (unless otherwise indicated by the prescriber), directions for use, date of dispensing, the name of the patient, and name and address of the hospital, together with appropriate auxiliary labels. Labels may be printed by computer automatically in systems where the necessary information has been input. The source and batch number of the medication should be noted on the prescription form to allow recall of defective material when necessary.

Medication errors

Normally the prescription sheet is not required elsewhere, as is necessary for supply to inpatients, and the treatment will not be changed until the patient's next visit to hospital. There are therefore no inherent disadvantages to this system of supply when a pharmacy department must in any case be manned.

However, when prescriptions for inpatients about to be discharged or psychiatric day-patients are sent to the pharmacy for dispensing, difficulties may be experienced on the ward in that it may be necessary to change other treatments or administer medicines according to the directions on the prescription

Dear Dr........................

Your patient (name)...

was discharged on ....

It is recommended that the following medicine treatment be continued.

A 3/......... days supply has/has not been dispensed.

Medicine and type of preparation	Dose	Times of administration	Method of administration	Quantity supplied

Medicine sensitivity

Pharmacist's initials ....

Date dispensed...........

OTHER TREATMENT AND COMMENTS:

....

A discharge letter will follow.   *House Officer*

Fig. 10.1 Combined discharge note/medication prescription. From Scottish Home and Health Department (1973).

sheet; second prescription sheets may have to be raised without knowing all current treatment on the first, or medicines fail to be given to the patient. These disadvantages can be minimised by nursing staff carefully selecting times for prescriptions to be sent to the pharmacy department. Alternatively, for medicines to be taken out on discharge (so-called 'TTOs') a separate prescription form may be used. Some designs for these combine the prescription for discharge medication with a discharge note to the patient's general practitioner (Fig. 10.1). Three copies are produced; one copy is sent to the general practitioner, a second to the pharmacy and the third copy retained in the patient's case notes until a discharge summary is completed. The advantages of this type of prescription must be balanced against the need for a comprehensive document containing details of all the patient's drug treatment.

Because outpatients are responsible for their own treatment, the majority of problems and medication errors (discrepancies between the prescriber's intentions and the patient's actions) are likely to occur away from the hospital. The pharmacist's potential role in alleviating these by patient interviews, etc. are discussed in the following chapter. It has been suggested (Anderson & Taryle 1974) that the drug distribution function and the direct patient care function may best be served by two different types of pharmacy practitioners.

Alternative methods of supply

Where outpatient prescriptions cannot be dispensed in a hospital pharmacy department, whether because (i) the hospital is too small to justify the provision of a separate department, (ii) the number of prescriptions is too small to justify manning it during the clinic times, (iii) pharmacy staff shortages require priority to be given to other activities, or (iv) a patient is to be discharged at short notice or a casualty patient presents in the evening or at a weekend when no 24-hour service is available, the following alternatives are available:

1. Prescriptions may be written on form FP10(HP) for dispensing to outpatients at a general practice pharmacy. Regional and Area Pharmaceutical Officers must be notified before these are used for the first time at a clinic.
2. Suitably labelled prepacked medicines for standard treatments may be issued to wards or departments for medical staff to insert the patient's name. Strip packaged tablets and capsules stapled into card wallets are particularly suitable for this as the maximum number of dose units likely to be required can be provided in each wallet and unwanted tablets, fully labelled and hygienically packaged, can be torn out for return to the pharmacy before issue to the patient.
3. Medicines may be posted to the patient or delivered by other health personnel.
4. The patient may be referred to his general practitioner for a prescription of the recommended treatment.

Nursing staff should not be called upon to dispense medicines to outpatients.

Medicines and other pharmaceutical preparations for use within the outpatient department are issued by one of the systems for stock items described below.

SUPPLY TO INPATIENTS

The relatively straightforward supply methods for outpatients are complicated in the case of inpatients for the following reasons:

1. The prescription sheet may be required simultaneously by the doctor for prescribing, the nurse for medicine administration and the pharmacist for dispensing the treatment.

2. The patient is not normally responsible for his own treatment, administration of medicines usually being carried out by nursing staff who centralise the holding of these in ward cupboards or medicine trolleys.

3. So-called 'regular' treatment may in fact be changed fairly frequently, especially in acute wards, and a number of medicines may be prescribed to be given once only.

Medication errors

Unless specific action is taken to avert their likely occurrence, the rate of medication errors in this situation can be high. Barker and McConnell (1962) found that the average nurse in the American hospital studied made approximately 18% errors, or one error for every six medications given. Similar levels of error were later reported in Britain by Vere (1965) and Crooks *et al* (1965). Some of the factors contributing to this high incidence were given in the Report of a Subcommittee of the Standing Medical, Nursing and Pharmaceutical Advisory Committees of the Central Health Services Council (DHSS 1970) and are quoted below:

1. Misinterpretation of the prescription due to:

    a. Bad handwriting.
    b. Poor design of the prescription sheet.
    c. Incomplete or insufficiently clear instructions.
    d. Alterations on the prescription sheet.

2. Failure to review treatment or to cancel a prescription.

3. Failure to adopt a uniform system for prescribing, dispensing, and administering drugs in the metric system.

4. Duplication of drug administration.

5. Failure to identify the individual patient correctly.

6. Absence of the prescription from the ward when required.

7. The required drugs not being available.

8. Transfer of drugs from one container to another on the ward.

9. Setting out the doses in advance of the medicine round.

10. Variation in the timing of medicine rounds.

11. Errors in prescribing including incompatibilities and failure to take account of previous drug treatment.

12.   The large variety of drugs used.

13.   The increased mobility of patients within the ward and within the hospital.

14.   Patients taking their own drugs into the hospital.

15.   The number of doctors who may prescribe for any patient.

16.   The large number of nurses involved in the administration of drugs as a result of shorter spans of duty, part-time and shift working.

17.   Alteration to or inadequate labelling of drug containers.

A number of these factors are related to the design of the prescription sheet, which is outside the scope of this book. Principles to be followed in the design of new sheets (to be combined with administration records) are given in this Report and the corresponding Report published by the Scottish Home and Health Department (1972, 1973) including specimens of recommended prescription and recording sheets. The results of a survey of prescribing and administration records were published by Booth and Ellis (1973).

Other opportunities for error listed may be minimised by the pharmacist seeing all prescriptions and annotating them where necessary, but if this is achieved by prescriptions being sent to the pharmacy, another factor (**6** in the list) is introduced. Even where the pharmacist is able to ensure that the prescription sheet is available for main medicine rounds on the wards, administration of those drugs to be given at non-standard times may be omitted in error. In addition, the doctor may at any time wish to review the patient's treatment; in the absence of the prescription sheet he may use a second document, leading to subsequent confusion and error. Transcription of information from the prescription sheet to a separate list to be used on the ward while the prescription sheet is in the pharmacy or vice versa may lead to errors, as would use of a copy of the prescription sheet as new drugs may be prescribed on the original copy without the knowledge of the pharmacist. Annotations made by the pharmacist on his copy may fail to be transferred to the original copy, or again transcription errors may be made. These considerations are central to an understanding of the distribution systems described below. Their multiplicity testifies to the absence of an 'ideal' solution; rather, each is aimed at achieving the correct balance or compromise of opposing factors often influenced by local circumstances such as availability of particular grades of staff or layout of the hospital.

Other potential sources of medication error are described under the individual distribution system concerned.

Ordering of ward stock items

In all medicine distribution systems there are a varying number of items treated as ward stock, which are supplied without directions for use or an individual patient's name. They are issued without reference by the pharmacy department to a prescription sheet. Under the so-called 'complete stock system' this operates for all, or virtually all medicines used on a ward. In most other systems *regular* oral and parenteral medications are treated separately. Ward stocks usually include disinfectants, antiseptics and other liquids for external use, infusion fluid solutions (unless a drug-additive service is being operated), reagents and medicines to be given once only or as required. Ordering systems used for stock items are listed below. Hospitals may use different systems for different categories of items; for example disinfectants or infusion fluid solutions may be supplied by 'topping up', other items supplied on a 'full-for-empty' basis.

Handwritten requisitions in pharmacy boxes

Very little structure is given to the forms, normally only spaces for hospital, ward or department, date, and signatures of the nurse in charge (with designation), the person making the supply in the pharmacy and the nurse receiving the medicines, with a final space for date of receipt. Columns are arranged for quantity required, preparation, strength, quantity issued and any costing information required. The forms are serially numbered. Ellis (1972) recommends that the forms be raised in triplicate and gives reasons for this choice. The advantage of the system is that it is easy to implement, the disadvantages being that forms are often difficult to read, items are listed in an order which bears no relationship to the organisation of the pharmacy with consequent time wastage in processing. Time is taken up by the nurse in deciding what is required and, in writing the order, and she has probably no knowledge of pharmacy pack sizes and so may overorder. Controlled drugs are ordered by this system in a standard requisition book which is used nationally.

Preprinted requisitions

The most commonly used stock items are preprinted on to the form, together with the pack size or unit of issue and, if considered necessary, costing codes. Some designs also incorporate a column for the normal maximum number of prepacks held on the ward to further assist the nurse in ordering the correct quantities. For these preprinted items the nurse need only enter the number of packs required. Additional lines must be left for the nurse to enter those items required which are not already printed on the form. Spaces for signatures etc. are required as described above. If too many names are listed on the form the nurse may take longer to locate the required item than to write it out in full; if too few items are listed the advantages of the system are lost. This problem may occur because differences in the prescribing patterns between wards or between medical specialties is very great. Some pharmacists have designed forms capable of being used daily for a week. This allows easy assessment of usage patterns. Design of different forms for particular specialties may partially solve this problem but the normal variation in prescribing patterns between doctors must be remembered (Barnett & Calder 1969).

This ordering system takes longer to initiate, the nurse must still take some time to prepare the order, but other disadvantages of the handwritten system have been minimised. Although the requisitions are normally sent in the pharmacy box for processing in the department an alternative is to take a trolley holding standard stock items to the various wards, for issue to be made against a preprinted form filled in by nursing staff and left in a suitable location on the ward. The possibility of better planning of the working day for both pharmaceutical and nursing staff is the main advantage quoted by Lockwood and Williams (1974), who found that pharmacy technicians and assistants working in two teams of two could service a 670-bed hospital in $2\frac{1}{2}$ hours on each of the three mornings of a week that the system operated.

Full-for-empty system

Ward stock levels are initially agreed and supplied, then all subsequent empty containers are replaced by corresponding full ones, either on the ward from a pharmacy stock trolley (Victorine 1958) or in the pharmacy department. Requisitions are necessary for medicines whose supply is restricted by law and for those preparations where return of an empty container is not appropriate (e.g. ointment tubes). Costing of issues is difficult and the system is not appropriate for preparations liable to abuse unless the pharmacy staff themselves raise a requisition for what has been supplied. This may appear to defeat the objective of saving time but does allow transfer of duties from nursing staff to, for example, pharmacy assistants. Although ward overstocking or understocking should not occur, in practice this may be found because of borrowing between units. If stock levels are inadequate there is an obvious temptation for a nurse to provide an empty container for the pharmacy by transferring its contents to another container, with consequent inadequate or absent labelling on this second bottle; this may in any case be essential if the preparation is to be used on the ward while the container is absent in the pharmacy. It should be noted that this hazard can also occur in any of the other ordering systems when it is insisted that empty containers must accompany an order but ward stocks are inadequate. The intention behind this insistence is usually to prevent overstocking.

Topping-up system

Under the three systems described above, stock lists may be prepared by joint consultation between nursing and pharmaceutical staff as a guide to the former. Pharmacists or pharmacy technicians or assistants may check ward cupboards against these at regular intervals to withdraw excess stock or point out understocking. Under a topping-up system this check by pharmacy staff is an integral part of the method of supply. The checks are usually made at least weekly and may also include examination of expiry dates and storage conditions. Pharmacy technicians are the grade most frequently employed on this task.

The number of prepacks required to bring the stock up to the agreed level is noted on a preprinted form, which may also serve as the ward stock list (Hetherington 1972). The form may then be taken to the pharmacy for the supply to be made later by locked box, the technicians returning to the ward to replace the new stock correctly in the cupboards, as described by Gaunt and Riley (1971). Alternatively a pharmacy trolley containing the stock items may be taken to the ward, as described by Hassan (1960). In either case, nursing staff do not have to be involved in the ordering system, apart from assisting in the drawing up of stock levels and in their periodic review. Overstocking should not occur, and other valuable checks can be incorporated into the system. In addition a check of empty containers returned against number of packs required to restore the stock level may be a guide to possible cases of abuse of medicines. Whether there is an increase in the time spent by pharmacy staff on the distribution system is likely to depend on local circumstances such as the layout of the hospital.

Pharmacy requisition card system

The ward is provided with a separate pharmacy requisition card for each item held in stock. These are pretyped with the ward's usual requirements for a week's supply of the required medicine and may be coded by colour and number to indicate the location of stocks on the ward and also in the pharmacy. The cards may be held in wall panels, along with fixed drug information cards. When requisitioning drugs the nurse removes from the panel the cards for the medicines required and sends these to the pharmacy. The cards for restricted medicines must be signed and those for controlled drugs must be accompanied by a standard requisition form. Supplies may then be made in the traditional manner, by pharmacy box, the cards being stamped with the date of issue. The use of these cards, the drug information cards and the associated pharmacy purchase and costing systems were described by Tyrrell *et al* (1970) and Lidgate (1970). The major disadvantage of the system would appear to be the time in setting it up. Where a computer is available specially designed cards which may be prepunched with information such as drug name and ward number may be used. These can be processed electronically (after their use in requisitioning) to provide statistics on drug usage or to record the issues from the pharmacy as part of the total stock control system. If the batch number of the preparation is recorded at the time of its issue from the pharmacy the computer can provide a list of wards holding stocks, should a product-recall be necessary. Similarly, if expiry dates are entered, the computer can alert the pharmacy each week or each month to those wards or departments which may be holding stocks in need of replacement.

Medicine distribution systems

Three basic systems are in general use:

1. Complete ward stock.
2. Complete individual dispensing.
3. A combination of 1 and 2.

These are described below, along with refinements to each. However, although unit dose medication systems may be regarded as refinements of the complete individual dispensing system these are described separately, as are computer applications. The advantages and disadvantages of each system or its refinements should be considered in relation to the objectives for medicine distribution systems given in the introduction to this chapter. Where a system involves the ordering of ward stock, this may be by any one of the methods described in the preceding section, based on descriptions of refinements to the basic systems appearing in the literature this usually includes the stock ordering method involved, but it is not normally essential to adopt this in order to take advantage of the fundamental improvement proposed.

Complete ward stock system

Each ward or department holds a basic stock of those medicines most likely to be required. The labels of containers include all legal and pharmaceutical requirements but do not show any patient's name or (normally) the dose to be administered, since this should be read by the nurse on the prescription sheet at the time of administration to each individual patient. Stocks are normally replenished by bulk requisition on the pharmacy. When a preparation outside the normal list is prescribed it also is supplied to the ward in the manner described but may be regarded by ward staff as 'temporary stock' for return to the pharmacy when the treatment has been discontinued. Thus if there is more than one patient on a ward on a particular medicine, all receive their treatment from the same container.

Where patients are to pay for their treatment a distinction may be made between 'charge' and 'non-charge' stock medicines, the former being charged to the patient's account after they have been administered to him, the cost of the latter being included in the daily cost of the hospital room. In British hospitals stocks are usually regarded as 'non-charge', but many American hospitals use both systems, classification depending on the cost of the preparation, and the frequency and quantity used.

The advantages of the complete ward stock system are:

1. Medicines immediately available to the patient.
2. Minimal pharmacy workload with full scope for prepacking or use of manufacturers' original packs and ease of costing.
3. Not essential for prescription sheets or copies to be sent to the pharmacy department with attendant possibility of medication errors (particularly important in supply of medicines from a main pharmacy department to other hospitals which may be some distance from it).
4. No requirement for all patient's unused medication to be returned to pharmacy department for relabelling (and consequent possibility of error) when treatment is discontinued.
5. All information on labels can be preprinted and therefore easily read.
6. The nurse and a witness have to check the prescription in order to know which medicine to give to a particular patient and must read the name of the preparation on the container label. Inclusion of patient's names on bottles may encourage failure to apply these safeguards. A criterion in the design of drug approved names is that they should not be readily confused with others; no such consideration applies to patients names.
7. Use of pharmacy assistants for supply from pharmacy as issue of prepacks against a requisition is not a dispensing act.

The following are stated by the American Society of Hospital Pharmacists (1974) to be some of the disadvantages:

1. Increased potential for medication errors resulting from lack of review by the pharmacist of each individual patient's prescription.
2. Financial loss due to misappropriation of medication by hospital personnel and the administration of medication to patients without initiating charges.
3. Increased stocks of medicines (compared with other distribution systems).
4. Increased cost of loss due to obsolescence and deterioration.
5. Limited capacity for proper storage facilities on the nursing units in many hospitals.
6. Increased danger of unnoticed drug deterioration jeopardizing patient safety.

Because of these disadvantages this system of distribution is 'strongly discouraged' by the ASHP. Ellis (1973) gives a further disadvantage as being the heavy responsibility placed on the nurse when she operates this system because an error in the interpretation or transcription of the item prescribed to the order will be perpetuated by the pharmacy. It may be argued against this that because the patient's name is not placed on the bottle label, the error of transcription or interpretation should be detected at a second reading of the prescription, especially with another nurse acting as witness on the medicine round. However, it must be accepted that when a nurse makes the selection of drug from a large ward stock, without any form of preselection by a pharmacist, an increased potential for medication error exists because of the different extent of training on drugs for these two professional groups. The lack of pharmaceutical control which exists when pharmacists do not see prescription sheets, but are acting only as storekeepers in supplying items against the nurse's requisition is illustrated in Fig. 10.2. Ellis (1973) further states that unless information is available as to correct usage of the medicine, possible side-effects, or precautions necessary in administering the drug, a casual attitude to medication is encouraged and no doubt contributed to the high initial rate of administration errors reported, 13.8% and 20.2% in the two hospital situations which she studied.

Attempts by pharmacy staff working in the department to reduce the accumulation of ward stocks by insisting on the provision of an empty or nearly

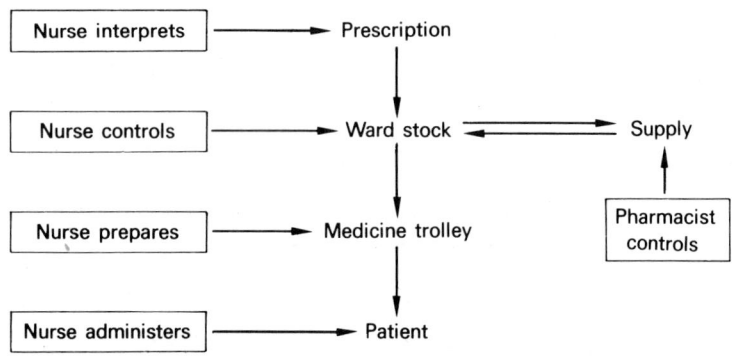

Fig. 10.2   Extent of pharmacist's control in 'traditional' complete ward stock system.

empty container before a full one is supplied may result in further problems for nursing staff if only one bottle of the preparation is held. If a dose of the medicine is to be given to the patient before the full bottle is supplied from the pharmacy this must be transferred to some other type of container and 'unofficially' labelled. Again the potential for medication errors to occur is increased. Unless a careful check is maintained on ward stocks, however, supply 'on demand' can increase the opportunity for appropriation of medicines by hospital staff. A further disadvantage given for the system is the possible risk of cross-infection, but this has not been proved.

The majority of these disadvantages can, however, be eliminated or greatly reduced if a pharmacist makes regular and frequent ward visits to see all presciption sheets and pharmacy staff check ward medicine stocks. The opportunities for medication error are further reduced if the pharmacist is able to make the selection of the medicine required for current treatments on the ward, and minimised still further if this selection can be made for each individual patient's medication, although this clearly involves progressively more pharmacist's time. The pharmacist is then carrying out one of his most important functions by selecting the correct pharmaceutical preparation which is the proper interpretation of the drug the prescriber requires and is ensuring, at the point of use, that it is in a proper condition to be used.

These were the reasons for the further development of the complete ward stock system (traditionally used in Scotland) which later became known as the 'Aberdeen system'. Initially the possibility of all prescription sheets or copies being sent to the pharmacy was considered but rejected as a potential source of error. The pharmacist, therefore, had to go to the ward and, in the pilot study (Report of Scottish Hospital Pharmacists' Conference 1966) supervised a technician dispensing sufficient of each medicine currently required on the ward to last 24 hours (72 hours at weekends). Only one bottle was supplied irrespective of the number of patients involved, although it was found that at least 50% of all medicines were for the use of only one patient, the average being about 75%. The medicines were laid out initially on medicine trays for storage in cupboards, later in lockable medicine trolleys. The medicines were dispensed from a pharmacy trolley by direct reference to the original prescription sheets, bottles being labelled in the normal manner for stock preparations. The ward medicine cupboard contained only such medicines as would reasonably be expected to be required in emergencies, or for 'once-only' doses which are supplied by the ward pharmacist as required. The ward sister ceased to order any pharmaceutical preparation other than controlled drugs, saving a considerable amount of nursing time (approximately 8 minutes per day in ordering medicines and 20 minutes per day in preparing medicine trolleys for each ward of 20 beds). Further development (Calder & Barnett 1967) increased the efficiency of the supply arrangements without reducing the overall benefits of the system, largely by the introduction of standard pre-packed units designed to last approximately 1 week. A ward pharmacist working $2\frac{1}{2}$ hours each week-day could serve 200 acute beds with additional assistance from pharmacy technicians. Investigations in two geriatric long-stay hospitals (each $2\frac{1}{2}$ miles from the base hospital) indicated that, because of the relatively few changes in prescriptions, weekly visits only were required by the ward pharmacist alone. Including travelling time, reading prescriptions, checking stock, initiating supply of medicines and discussions with medical and nursing staff, 2 hours were required to cover 84 beds. The pharmacy stock trolley could not be taken to these hospitals, the pharmacist instead completing a preprinted requisition form for subsequent supply from the pharmacy. Use of this trolley was eventually discontinued in the acute wards in favour of the pharmacist taking the preparations required for the medicine trolley from the stock cupboard, with replacements being sent to the ward later by pharmacy box for nursing staff to put away. In the final phase of development of the 'Aberdeen system' (Calder & Barnett 1971), each patient's medicines were placed in the medicine trolley in a box labelled with his name (Fig. 10.3)

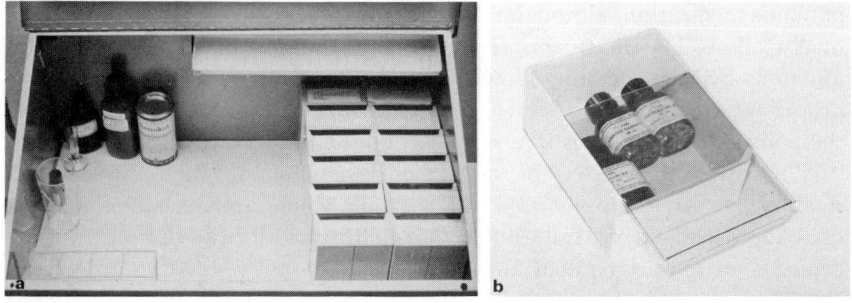

Fig. 10.3 (a) Medicine trolley showing the individual boxes for each patient's medicine. (b) Box containing the different medicines for one patient.

The patient's name was *not* included on individual bottles so that the sequence of medicine selection was as follows:

1. Patient identified with prescription sheet.
2. Appropriate box selected according to patient's name.
3. Medicine selected from the box by reference to the prescription sheet and the name of the preparation on the bottle.

If similar patient names caused the wrong box to be selected, this would be immediately obvious in that the appropriate medicines would not be present. It was considered that in the above sequence the name of the patient on the final medicine container would increase the possibility of error (administration by patient name rather than by drug name) and further complications would arise if the drug were put back in the wrong box. Final selection by drug name meant that a preparation put into the wrong box by a nurse was ignored in that box and was replaced from ward stock at the next medicine round for the other box. This final refinement was found to take more pharmacist's time only when many changes in patients and/or prescriptions had taken place and was considered to approach as closely as was possible, within

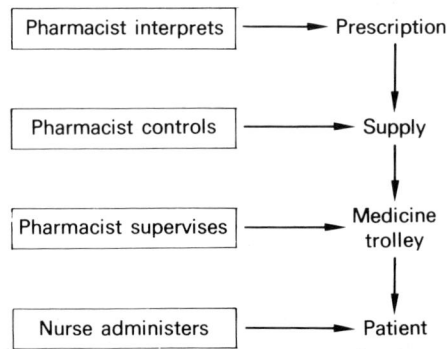

Fig. 10.4 Extent of pharmacist's control in 'Aberdeen' complete ward stock system.

the staffing levels at the time, the ultimate system where the nurse would be handed one dose for one patient at each administration time.

The extent of the pharmacist's control under the 'Aberdeen system' of supply of complete ward stock is illustrated in Fig. 10.4. The supply of medicines for regular prescriptions was essentially done by 'topping up' by pharmacy staff against the prescription sheet rather than the ward stock sheet. A system of the latter type, operated by pharmacy technicians but incorporating a method of ward pharmacist-initiated supply (and if necessary, return) of 'temporary stocks' was described by Gaunt and Riley (1971). In the system incorporating a ward pharmacist described by Lockwood and Williams (1974) an accurate list of ward stocks and temporary stocks is maintained in a convenient, easily portable form for checking the needs of the ward; this would also clearly provide an additional safeguard against misappropriation of medicines, particularly if this is checked at irregular intervals by the ward pharmacist against the administration record made by the nurse.

Complete individual dispensing system

In this system virtually all medicines required for 'regular' treatment are dispensed in the pharmacy department either by, or under the direct supervision of a pharmacist, labelled with the individual patient's name and sometimes the instructions for dosage. The prescription sheets are normally sent to the pharmacy as other methods would involve transcription or direct copies; non-prescription pharmaceuticals are held as ward stock and ordered by one of the methods already described. The system has been traditionally used only in the small and/or private hospital, mainly in North America because of the large pharmacy workload involved and the preference in these institutions for individualised service.

Advantages of the system include:

1. All prescriptions are directly reviewed by the pharmacist who can annotate them if necessary to assist the nurse and is also able to specify the dosage form given.
2. Opportunity for close liaison between pharmacist, nurse and physician in pharmaceutical matters as a result of **1.**
3. Provides potential for close control of stock if all treatments for discharged patients are returned to the pharmacy.
4. Facilitates charging of private patients.
5. Enables investigation of possible medication errors if too many or too few doses appear to have been administered.
6. The name of the medicine, whether approved or proprietary, appearing on the patients treatment can be the same as that used in the prescription, avoiding confusion of nursing staff.
7. By limiting the supply in each bottle the pharmacist can ensure that

treatment is not continued indefinitely without review, (for instance, only 5 days' treatment of an antibiotic preparation may be supplied at any one time).

The following are given by the ASHP (1974) as some of the disadvantages:

1.   Increased potential for medication errors due to the lack of checks in the distribution of medication doses and to the inefficiencies inherent in the procedures used to schedule, prepare, administer, control and record during the drug distribution and administration process.

2.   Consumption of excessive nursing manpower in the preparation of medication doses and in conducting other medication–related activities.

3.   Increased potential for drug loss due to waste, obsolescence and deterioration.

The ASHP state that 'while not as disadvantageous as the complete floor (ward) stock system, this method of drug distribution is also discouraged'.

Disadvantages **1** and **3** would appear, however, like those of complete ward stock systems to be at least partly related to the way in which the system is operated, rather than inherent to the basic system. The second disadvantage has been reduced, if not eliminated in the refinement described by Ross (1966) and Walsh (1969) (see below).

The 'traditional' individual dispensing system is undoubtedly more time-consuming for pharmacy staff than the complete ward stock system relying on nurse's requisitioning. The refinements of each are more difficult to compare but if it is desired to incorporate ward visits by the pharmacist, individual dispensing may take slightly longer because of the time taken to incorporate the patient's name on the label. The return of individual patient's treatment to the pharmacy after discontinuation or discharge also involves an additional workload, particularly for pharmacy staff, although use of strip-packaged material attached to cards or wallets could also considerably reduce this by allowing easy removal of the patient's name ready for reissue, also eliminating any possibility of cross infection, mixing of batches etc. The requirement for prescription sheets to leave the ward is a particularly important disadvantage in hospitals supplied from a central pharmacy elsewhere. Retention of the system may thus prevent centralisation, designed to produce staff economies and thereby allow scarce pharmacist manpower being employed on other activities where his professional training may have greater benefit to patients. The pharmacy service must be prompt and reliable and, if the system is to be strictly adhered to, provided over 24 hours for 7 days each week. Where more than one patient on a ward is being treated with a particular medicine, busy nursing staff may be tempted to administer doses to the second patient from the others bottle. The pharmacist may then not have the opportunity to review this second patient's sheet, and the checks on medication errors are also lost. The refinement initiated by Ross (1966) described below obviates this disadvantage.

A large number of containers are required on the ward under this system and this may cause increased potential for medication error unless they are placed in a trolley with drawers labelled for individual patients. The dispensing of all these treatments also increases the opportunity for pharmacy error unless a prepacking system is used. Serious medication errors may arise if the dosage instructions are included on the label of the dispensed medication, since the nurse may then administer the medicines to the patient without any reference to the prescription sheet and any changes or cancellations on this document may not be seen. This may account for an error rate reported to be as high as 41% in a psychiatric ward of 40 patients, although caution should be applied in comparing published rates as the definition of an 'error' and the clinical significance of these may vary.

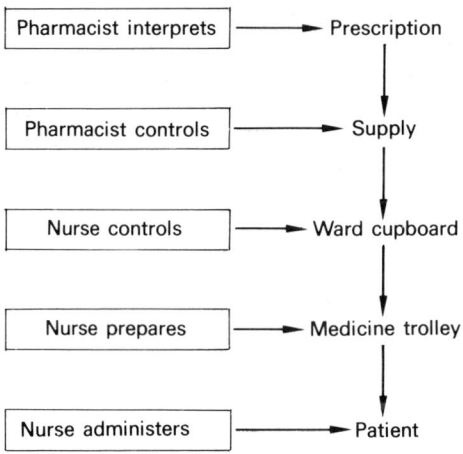

Fig. 10.5 Extent of pharmacist's control in 'traditional' complete individual dispensing system.

The extent of pharmaceutical control existing in the system as traditionally operated is illustrated in Fig. 10.5. This can be seen to be better than that under the traditional ward stock system (Fig. 10.2) but not as extensive as that in the Aberdeen refinement of this (Fig. 10.4).

In the refinement described by Ross (1966) each patient's treatment (sufficient for 1 week, normally) is contained in a small drawer of the medicine trolley labelled with his name. On the medicine round the trolley is taken to the patient's bedside, the appropriate drawer removed, the prescription sheet checked to find the doses required, and these are then removed from the appropriate bottles. Lockable cupboard doors fitted to the front of the trolley and the facility to lock the trolley to the wall ensures security of the medicines. New supplies are obtained by sending the prescription sheet to the pharmacy. The nurse thus no longer has to sort through large numbers of bottles at each medicine round, and is encouraged to obtain and use separate containers for each patient, allowing checks on medication errors, minimal opportunity for misappropriation and review of all prescriptions by the pharmacist. Medicines are easily returned to the pharmacy when the need for them has passed because no searching on the part of the nurse is necessary, there is also incentive in that space in the drawers is needed for other items. Ward stocks were retained in the pilot study only for 'sister's medications'—antacids, laxatives, mild analgesics and cough suppressants and expectorants which were not normally written up if only an occasional dose was involved—infusion fluids because of their bulk and controlled drugs and unstable preparations because of their special storage requirements. External preparations were not included in the new system. It should be noted that many in the medical, nursing and pharmaceutical professions consider that the occasions when hospital nursing staff administer drugs without a written prescription for the patient should be very rare or totally absent because of the risk of interactions with other medicines given concurrently. Medicines required when the pharmacy was closed were obtained from the hospital emergency cupboard. Ross found the medicine round more time-consuming compared with the previously used combined stock/individual dispensing system (see next section). However, a number of other changes were introduced to the nursing procedures which may have accounted for this, since Walsh (1969) applying the system in a different hospital on a larger scale, found a saving of about 40% on nurses' time spent on medicine rounds compared with the 'old' system (unspecified), and McMullan (1975) reported similar figures in changing from the combined stock/individual dispensing system. Both Ross (1966, 1967) and Walsh (1969) minimised the pharmacy workload by a system of prepacking and prelabelling, only the name of the patient and date (Ross) or these details plus ward and directions for use (Walsh) being written at the time of dispensing. In neither case were significant problems encountered with prescription sheets leaving the ward. However, the pharmacy was in the same hospital as the wards into which the system was introduced; Ross dispensed the prescriptions immediately, and Walsh used a system of photocopying the sheets after they had been checked (and annotated if necessary) by a pharmacist so that the originals could be returned to the ward almost immediately, dispensing being carried out from the copies.

If the dangers of including the dosage directions on the label are accepted, the main reason for including the patient's name on the *bottle* in the Ross system would appear to be to allow the nurse to place the medicine in the correct drawer when it is sent to the ward from the pharmacy. If the system is combined with ward visits by a pharmacist therefore, this step, which is time consuming in itself and also creates an additional workload in relabelling unused medication, can be avoided without any loss of advantages. The method would then be identical to that final refinement of the Aberdeen system described in the previous section. Thus, although Walsh considers the 'Ross system' as an alternative to ward visits by a pharmacist, comparing the time taken by each, the advantages of both can be realised without excessive pharmacy workload. Although McMullan (1975) describes the use of the 'Ross trolley' in a ward visited regularly by a pharmacist, it is not clear whether or not the patient's name is included in the label.

The times taken by pharmacists on the wards of various United Kingdom Hospitals in checking prescriptions at least once daily and carrying out any functions associated with the medicine distribution system were found by Walsh (1969) to vary between 2.5 minutes per patient per week and just over 4 minutes per patient per week, the shorter visits occurring when only new prescriptions were checked.

A system which may be considered to form a logical step between that described by Ross and unit dose dispensing has been used in a Canadian hospital. Medicines were individually packaged in labelled, heat sealed 2-inch square plastic bags; a 5-day supply of these was placed in a cardboard box labelled in the traditional manner and kept in the individual patient's drawer. This system allows the pharmacy staff to preselect the patient's doses, perhaps reducing errors where, for example, two tablets of a drug are required to be given at a time; to be balanced against this is the risk of error if doses are changed during the 5-day period. This system was adopted in preference to unit-dose because it did not require a 24-hour pharmacy service.

Mechanical dispensing

So-called 'mechanical' dispensing may be considered to be individual dispensing, since the machine produces a label containing the patient's name for attachment to the package which it releases. An example is the 'Brewer system' described by Manzelli (1961), the main feature of which is the 'drug station', an electronically controlled device which only releases the appropriate prepacked medication when three identification plates, for the patient, desired medication and nurse, have been inserted. The label printed includes the name and strength of the medicine, the patient's name and the identification of the nurse. Simultaneously a similar record is made within a locked compartment of the machine for control purposes and a charge ticket is produced to allow charging of private patients. The machine holds up to eight packages of each of 96 different medicines and incorporates various 'fail-safe' mechanisms to avoid errors. A 'drug cart' is used in conjunction with the drug station; a medicine trolley which has amongst its features lockable individual patient drawers for the individually dispensed medicines. Advantages claimed for the drug station include:

1. Maximum control of medicines in each nursing unit.
2. Reduction of pharmacy time in pricing and labelling and in replenishing nursing station supplies.
3. Reduction of pharmacy stock.

4.　　Financial accounting facilitated.
5.　　Ready availability of medications to nursing staff.

The major disadvantage of the unit is its cost. Use in Great Britain is likely to be restricted because of this, and because the accounting advantages are not directly applicable, although a trial of one unit has taken place in a psychiatric hospital for 'emergency' supplies when the pharmacy is closed.

Combined stock individual dispensing systems

Under this system, medicines are supplied either as ward stocks for those drugs in more or less frequent use or individually dispensed items for all others. The distinction between this and the previously described individual dispensing system where some ward stocks were still necessary is basically one of approach. In the individual dispensing system the aim is to provide the maximum number of treatments as individually dispensed items, whereas in the combined system a positive decision is made to restrict these, usually to minimise

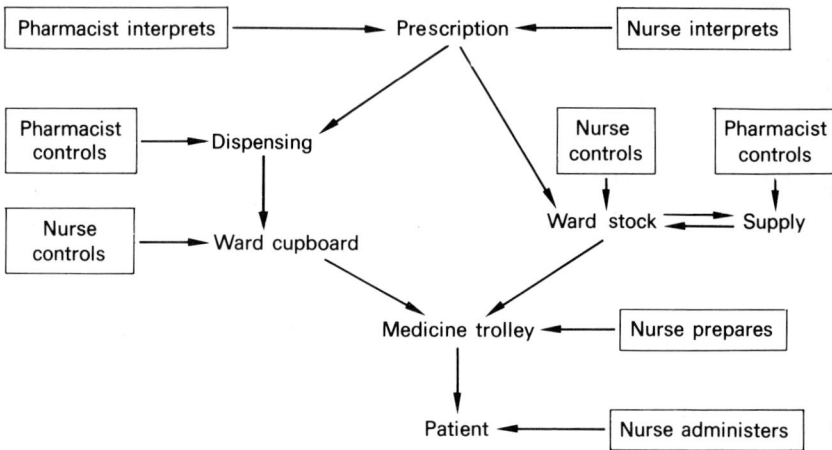

Fig. 10.6　Extent of pharmacist's control in 'traditional' combined stock/individual dispensing system.

pharmacy workload but also because, without a 'Ross-type' trolley, medicines to be administered to more than one patient are often taken from one patient's bottle anyway, and provision of these items as stock takes account of this. Problems may arise, however, for both nursing and pharmaceutical staff if the range of stock items is not standardised and the same medicine is treated as stock on one ward and individually dispensed in another. The extent of the ward stock varies considerably in the application of this system to different hospitals. The advantages and disadvantages of this combined system (which has been traditionally used in England and Wales) are similar to those of the complete ward stock and complete individual dispensing systems already described in proportion to the ratio of stock to individual prescriptions, the optimum sought being that which realises the best features of each. The extent of the pharmacist's control in the system as traditionally practised is shown in Fig. 10.6. It will be appreciated that this diagram, like those previously given, is in fact only the briefest of summaries of the various steps and checks involved which can make medicine distribution systems very time consuming for the professions involved.

In the refinement to the traditional system developed at Westminster Hospital, London (Baker 1967) the proportion of stock items still to be requisitioned by nursing staff was increased to 90% (except for disinfectants and infusion fluids which were 'topped up'). This was aimed to minimise visits to the pharmacy for individually dispensed items. By supplying stock items as prepacked units there were sufficient savings in pharmacists' time to allow them to visit wards twice daily. They were then able to check all *new* prescriptions, annotating them where necessary and, if the medicine was not carried by the ward as stock, write a label for individual dispensing, including sufficient detail to allow completion of the dispensing in the pharmacy. The medicine would then be delivered to the ward before the next medicine round. When repeat supplies were required the empty bottle and a nurse's requisition were sent to the pharmacy. Each pharmacist required only approximately 1 hour per day to provide a service for 150 beds, the system therefore becoming widely accepted as a considerably improved pharmacy service despite the then current recruitment problems in hospital pharmacy. A criticism made has been that in writing the labels on the ward these may not be so clear as typewritten labels produced in the pharmacy. No attempt was made to preselect the medicines required by the nurse for current treatments.

As already described, Ross started from the same traditional system but, in contrast to Baker, placed the emphasis heavily on individual dispensing without introducing ward visits by pharmacists. The system described by McMullan (1975) in which a Ross trolley is used and a pharmacist visits the ward regularly to see new prescriptions is to a certain extent a link between these two refinements.

Unit dose systems

In all unit dose systems the pharmacy delivers medications to wards in single unit packages just prior to the time of administration, the doses being as ready as possible for administration to the patient. A single unit package has been defined (ASHP 1974) as 'one which contains one discrete pharmaceutical dosage form, ie. one tablet, one capsule, one 2 ml volume of a liquid, etc. It is a unit dose or single dose package if it contains that particular dose of the drug ordered for the patient. A unit dose package could, for example, contain two tablets of a drug product.' The medicines are delivered to the ward at least once daily, the number of doses being sufficient until the next visit. As far as possible doses of liquid medicines are packaged in individual containers, injections are reconstituted or diluted if necessary and drawn up into the syringe, and tablets and capsules are supplied individually wrapped in foil or cellophane; each package is fully labelled with its contents (but not the patient's name) allowing positive identification of the contents up to the time of administration to the patient, thus reducing the possibility of medication errors.

The medication doses for the next 24 hours or less are prepared by a technician, who places them in the patient's individually labelled drawer in a medicine cabinet, trolley or cassette for subsequent checking by a pharmacist. Where the supplies are for more than one medicine round, the drawers may be subdivided into compartments for each time with an additional compartment for medicines to be taken 'as required'. Medicines required immediately are also supplied in single unit packages but are not, of course, placed in the drawers. An American investigation (Silverman et al 1974) revealed that approximately 7.8% of new prescriptions or prescriptions for a change in dose required the pharmacy to immediately send an initial dose to the ward (a smaller number than anticipated). As this filling operation is normally carried out in the pharmacy the problems of medicine trolleys and prescriptions being away from the ward have to be overcome. Two trolleys may be used for each ward, one being prepared in the pharmacy, then taken to the ward for exchange with the other used for the preceding period (an initially expensive method which also requires considerable floor-space in the pharmacy). Alternatively, only drawers may be exchanged on the ward, or a compromise between the two, cassettes of drawers may be taken to the wards on a transfer trolley; if this trolley is designed to carry medications for several wards it may become unacceptably heavy, but otherwise this system works well (Ellis & Ford 1972). The problem of prescription sheets leaving the ward is more acute under unit dose systems because of the frequency with which the pharmacy staff must have access to them. Nursing staff may send a copy to the pharmacy (produced by carbon or non-carbon-requiring paper) as soon as a new treatment has been prescribed, or pharmacists may make frequent ward visits to collect these. However, it is normally found necessary to make abstractions to maintain a comprehensive record of the patient's treatment, thus involving potential transcription errors in addition to the difficulties already described inherent in the use of copies of prescription sheets. The method used by Ellis et al (1973) overcomes this; the pharmacist visits the ward 1 hour before each medicine round (except that at 6 a.m.) to see the original prescription and to transcribe any new prescriptions or alterations to existing treatment to a pharmacy profile which is used for compiling statistics on drug usage and checking drug interactions in addition to its principal function of showing when doses are to be dispensed; transcription errors are detected because the pharmacist checks the trolley contents against the original prescription before the next medicine round (Fig. 10.7).

On the medicine round the nurse takes the trolley to the bedside, checks the patient's identity and removes the required medicines from the appropriate drawer, comparing the labels with the prescriptions before opening the wrapping, and administering the dose, if possible directly from the package. Finally, a record of the administration is made; in one Dutch hospital this is done by removing the self-adhesive label on the package and attaching it to the medication form. Ward stocks can be drastically reduced as for all medicines supplied as single unit packages only sufficient doses are required to cover the period whilst the pharmacy is closed. Other preparations are supplied as stock in the normal manner by requisition.

Unit dose systems may be described as either centralised or decentralised according to whether the preparation of patient medication drawers is carried out in a central pharmacy or in two or more smaller 'satellite' pharmacies

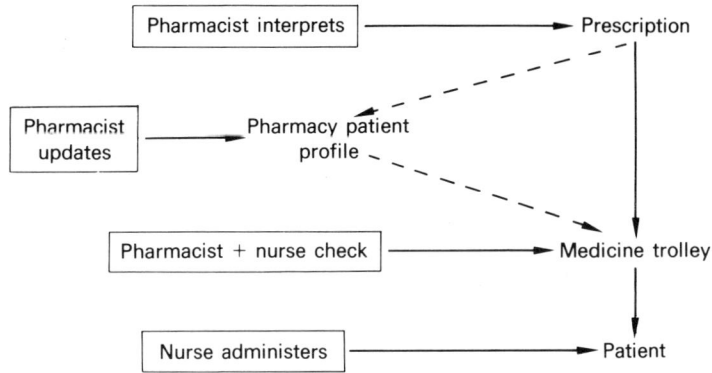

Fig. 10.7 Extent of pharmacist's control in a unit dose system.

serving perhaps 100 or 200 beds and located in or near the patient care areas of the hospital. The physical layout of the hospital is an important factor in determining which alternative is adopted. The centralised system allows greater management efficiency and control and may facilitate mechanisation and computerisation of the processes involved; pharmacy staff may, however, feel detached from ward activities, and physical difficulties in transporting the drawers throughout the hospital and supplying medicines for immediate use between trolley deliveries may be important. The advantages and disadvantages of the decentralised system are the converse of these but total stocks of medicines in the pharmacy organisation are much higher. However, decentralisation, according to Ellis and Ford (1972), 'seemed to provide the greatest satisfaction to all the pharmacy staff, because their close proximity to the ward situation made every task meaningful and enabled them to play a real part in the health team'.

Newer hospitals in America have pneumatic tubes or dumb-waiter facilities which reduce the problems of centralisation. The classification of unit dose systems in this manner may, however, be misleading as all the functions associated with the supply may have been either centralised or decentralised and, moreover, a centralised system in a small hospital may have the characteristics of a decentralised system in a larger institution. Floor plans for a decentralised pharmacy are given by Smith and Mackewicz (1972).

Unit dose dispensing systems have been adopted or are being developed fairly extensively in North America and most European countries, but to only a very limited extent in the United Kingdom, although use of single unit packages (particularly for tablets, capsules and eye preparations) has increased (Anon 1973); this is generally regarded as an essential step in the introduction of the full system. An American survey in late 1973 revealed that one in three hospital prescriptions were dispensed in unit dose containers.

Use of single unit packages in any medicine distribution system will reduce the possibility of medication errors, reduce contamination, save nursing time, reduce wastage by allowing unused doses to be returned to stock, and facilitate stock control. Unfortunately, packaging of oral liquids and provision of prefilled syringes has proved difficult, and these may be the areas where maximum benefit in terms of reduced medication error is likely to occur. Barker *et al* (1966) found that intramuscular and subcutaneous injections were three times more liable than the average to dosage errors ($> \pm 5\%$ of the ordered dose) and over one and a half times as likely to be given unordered. A wider range of ampoules is, however, available in Britain. Mehl (1968) considers that only injections requiring the mixing of two or more drugs need be prepared in the pharmacy, and that the increased pharmacy workload involved in prefilling syringes from single unit vials would not be justified. Oral liquids were found to be involved in significantly more errors (of all types combined) than any other dosage form.

Adoption of a full unit dose system should, however, produce greater advantages:

1. The opportunity for medication errors to occur are reduced still further because the dosages are preselected and checked by pharmacy staff before the nurse again checks the medicines supplied against the patient's name on the drawer and each labelled dose against the prescription. Ellis *et al* (1973) found that the introduction of unit dose dispensing to replace a complete ward stock system reduced the rate of administration errors by 54.4%. The contribution to this reduction made by the packaging system alone was not identified. The definition used for an administration error was 'any variation from the written prescription during the administration of the drugs prescribed or the recording of those administrations' but intentional variations for the benefit of the patient or patient refusals were not included. Medication errors resulting in doses remaining in the drawers can be readily detected under this system. Moeys (1968) however, states that 'in our opinion the training of the qualified nurse in Holland is such that she generally will be quite able to understand the doctor's instructions and carry them out correctly'. He therefore adopted a total stock, in preference to unit dose system.

2. Reduced stocks of medicines on wards, with increased control and decreased opportunity for wastage and misappropriation of those remaining. Withdrawal of stocks because of a reported defect is also facilitated.

3. Saving in nursing time. Figures quoted should not be extrapolated uncritically from one hospital situation to another as variations in procedures before and after introduction of the system are considerable. The results of Ellis *et al* (1973) are likely to be the best guide to United Kingdom trends, the overall saving amounting to an average of 24 minutes per ward per day, a 26% reduction in the time normally spent on drugs and 4% overall saving.

4. In American hospitals the system has allowed reduction of documentation, more accurate charging of patients for medicines and minimisation or elimination of the need for credits for unused doses, advantages not directly applicable to British hospitals.

5. Greater involvement of the pharmacist in drug therapy. Although it is feasible to operate a unit dose dispensing system without ward visits by pharmacists, the overriding advantages of these in terms of review of the doctor's original prescription and general coordination of the system have facilitated his acceptance in the clinical role in American hospitals. This, coupled with a shift of workload from pharmacist to technician in handling medications, allowing more time for this new clinical role, has presented advantages to American pharmacists which go beyond the 'nuts and bolts' of the distribution system. These advantages can, however, be achieved in less elaborate systems already described, although there may be longer delays before the pharmacist sees new prescriptions. Where the pharmacist has gained acceptance of his role on the ward with minimal linkage with medicine distribution, adoption of unit dose systems may actually reduce his clinical involvement.

6. Reduction in nursing time spent maintaining controlled drugs records by centralising documentation in the pharmacy.

7. Because of the extended pharmacy service the patient may receive his treatment more promptly.

8. Easy adaption to computerisation and automation (see last section of chapter).

Claims that the overall cost of medicine distribution is reduced under this system, based on American findings, may be misleading in relation to British hospitals and require detailed investigation based on the systems already in use in this country.

Disadvantages of the system are:

1. A considerable increase in pharmacy establishment is likely to be necessary in United Kingdom hospitals. It may be argued that this increase is due to the workload of handling, selecting and measuring the medicament being carried out entirely in the pharmacy. From the experience of their study, Ellis *et al* (1973) suggest that 'two pharmacists and a technician, working as a team, could be responsible for a unit dose distribution service to 150 acute beds and still have time to extend the clinical pharmacy aspects of the service', the latter being then mainly confined to regular prescription checks without reference to patient's notes or medical and nursing staff. The cost of a technician and an additional pharmacist required in introducing the system could only partially be offset by the saving of the equivalent of one nurse's time, even if that post could be released. A number of American studies (e.g. MacPherson *et al* 1973; Austin 1973), have shown that the physical layout in the pharmacy and the design of the profile can make a considerable difference to the time required in the pharmacy to prepare the patient's medication drawers.

2.   An extension of the hours of service by the pharmacy is necessary, usually consisting of two shifts for smaller hospitals, with an on-call system through the night, or a full 24-hour service in larger hospitals in both cases for 7 days each week. This is because of the reduction in ward stocks and requirement for provision of non-routine reconstituted injections, starting doses for new prescriptions etc. Whilst this second disadvantage (ie. working 'non-social' hours) provides recruitment problems in addition to those inherent in an increase in establishment, it should be noted that other services such as provision of intravenous drug additives may also be made possible or extended because of this move. Pharmacy staffing levels in American hospitals, relative to the number of beds served, are consistently higher compared to this country. For example, the pharmacy service, which includes unit dose dispensing, for a 300-bed private hospital described by Pang (1973) required five pharmacists, an intern, a messenger and five technicians.

3.   Conversion to single unit packages may require additional storage space in the pharmacy department. This problem can, however, often be reduced or eliminated if outer containers for the new units are organised so as to make use of the 'dead' space normally wasted above the conventional bulk packs on store shelving; in addition, space for empty containers and bottle washing may no longer be required.

4.   Additional cost of the purchase of medicines in single unit packages or for repackaging. To be set against this are the savings gained in eliminating conventional containers, prepackaging, bottle washing, medicine cups and spoons, syringes etc.

5.   By reducing the amount of thought required there is a loss of interest for nursing staff in the administration of medicines. This may lead to a tendency for the nurse to carry out the important final check of medicine supplied against prescription in a somewhat superficial manner.

6.   Loss of interest for technicians may occur unless they have some contact with wards and patients. This may lead to inefficiency and inaccuracy in the filling of medicine trolleys.

7.   Implementation difficulties would arise in small particularly rural, hospitals.

The attitudes of the various groups of staff involved are also relevant. The concensus opinion of American pharmacists who have implemented the system has been described. Nursing staff in American hospitals also appear to favour unit dose systems. This was shown, for example, in the detailed study by Moody et al (1970) carried out 4 years after introduction of such a system; it was found, on the other hand that 60% of the residents and interns were indifferent or did not favour it, in contrast to earlier findings on pilot projects by other workers. The medical and nursing staff involved in the Leeds trial (Ellis *et al* 1973) were dissatisfied with the quality and method of supply of prefilled syringes and with the packs of oral liquids, which were all in the developmental stage; they wished to restrict the service to oral doses until improvements could be made but despite this none wished to return to the old system.

Implementation of unit dose systems requires the introduction of agreed times for medicine rounds, if this has not already been done, as both nursing and pharmacy staff must work to these. The nurse must inform the pharmacist if there is to be any deviation. In addition, the pharmacist must be aware of patient admissions, operations, discharges and transfers.

A unit dose method is the most complex medicine distribution system to implement and requires even closer cooperation between medical, nursing, pharmaceutical and administrative staff to achieve this than any of the other alternatives already described. A formal committee to back up and coordinate informal discussions and decisions at ward level is probably necessary. Other factors affecting the design and implementation of the system will include the availability of the medicines in single unit packages, the staffing levels, hours of operation, dimensions and location of the pharmacy, the size and layout of the hospital, and the finance available for purchase of trolleys. A publication *Unit Dose Distribution Systems* (ASHP 1972) gives the collective experiences of a number of authors in planning and initiating systems in American hospitals and may be of use to British pharmacists.

Unit dose systems have been implemented in a number of specialised hospitals. Mathieson and Rawlings (1971) described the introduction of a unit dose system into a nursing home by a general practice pharmacy. Introduction into a paediatric hospital is described by Durant and Herrick (1970). Although more difficult in a childrens hospital because of problems of dosage calculation, use of non-standard treatments, and the greater proportion of liquid preparations with varying dose problems, implementation of unit dose systems consequently bring correspondingly higher benefits. Prepackaging is often not applicable, the pharmacist often being called upon to provide doses extemporaneously. McLeod *et al* (1971) describe a unit dose system in a mental retardation centre and believe it to be feasible for all mental institutions. Although doses were initially prepared for a 24-hour period, it later proved practical to extend this to 48 hours. A unit dose system for distribution of respiratory therapy medication is described by Warren (1975). Each ward is provided with a unit dose trolley containing the medicines for respiratory therapy and equipment for its use.

Self administration

Self administration whereby the inpatient is given responsibility for taking his own individually dispensed treatment at the proper times, would appear an obvious means of reducing nursing workload (particularly in non-acute units) and educating the patient in the manner in which his medication should be taken, or identifying problems such as overcomplicated regimes or packaging which the patient cannot open. However, in practice many patients, because of their illness, are physically or mentally unable to accept this responsibility; moreover, for others the relatively frequent changes in medicine and dosage occurring in hospital would be confusing and, perhaps, worrying. The hospital takes responsibility for any drug administered to the patient, whether self administered or given by the nurse, and there may therefore be medicolegal implications in the adoption of this system, which should consequently be approached with caution.

It is normal hospital practice to discourage uncontrolled self administration by taking away from the patient on admission those medicines which he has brought with him. It should be explained to the patient that it may be necessary to give him different drugs in hospital. If his own medicines are not suitable on discharge, his permission is obtained for their destruction. Because the conditions of storage of the patient's drugs before bringing them into hospital are not known, and because their identity cannot be guaranteed, no attempt should be made to reuse them.

The problem of patients failure to take medicines correctly has been shown to occur over all ages and types of therapy, and is by no means restricted to the very young, the elderly and those on complex and multiple therapy. Sex, intelligence, knowledge of disease or treatment, type of therapy and incidence of side effects do not appear to have a significant effect (Horan 1973). Error rates can be high; an informal survey of outpatients at an American hospital revealed that nearly 40% of them exhibited errors in the way they were taking their medicines, the highest proportion occurring where the treatment was to be taken 'as directed' and the patient received more than one prescription. Failure to understand instructions and premature termination of treatment because the patient is feeling better were common causes of error revealed in the literature search by Horan. These findings have been used both to support and criticise self-administration schemes, since on the one hand patient education is clearly necessary, and taking the medicines first under careful supervision in hospital will facilitate this, but against this the high failure rate in outpatients would indicate that this would also occur in an inpatient self administration scheme, with perhaps prolonged hospital stay and possible legal implications. The necessity of careful instruction of the patient in the use of his medicaments, whether he be outpatient or inpatient about to be discharged, is clearly necessary and is undisputed. The pharmacist is in a good position to give this advice to outpatients and, where ward visits by the pharmacist are initiated, to inpatients also. Hassan (1974) reviews the literature on self-administration schemes (including those in a psychiatric hospital, a physical rehabilitation hospital, an extended care facility, a geriatric ward and a cardiology unit) and finds that most are believed to be successful.

The ASHP (1974) states that inpatient self-administration medications should be labelled as for outpatient prescriptions. The normal policy of the person administering the medicine remaining with the patient until the dose has been taken is relaxed in the case of self administration, when the medications may be left at the bedside upon the physician's written order for self administration. They recommend that a system should be implemented for checking that the patients are taking their medications correctly.

In the study conducted by Horan (1973) patients in a minimal care unit of Westminster Hospital, London, (in the last 7–10 days of their hospital stay) were provided with medications which were not labelled with the instructions for use until the time of discharge. Instead, while the patient was in the unit he used a two-part medication card, one section giving the instructions for use, the other forming a simple recording chart which he ticked after taking the dose. Each week a pharmacist checked the residual tablets and the medication card to assess performance and interviewed the patients to discover whether they understood how to take their treatment. The recording section was found to be of little value as most patients completed them at the end of the day and whilst some found the method of providing instructions useful, especially those beginning long-term multiple therapy, others put their own instructions on the bottle label. It was shown that, with careful explanation, patients will take their medication correctly within certain tolerance limits, and that some patients persistently fail because they fail to understand either the instructions themselves or the importance of following them.

The self-administration system for obstetric patients in the Ohio State University Hospital, USA, is co-ordinated by the clinical pharmacist who reviews medication orders, assigns patients to the self-administration programme, instructs them about their medication and monitors their performance (Lucarotti *et al* 1973).

If instructions for use are included on the labels of medication for self administration, care must be taken to see that these are amended if the physician wishes to alter the dose. Consideration must also be given to the security of drugs in this type of system.

ADDITION OF DRUGS TO INTRAVENOUS SOLUTIONS
AND OTHER SPECIAL COMPOUNDING SERVICES

Every general hospital provides an intravenous solution additive service ('i.v. additive service') but with few exceptions, even in the USA this is provided by nursing rather than pharmaceutical staff. Similarly ward nursing staff are often responsible for the preparation of solutions by reconstitution or of suspensions from powdered tablets in order to facilitate drug administration.

Provision of these services by pharmaceutical staff can be regarded as an extension of the unit dose philosophy in that doses are being prepared as ready as possible for administration to the patient and are normally delivered to the ward in single unit packages just prior to the time that they are required. However, because of the additional hazards of microbial and particulate contamination; drug-to-drug, drug-to-fluid and even possible drug-to-container incompatibilities; reduced stability of the medicaments; increased complexity of dose calculations, with correspondingly increased opportunity for medication errors, together with possibly inadequate labelling and mixing, all so obviously requiring the expertise of the pharmacist in his traditional dispensing role to minimise the risks, the introduction of pharmacy i.v. additive services has usually been given a higher priority than other aspects of unit dose systems.

The design of the form used for the prescription and recording of administration of infusion fluids/added drugs, and the manner of its completion, may also be a source of hazard to the patient if the prescriber's intentions cannot be clearly and unambiguously interpreted by the person administering the medication. The design of prescription sheets is outside the scope of this book but the pharmacist has a contribution to make in this respect. The pharmacist should also examine all prescriptions for legibility and completeness before administration to the patient is commenced.

Although described with particular reference to additive services, including preparation of hyperalimentation fluids, many of the considerations in this section apply equally to drug reconstitution services (which may be for sterile injectables or non-sterile products), addition of drugs to irrigation and peritoneal dialysis solutions, provision of injections in prefilled syringes and dilution of allergenic extracts for sensitivity testing. Some American authors use the term 'intravenous additive programme' to embody not only the aseptic preparation of the solutions (the additive service) but also the policies and procedures concerned with their administration.

Drugs may be added to infusion fluid solutions although other routes may be more appropriate and less hazardous. The intravenous route should be avoided if intramuscular or oral administration is feasible. D'Arcy and Thompson (1974) suggested that 'before any drug is added to any infusion fluid container the following questions should be asked:

1.   Is it necessary that the drug shall be given in this way?

2. Is the stability of the particular drug in the selected infusion fluid firmly established?

3. If multiple additives are intended, is the stability in the selected infusion fluid of each drug in the presence of the other firmly established?

4. Will the drug(s) have the intended therapeutic effect if given in high dilution over a period of hours?

5. Since many drugs decompose slowly in infusion fluids, will the interval between drug addition and use of fluid be kept to a minimum? Also, if the duration of the actual infusion is kept short, will it be compatible with the treatment regimen?'

The authors suggest that unless all these questions can be answered in the affirmative the drug or drugs should preferably be given by another method.

Positive indications for continuous infusion are where the drug must be well diluted and given very slowly to avoid irritant or toxic effects (e.g. potassium chloride) or where it is required to achieve a sustained therapeutic effect (e.g. lignocaine, Heparin or oxytocin). Some antibiotics are given by continuous infusion because they are too toxic or irritant to be given by intermittent intravenous administration but the latter method is usually preferred for the remainder if this is the only means of achieving high drug levels in the blood.

Intermittent intravenous administration via an infusion fluid may be accomplished in the following ways:

1. A solution of the drug is drawn into a syringe and given through an injection site on the administration set tubing. Alternatively it may be injected into a fixed needle or cannula or through a diaphragm in the side arm of a three-way tap. The administration time is usually 1–2 minutes. This method is commonly referred to as 'i.v. push' in American literature. If this method is not suitable because of the type of solution or dose of the drug either **2** or **3** are used.

2. In the 'piggyback' system the prescribed dose of the drug is transferred to a small volume of infusion fluid (usually 50 ml) in a second infusion container and is then given by use of a Y-type set or by inserting the needle from the administration set for the small volume bottle into an injection site on the main set. Administration is normally over 5–15 minutes or at the same rate as the large volume solution.

3. Use of 'volume control' sets. A special volumetric i.v. administration set with a calibrated chamber is used in place of the routine set; 25–50 ml of solution from the main bottle is run into this chamber and the prepared dose of the drug injected into it from a syringe; after mixing the diluted dose of the drug is administered to the patient before restarting the primary infusion solution. It is generally recommended that this method be restricted to paediatrics and special situations where very accurate measurement of fluid or drug administered is required.

The relative advantages and disadvantages of three methods for intermittent therapy are discussed in detail by Paxines and Samuels (1975) who also describe a combined volume control set/piggyback system. A 'retrograde technique' designed to reduce nursing time taken by use of the piggyback system is described by Eling and Brissie (1974).

It will be seen from the above that use of intermittent rather than continuous intravenous therapy does not necessarily remove the requirement for pharmaceutical involvement. Disadvantages with the technique may include:

1.   Where hospital policies still require only medical staff to carry out direct intravenous injections, an unacceptable additional workload may be created for them.

2.   Repeated use of the injection site on the administration set could increase the possibility of contamination.

3.   Insufficent time may be allowed for the administration of the bolus.

4.   A concentrated solution of the drug may react with the solution in the giving set, when the incompatibility would be difficult to detect. In any case, the concentration of the drug and the vehicle for the solution must be selected with care.

Since there is a risk of microbial contamination when drugs are to be added to sterile products, wherever possible they should be incorporated along with other constituents of the fluid before final sterilization. Potassium chloride, often the drug most frequently added to infusion fluids, and lignocaine, are stable to autoclaving and, with relatively few exceptions, need not, therefore, form part of an additive service. Heparin in Sodium Chloride Injection can be autoclaved and may also be supplied as a ready prepared solution where a standard strength is indicated; it is preferably administered by infusion pump. The increased range of sterile products required may cause storage problems but there is often scope for considerable rationalisation, using commercially available fluids where possible; the clinical pharmacist can play a key role in this. Thus, by supply of ready prepared solutions where possible and advice to medical and nursing staff on pharmaceutical aspects of procedures, the potential demands on an i.v. additive service (whether it be provided by medical, nursing or pharmaceutical staff) may be considerably reduced from the level indicated by the D'Arcy and Thompson (1974) survey when 39.2% of all infusion fluids were found to contain additives.

The education and training role of the pharmacist need not be restricted to advice on choice of route but may be extended to cover advice on the procedures to be followed in carrying out the drug additions where these must be done on the ward (aseptic technique, mixing procedures, storage if necessary, inspection and labelling records) and in fitting sets to the infusion container etc. The recommendations of a National Coordinating Committee on Large Volume Parenterals (1975), an American reference, gives a usefully comprehensive guide to the techniques and policies to be followed.

A 6-month educational programme consisting of symposia on the problems of administering drugs by continuous intravenous infusion, and the introduction of an incompatibility chart printed on the reverse of the fluids chart was described by Brodlie *et al* (1974). Following this programme there was a tenfold decrease in the number of times antibiotics were administered to surgical patients by continuous infusion and a sevenfold decrease for medical patients. The combined effect of the programme and the introduction of ready made infusion fluids containing potassium chloride was to reduce the number of additives by 62%. For surgical patients the incidence of incompatibilities occurring between a drug and the fluid or between drugs fell from 15% in the 2 months immediately prior to the programme to 2% in the 2 months immediately following it; no recognised incompatibility was found in a further 2-month period. An incompatibility may result in embolism, granuloma or other adverse effects, blocked administration sets or a reduction or total loss of therapeutic effect. Research and documentation of possible physical or chemical incompatibility between added drugs or between them and the infusion fluid presents very great problems because of the large numbers of combinations possible. There are more than 11 000 possible combinations or pairs, threes and fours using only 24 drugs commonly added to infusion fluids. Although D'Arcy and Thompson (1974) found in their Northern Ireland survey that 96% of infusions with additives had only one drug added, 2.8% with two drugs, 0.9% with three drugs and 0.3% (one bottle) with four, an Israeli survey revealed 21% with four or more drugs added, the maximum number of additions to one container being seven. Clearly, multiple additions to a single fluid should be avoided if at all possible in order to minimise the risk of drug interaction.

The incidence of incompatibilities is relatively high; for example, in one trial 23 out of 207 pairs of drugs were incompatible when added to 5% dextrose in water. The evidence that an incompatibility exists may be visible when precipitation, haziness, crystallisation or discoloration may be seen but in other combinations invisible changes may take place which can only be detected by prior laboratory investigation. Even visible changes may take some time to develop. Drugs may be compatible at one concentration but incompatible at another. Incompatibilities may not be due to the drug itself but arise from the stabilisers, etc used in the formulation. Variations may therefore be found between brands of the same drug, between the charts produced in different countries and even within the same brand with a change in formulation. The order of mixing may be important in determining whether or not an incompatibility occurs. These points are discussed in detail by Neil (1977). Similarly there is often a lack of specific information concerning the stability of a drug under varying conditions; even pharmaceutical manufacturers may be unable or unwilling to assist (Jacobs 1970). This information is necessary to determine whether the drug will deteriorate to an unacceptable degree during the period of the infusion. Even when detailed stability data is available this decision as to acceptability must be arbitrary but the criterion proposed by Carlin and Perkins (1968) of not more than 10% loss in potency during the period of the infusion has become tacitly agreed in recent years (Ashwin & Lynn 1975). With adequate data it should also be possible to establish the maximum acceptable storage time under refrigeration prior to administration for the solution and additive. This information may be essential for the assessment of the requirements to be met by a central pharmacy i.v. additive service.

This lack of adequate data on compatibility and stability of drugs in infusion fluids highlights the need for continuing extensive research in this field by pharmaceutical manufacturers and hospital pharmacists. It should not, however, inhibit pharmacists from communicating the available information to medical and nursing staff by the most effective methods possible as they are unlikely to receive it from other sources.

Because of the variation in prescribing practices, a number of pharmacists have carried out local surveys to determine which drugs are most commonly added to infusion fluids (e.g. by studying drug additive labels on returned infusion containers) and have then drawn up charts based on those incompatibilities most likely to occur in their hospital. The size of the chart and the amount of information to be contained on it are then not excessive. In the survey by D'Arcy and Thompson (1974), for example, ten drugs (including potassium chloride, heparin and lignocaine) accounted for 95.8% of all additions to infusion fluids. A statement is usually included to the effect that the pharmacy should be consulted if further information is required or any doubt exists; despite this 'disclaimer' type statement, however, medical and nursing staff must assume to some extent that if an incompatibility is not listed it is safe to mix the two or more drugs under consideration. There is thus no 'fail safe' mechanism which would be inherent in a list of *compatible* drugs and fluids, when the pharmacy could be consulted if it was desired to use a combination *not* on the list. Nevertheless, introduction of such charts, together with an educational programme aimed at reducing the incidence of multiple drug additions to a single fluid has been shown to be successful. The chart may also include recommended procedures to be followed in the addition of drugs to infusion fluids, the properties of intravenous infusion fluids in relation to drugs added and an indication of the period for which frequently used drugs are 'stable' in common infusion fluids (using the 10% criterion described above). Jacobs (1970) also suggests a table giving the data required to prepare a solution from the powder form of a drug (the solvent to be used and its volume to give a specified final concentration), the rate of administration (based on manufacturers' recommendations) and the optimal storage conditions for the reconstituted solution.

Publications useful for their content and also as sources for further references when preparing such charts include those by Jacobs (1970), Neil (1977), Grayson (1971) who gives an extensive table of previously published information on incompatibilities, Ashwin and Lynn (1975) for stability of semisynthetic penicillins, Kramer *et al* (1972) and Carlin and Perkins (1968) for American literature on incompatibilities and Ho (1972) for the prediction of pharmaceutical stability of parenteral solutions from basic kinetic studies. Having produced a chart it is essential that it be updated as necessary and that it is brought to the attention of all new members of staff. Wall charts and/or pocket-sized leaflets may be used.

The risk of microbial contamination is often quoted as a reason for providing a pharmacy central i.v. additive service since better facilities can be provided for use by staff specially trained in aseptic techniques; at present the majority of additions are carried out by nursing staff (97.5%; the remainder by medical staff; D'Arcy & Thompson 1974) in ward utility rooms or at the patient's beside. The majority of standard infusion fluids will allow survival of the contaminant and some are almost ideal for supporting growth of microorganisms, particularly Gram-negative bacteria. Since 1 litre containers may be in position for up to 24 hours, any contamination could reach levels which may cause pyrogenic reactions or even clinical sepsis. Moreover, unless the administration set is changed every 24 hours these contaminants may persist for many days after the bottle has been changed.

It must be stressed, however, that addition of drugs is by no means the only potential source of contamination of fluids and sets; the influx of unfiltered air into the container during administration and faulty technique in fitting sets to the infusion bottle or bag may be at least as important. The importance of applying aseptic techniques from the time the infusion container was removed from its carton to the completion of administration was emphasised by the investigation by Pinckney *et al.* (1973).

Experimental evidence of the risk of microbial contamination on the addition of drugs to infusion fluids is to some extent conflicting and at variance with what might be expected from theoretical considerations (D'Arcy 1976). One investigation, in which the residual fluid remaining in 101 containers after administration was examined, indicated that 55.7% of solutions which contained additives were contaminated compared with 12.5% for those which contained none. Another survey in which a larger number of containers (1003) were examined, again indicated a higher percentage contaminated when additions had been made (6.69% compared to 3.61%) but the highest levels of contamination were observed in the residual fluids which contained no additives. A third independent study on 183 containers showed 3.3% to be contaminated when drugs *had* been added compared with 5.5% when they *had not*; it was specifically stated that only one bottle contained an antibiotic. Little or no experimental detail was quoted in any of the reports. In another study, based on a monitoring programme for a pharmacy i.v. drug additive service, 4% of 155 solutions were found to be contaminated with organisms indicative of a break in aseptic technique, although all solutions with more than one addition were found to be sterile; it was concluded that operators may have a false sense of security in using a laminar air flow hood but take greater care with those solutions known to be associated with a higher risk.

A membrane filter unit of 0.45 μm pore size for attachment between the end of the fluid administration set tubing and the cannula entering the patient's vein is now commercially available. This is said to increase patient safety by reducing the risk from both bacterial and particle contamination and a number of studies have also shown reduced incidence of phlebitis. The main disadvantage appears to be the cost of the units themselves and of new giving sets to be used after administration of blood and associated products. Unless the pharmacy is providing a *complete* i.v. additive service, labels should be provided for attachment to the container by medical and nursing staff; these should have spaces to enter at least the name of the patient, name and dose of drug added and the date and time of the addition.

A committee with representatives of the medical, nursing and pharmaceutical professions should be formed in each District or Area to establish and implement policies and procedures on the addition of drugs to infusion fluids, including definition of areas of responsibility and training needs; such policies would be required to be approved by the Area Health Authority as the employing authority and as the body responsible for the care and welfare of the patient. Whether these measures are considered sufficient or whether a complete service should be provided with pharmaceutical staff carrying out the additions themselves may be regarded as to some extent controversial and in any case can often only be decided according to local circumstances. For example, where acute beds are scattered between several small hospitals some distance apart in a rural area, the logistical difficulties may be almost insuperable. Even in Central London it has been found that special problems in collection, preparation and delivery of intravenous drug additive orders in time for administration were sufficiently great to cause the abandonment of an experimental, daytime additive service to a large peripheral hospital with a twice daily ward pharmacy service. Because of the limited stability of many of the added drugs in the infusion fluids an extended-hours or 24-hour, 7-day service from the pharmacy is essential if all but emergency additions are to be carried out. The survey by D'Arcy and Thompson (1974) revealed that approximately half the total number of drug additions were made between 5 p.m. and 9 a.m., with approximately 40% of these between midnight and 9 a.m.; no attempt was made, however, to assess the proportion where the stability of the drug would allow preparation at more convenient times. Although the additional pharmacy staff required to provide this may also enable introduction of a full unit dose service at the same time and nursing time will be freed for other duties, an overall increase in costs is almost inevitable. A part-time (9 a.m. to 5 p.m.) service has been advocated as an interim measure to minimise the risks associated with at least a proportion of the additions to be carried out, although again increases in the pharmacy staff establishment will be likely.

Preparation of the final product under aseptic conditions should be a significant advantage for a pharmacy i.v. additives service provided the staff involved remain sufficiently highly motivated to maintain full precautions. Provision of near-ideal facilities may be feasible for only one location where it would be uneconomical to provide these for each ward (although in some American hospitals 'decentralised' pharmacies associated with unit dose supply systems may have a room set aside for i.v. additions). The smaller number of individuals involved when a pharmacy service is operated reduces time spent training and supervision. Fully comprehensive and continously updated information on drug stability and incompatibility should be available in the pharmacy whereas it may not be feasible to provide this to all wards. Again, motivation to use this information at both ward and pharmacy levels is important. Pharmacists can more easily ensure that the available knowledge is applied in practice when they are themselves directly responsible for provision of the service. Calculations and adequate mixing can be correctly carried out and fully comprehensive standardised labels prepared by trained staff familiar with the work and away from pressures of other ward activities. Medication errors such as use of the wrong drug or solution, the wrong dosage, or administration of an unordered drug should also be avoided or minimised. Where pharmacists do not see fluid and additive drug prescriptions on the ward, the provision of this service enables dosages etc to be checked. Complete records of drugs added or batch numbers can also be ensured.

Pharmacy operated intravenous additive services are rare in Britain but have been described by Hetherington (1971), Goldberg (1974) and Birch *et al* (1974). The principle components of a pharmacy operated i.v. additive service are as follows:

1. A prescription for the fluid and additions. Ideally this should be the document used in the pharmacy for the preparation of the solution with additives. The intravenous infusion request form described by Goldberg achieves this, but a large number may be accumulated for a single patient on prolonged treatment, possibly causing some difficulty when subsequently filed in case notes. In the system described by Birch *et al*, requests for additions to fluids may be received from ward pharmacists, by telephone, or as written requests from nursing staff, but in all cases before administration is commenced the original doctor's prescription is seen and initialed by a pharmacist. Other systems described use an NCR copy of the prescription.

2. Check dosage and check absence of known incompatibility etc.

3. A typed label. Details which should be included are:

    a. Patient's name, hospital number, ward and physician's name.
    b. Name and volume of fluid.
    c. Names and amounts of additives.
    d. Bottle sequence number.
    e. Initials of technician and supervising pharmacist.
    f. Preparation date and time.

g. Expiry date and time.
h. Prescribed administration time and flow rate.
i. Any relevant warnings.
j. Initials of nurse setting up bottle for administration.

4. 'Scheduling' of order where the prescription is for more than one container; details are entered on a schedule to indicate when further solutions must be prepared (usually 1 hour before administration). A card system is often used since this allows filing of all patient's requirements in the order of their time of preparation. A 'day book' record may also be maintained.
5. Assembly of additive(s) and solution. The techniques, accommodation and equipment for carrying this out are beyond the scope of this chapter. A new overseal is applied to the container which has been checked for particulate contamination and colour change before the label is applied (upside down to facilitate reading when the container is hung from a drip stand). Further checks on the label, the contents and the calculations may be made by the pharmacist. In some American hospitals the first bottle each day for a patient is sent to the ward with the administration set already inserted in order to ensure that the sets are changed every 24 hours; this procedure is controversial as there may be a risk of contamination arising during delivery to the ward.
6. Delivery and ward storage. If storage of the final solutions is necessary, either in the pharmacy or on the ward, refrigeration is essential.
7. Final check by nurse for absence of particulate contamination or colour change and that the solution is as prescribed.
8. Administration. Further checks for particulate contamination may be made.

The duties of clinical pharmacists at San Francisco Veterans Administration Hospital, Califoria, include documentation of clinical experiences from the administration of new drug additive combinations. Before setting up an i.v. additive service it is often considered necessary to carry out a survey of the quantities of fluids used, the proportion with additives, which drugs are added, and when. The survey should include intermittent i.v. administration if it is intended to provide a reconstitution service for this. Rather than attempt to survey all prescriptions, a specific percentage (e.g. 20%) on each ward each day for 3–6 weeks may be selected using a random sampling technique. The results will provide an estimation of the potential workload for the service, allowing assessment of staffing, equipment and accommodation requirements.

Two American studies have estimated the time taken to prepare each admixture. In one, although 2.7 minutes was required to carry out the addition, an average of a further 5.1 minutes was required as 'back-up' time in prepackaging, reconstitution, obtaining supplies, delivery, cleaning up and pricing. In the other study an average total time of 9.2 minutes was required to carry out approximately the same tasks. The proportion of the workload which can be delegated to technicians and the training of all grades of staff must be considered.

Sterility testing should be carried out on some of the solutions prepared by the pharmacy i.v. additive service in order to ensure that procedures are being carried out correctly. The samples should be selected randomly from those actually prepared for patients so that the operator has no prior knowledge that the solution is to be tested. A membrane filtration method (for example that described by Buth *et al* 1973) is often preferred. Routine monitoring of the environment is, of course, also essential. A disadvantage of a pharmacy operated i.v. additive service is that some wastage is almost inevitable because solutions have been prepared before therapy is changed. Good communications will minimise this but where it is unavoidable it may be possible to use these solutions in the sterility testing programme.

Whether or not the pharmacy provides a full i.v. additive service it will be seen from the considerations described in this section that the addition of drugs to infusion fluids constitutes an extremely important aspect of ward pharmacy; the pharmacist can use his knowledge of drug properties and therapeutic requirements in order to achieve safer and more efficaceous treatment for the patient.

The report of the working party on the addition of drugs to intravenous infusion fluids (DHSS 1976) summarises the pharmacists responsibilities as follows: 'Wherever possible, drug-infusion mixtures should be provided from the pharmacy. Pharmacists should advise on pharmaceutical aspects of policies and procedures concerned with the addition and administration of drugs via intravenous infusion fluids, and should ensure that doctors and nurses are alerted to specific problems which may arise. Pharmacists should not only provide for the training of their own staff but should also advise on the training of doctors and nurses in this area of drug therapy.'

URGENT AND EMERGENCY SUPPLIES

With any distribution system, unless the pharmacy is staffed 24 hours a day, 7 days a week, situations will arise where medicines are required when the department is not staffed. These occasions may arise as a result of a defect in the drug distribution system (failure of nurse to order or pharmacy to supply), but most frequently occur because it is desirable to start as soon as possible on a newly prescribed treatment which is not stocked on the ward. These urgent requirements may be met by:

1. Provision of central 'emergency' cupboards, for use by medical and/or nursing staff.
2. Access to pharmacy stocks by medical and/or nursing staff, as an alternative to **1.** or as additional back-up.

3. Pharmacist on-call, either by specific rota or by a list of telephone numbers and/or addresses at the hospital switchboard. This may be an alternative to **1** and **2** or as a supplement.

4. Pharmacy technician on-call.

Method **3** is preferred as dispensing is carried out by a pharmacist and pharmaceutical advice is available. However, unless there are several pharmacists on the staff of the department, a specific rota may be onerous to the individuals concerned, particularly as at present no payment can be made for these duties and allowance of time off duty for that spent on a call cannot compensate for the inconvenience caused. Payment can be made to pharmacy technicians so that, provided no dispensing is involved unless a pharmacist is present, with supplies restricted to prepacked items, their participation in a system of supply for urgent items may be considered. Prepacked items can be provided for method **1** but it may be difficult to avoid some dispensing by individuals other than a pharmacist when access to the pharmacy is allowed. Where medical staff only are allowed access to a cupboard or to the pharmacy the physician may be influenced to use a more readily available drug to accomplish the same purpose. The location of medicines in the pharmacy must be fully indexed if other staff are to have access to them. Problems with the security of drugs could also arise where medical and nursing staff have *unrestricted* access to the pharmacy out of normal working hours, particularly as there are a large number of partly used containers and the exact quantity in each is rarely known or checked each morning. An emergency cupboard containing only sealed prepacked drugs is to be preferred for this reason, although it is difficult to make these stocks sufficiently comprehensive, especially as some drugs require refrigerated storage. The Department of Health and Social Security, in circular HM (70)1 on *Security of Drugs Liable to Misuse* recommend in paragraph 6(b) : 'It should not normally be necessary for anyone except a pharmacist to have access outside working hours to the pharmacy or pharmacy store cupboards. Drugs liable to misuse (and other drugs) which may be required in an emergency and are not included in ward or departmental stocks should be kept in an emergency drug store cupboard which can be reached without entry to the main pharmacy. Access to the emergency drug store should be limited to authorised members of the medical staff who should be required to sign for the key(s) on each occasion.' Security arrangements should be such that only persons authorised by hospital regulations can gain possession of the keys. It is also recommended that separate alarm systems be provided to cover drugs in the main pharmacy and the emergency store cupboard.

The 'drug station' of the 'Brewer system', described on p. 295, can be used as a source of urgently required medicines. The patient identification plate is not used but an automatic record of which drug was withdrawn, and by whom, is recorded in the machine for reference by the pharmacist on the following day; this improves security and ensures correct replenishment. Handwritten records are usually requested from medical and/or nursing staff using conventional cupboards or when access to the pharmacy is permitted.

Retail pharmacies have been used to provide out-of-hours service in America. Greater cooperation between hospital and general practice pharmacists in this respect may also be possible in the United Kingdom.

The above considerations generally relate to urgent rather than emergency requirements. However, it is essential that certain drugs are always available for instant use on each ward or group of wards, for example those used in cases of cardiac arrest. These are usually placed in an emergency box or a tray covered with cellophane in an easily accessible place known to all ward staff. Although drugs required on an emergency trolley should ideally be stored in a lockable container attached to it, with the whole unit immobilised when not in use, it is generally acceptable to place the drugs in a sealed box which is itself inside a container fixed to the trolley frame, provided suitable safeguards against tampering by unauthorised persons are observed (Aitken Report; DHSS 1958). The contents of the box or tray should be periodically checked for completeness against an agreed written list. However, if a readily breakable seal is provided it will be obvious that drugs have been used and replenishment is necessary. This may be done by the pharmacy providing a replacement sealed box at the earliest possible opportunity after being notified by nursing staff. The box or tray should be clearly labelled with the expiry date of the product which will first reach the end of its shelf-life. The arrangement of the drugs should allow easy access and identification; plastic tool boxes, which on opening reveal several layers of trays divided into compartments, have been widely used for this purpose (an illustration is given by Lee *et al* 1971). The number of medicines contained in the box should be as small as possible to allow rapid selection and separate boxes may be provided for drugs for general emergency (circulatory collapse, allergic reactions, convulsions, bronchospasm) and for cardiac arrest.

Clinical pharmacists in some American hospitals have been included in the actual resuscitation team, their duties being to maintain all equipment and supplies in a state of readiness, be responsible for the preparation of medications for administration and record their use and the procedures performed, provide advice on dosages, incompatibilities etc, and participate in evaluation and teaching of cardiopulmonary resuscitation. Experienced pharmacists providing a 24-hour service are necessary before this can be attempted.

Pharmacy staff should also be responsible for ensuring that stocks of drugs and infusion fluids kept for major disasters are rotated as necessary. It has been suggested in some American hospitals that pharmacists should be available in such emergencies to prepare medications.

WITHDRAWAL OF DEFECTIVE MEDICINES

An efficient drug distribution system should also facilitate the withdrawal of products which have been found to be defective. Notification of a defect is normally received via a Regional 'clearing house' by telephone, with written confirmation, for the most urgent messages. The procedures followed by the District Pharmaceutical Officer or Principal Pharmacist in charge of the hospital(s) concerned in disseminating the information will again depend on the urgency of the withdrawal; they will normally be in writing and have been circulated to all staff concerned so that each member is aware of his or her responsibilities.

If it is known that the batch of product in question was never purchased, it may not be necessary to take any action. Recording of batch numbers on stock control cards is extremely useful in this respect provided that *all* medicines received in the hospitals concerned are recorded. It is most important therefore that, for example, medical samples of new preparations be left in the pharmacy by manufacturer's representatives for subsequent issue, if necessary, to the medical staff or wards concerned; the pharmacist is then also able to ensure that samples are not issued to unauthorised members of staff and that any unwanted medicines are destroyed in a safe manner. It is also most important that, after packing medicines for ward issue, the identity of the manufacturer and the batch number can be traced.

When it is known that the product and batch in question have been purchased, or if it is considered possible, subsequent action may be to telephone wards concerned with subsequent written confirmation, circulate a letter only, or arrange for pharmacists to personally withdraw the defective stocks; the action will depend on local circumstances and the urgency of the recall. All stocks returned to the pharmacy department must be carefully quarantined.

Follow-up of outpatients who have received a defective product is likely to be extremely difficult. If patient medication profiles are maintained which can be annotated with the manufacturer and batch number of medicines issued, these will normally be filed in alphabetical order of patient's name. If the information is recorded on the outpatient prescription, it may be difficult to identify which case notes should be examined for the drug in question.

When a serious defect, potentially dangerous to patients, is discovered on a ward there is normally a written hospital procedure to be followed based on Department of Health and Social Security advice contained in circular HSC(IS)41 (*Reporting of accidents with, and serious defects in medicinal products and other medical supplies and equipment*). For defects in infusion fluid solutions supplementary advice is contained in circular HSC(IS)118 (*Reporting of infusion incidents involving suspected contamination*).

The above procedures are in addition to the pharmacist's regular checking of ward stocks and withdrawal of material which has passed the expiry date.

WARD STORAGE OF PHARMACEUTICAL PREPARATIONS

All distribution systems involve some requirements for ward storage of medicines and other pharmaceutical supplies such as disinfectants and urine testing materials. The custody of ward stocks is normally entirely the responsibility of the nurse in charge or his or her official deputy. The domestic department may be responsible for the safe-keeping of certain disinfectants used by them.

The pharmaceutical department may assume responsibility for replenishment of these stocks, will advise on the type and location of cupboards, regularly inspecting them, and will assure the quality of the preparation at the time of use, but is rarely in a position to do more than this, as pharmacy staff do not administer or use the items stored. Thus the Aitken Report (DHSS 1958) recommended that nursing staff rather than pharmacists should be required to check the physical stock of dangerous drugs (now controlled drugs) on the ward against the record of doses given. It was recommended, however, that the pharmacist may be able to give technical assistance when an apparent discrepancy is being investigated and should also report any 'unusual features' observed in his contact with wards.

Each ward should normally have the following storage units:

1. Controlled drugs cupboard. Private hospitals and nursing homes holding stocks of schedule 2 or 3 controlled drugs (except certain liquids) must store them in a cabinet designed to meet the requirements of the Misuse of Drugs (Safe Custody) Regulations 1973. In wards in public hospitals the drugs are stored in an independently locked inner compartment to the poisons cupboard (see below), the whole unit being constructed to British Standard 2881:1969. The cupboard is so designed that it cannot be closed unless the inner door has been closed, locked and the key removed; a red warning light is provided to show when the outer door is unlocked and this can be wired in parallel with another light in the sister's office. A controlled drugs cupboard should not be provided in a department which does not have a person authorised to possess these drugs; this could apply, for example, to a radiology department. Controlled drugs supplied from a pharmacy department in a public hospital should be requisitioned on the design of form recommended by the Aitken Report and although not specifically required by the Misuse of Drugs Regulations 1973, the design of ward register recommended should also be used. Any individually dispensed controlled drugs, as well as ward stocks, should be stored in this cupboard.

2. Schedule 1 poisons cupboard. Although the Poisons Rules (1972) (with subsequent amendment) were repealed on 1 February 1978, so that the requirements relating to the supply and storage of poisons in hospitals and other health service premises cease to have statutory effect, the DHSS asked health authorities in Health Notice HN(78)4 (*Poisons: supply and storage in health service* *premises*) to 'ensure that the existing practices and procedures required by the Poisons Rules continue to be observed' until replacement provisions are made under the Medicines Act (1968). The Poisons Rules (1972) required that 'every substance included in schedule 1 kept in a ward in any institution shall be stored in a cupboard reserved solely for the storage of poisons and other dangerous substances'. An 'institution' means 'any hospital, infirmary, health centre, dispensary, clinic, nursing home or other institution at which human ailments are treated' or any family planning clinic as defined in the rules. No definition for 'dangerous substances' was given and some pharmacists argue that, since all medicines are potentially dangerous, no distinction need or should be made for schedule 1 poisons. The Aitken Report disagreed with this view, stating 'we think that the advantage of securing for the most potent drugs of all a degree of care which one could not hope to be accorded to every medicine outweighs the possible disadvantage of nursing and other staff inferring that the remaining drugs are less potent than they in fact are'. It was recommended, however, that 'the hospital pharmacist or consultant should have discretion to decide whether a new experimental drug should be treated as a schedule 1 poison', in which case it should be labelled 'Store in schedule 1 poisons cupboard'. Any schedule 1 poisons dispensed for an individual patient should be stored in this cupboard in addition to ward stocks, unless required in the medicine trolley.

3.   Medicines cupboard(s). For all those medicines not stored in the other units described, although infusion fluid solutions may be placed on open shelves. Construction should again be to the British Standard.

4.   Reagent cupboard. For all reagents, strips and tablets used in urine testings, etc.

5.   General disinfectants and cleaning materials cupboard. Normally the responsibility of the domestic department.

6.   Refrigerator. Where drugs requiring low-temperature storage are required to be stored on the ward, a lockable refrigerator reserved solely for medicines should preferably be provided. One of 1 cubic foot capacity will be found to be adequate for most locations unless it is required to hold a number of infusion fluid bottles. It may be necessary for several wards in a block to share a refrigerator. Where the ward kitchen refrigerator has to be used, the medicines should be kept on a separate shelf from any other contents, or in a locked box.

7.   Medicine trolley. This should be used solely for the medicines in current use on the ward, not as a permanent storage, and will not normally be used for controlled drugs. Such a trolley saves a considerable amount of nursing time as there is no need for medicines to be returned to their cupboards after every round and, especially where a pharmacist checks the contents of the trolley against the prescriptions, can reduce the chance of medication errors. Although its design is varied in different distribution systems, it must be capable of being locked, (perhaps with 'slam' locks, which do not require a key to lock them, in psychiatric hospitals), the section containing the drugs must be permanently fixed to the trolley frame, and the whole unit must be either locked in a cupboard or to a wall or floor when not in use. In some designs a separate schedule 1 poisons compartment is provided, but this is often so small that easy selection of the required medicine is difficult and may even encourage labelling of bottle caps by nursing staff and consequently mixing of caps may lead to a serious source of medication error; unless a uniform design of cap and container is supplied there may be a tendency to select on the basis of these characteristics rather than the contents of the label. Medicine measures, water, a box for used containers and, where injections are included, syringes, needles etc, may all be carried to avoid the need for the nurse to break the medicine round. If the top of the trolley is unsuitable for writing, a separate folding shelf is necessary. Where the physical layout of the ward or hospital makes use of a trolley impossible an easily portable cabinet or case may be feasible. It may not be considered worthwhile to have a medicine trolley in a paediatric ward because of the high usage of liquid preparations requiring refrigeration. However, where a unit dose system is in operation for this specialty and the pharmacy service is frequent, the extent of deterioration in a limited period at room temperature may be within acceptable limits; alternatively, a signal may be placed on the outside of the patient's drawer to remind the nurse to collect the refrigerated dose before commencing the medicine round.

The Aitken Report recommended that all the types of cupboard should be locked, as many of the contents were potentially harmful. The keys to the controlled drugs cupboards, the schedule 1 poisons cupboard and the medicine trolley should be kept *on the person* of the sister or nurse in charge of the ward; this requirement should not be allowed to encourage the keeping of patients' valuables in these cupboards, even as a temporary measure. The keys to the remaining cupboards should be available only to authorised personnel. Keys should be handed over with changes of duty, with the same set of cupboards used by night staff.

Where medicines for external use are to be stored in the same cupboard as those for internal administration they should be placed on separate shelves. However, the number of preparations to be kept in the general medicines cupboard is usually such that separate storage units have to be provided. The cupboard for internal medicines can then be more shallow with narrow shelves fitted to the door to give maximum storage space for a large number of small items whilst retaining the facility for the easy selection of the correct medicine. Drugs which may be required in an emergency may be stored independently of the above system.

Standardising the location and design of cupboards in all the wards of a hospital, where this is feasible, with a uniform system of arranging the contents, simplifies the work and training of nursing and pharmaceutical staff when their duties are rotated. The Aitken Report recommended that the dangerous drugs (now controlled drugs) cupboard, the schedule 1 poisons cupboard and the medicines cupboard should in general be sited wherever possible in such a position that 'the nurse can still keep an eye on her patients while she is at the cupboard ..., should be in a good light, both natural and artificial, at a suitable level and over or near a table or flap on which medicines can be prepared'. The medicine trolley is preferably stored adjacent to these cupboards when not in use. Storage of the majority of preparations within the same area of the ward increases the convenience for nursing staff. The cupboard for reagents is usually sited in the dirty utility or 'sluice' room of the ward, the cupboard for disinfectants and cleaning materials wherever this is most convenient. The pharmacist advising on location of storage facilities will check that the position of hot water and steam pipes, radiators etc, does not significantly increase the temperature within the cupboards.

The extent of the stock will vary considerably according to the medicine distribution system operated within the hospital and the medical specialty of the ward. The items to be stored and the quantity of each should be agreed between medical, nursing and pharmaceutical staff, perhaps after a preliminary survey of the ward usage; however, prediction of ward requirements may be difficult even when an attempt is made to do this objectively (Barnett & Calder 1969). Any changes may only be made by mutual agreement. Stocks of inflammable liquids such as ether should be as small as possible.

Stocklists may be provided for each ward, usually by the pharmacist. These may be in the form of a standard list of medicines normally held on all wards, but with deletions where a stock is considered unnecessary, together with a supplementary list of preparations which are the requirements of a particular ward. Where preprinted requisitions are used for ordering pharmaceutical preparations these may form the basis of the lists and also show the maximum stock levels. A cross-referenced list of contents which gives the approved name for the most widely known proprietary brand name and vice versa may be useful as will inclusion of cupboard and shelf numbers for each preparation, especially where a pharmacological classification is adopted (see below). One copy of the lists should be attached to the inside of the cupboard doors (where possible), a second should be available to the prescribing doctor (perhaps inside either the prescription form holder or the cover of the ward medicine requisition book), and a third retained in the pharmacy.

The contents of all the cupboards, including the medicine trolley, must be arranged systematically, with all labels visible, or overstocking or missed doses of a medicine may result. This may be facilitated by attaching the label to a narrow face of the bottle so that the containers can be packed closer together. Labelling in this way may, however, also result in the instability of the bottle when in racks on the medicine trolley. Medicines may be arranged in alphabetical order throughout or in broad pharmacological groupings in alphabetical order. The latter system has the following advantages:

1. It shows more easily which drugs are available from ward stock for a particular condition.
2. It reinforces nurse training.
3. It physically separates drugs with similar names but different uses, reducing the potential for medication error.

With this system, however, alphabetically arranged stocklists showing the shelf number for each item will be useful. The same system of arrangement should, as far as possible, be used throughout the hospital.

Pharmaceutical staff may have responsibility for the organisation of the cupboard contents and, for example, a pharmacy technician may check this weekly against the agreed list, also withdrawing all medicines which have passed their expiry date, those which are not stock items or are no longer in use. This check may be an integral part of a 'topping-up' system of stock supply.

The Poisons Rules require that 'all places in which poisons are kept in an institution shall be inspected at intervals of not more than three months by a pharmacist or other person appointed for the purpose ...' The Aitkin Report recommended that this inspection should always be carried out by a pharmacist, should extend to the other medicines cupboards, and should include advice to the sister on storage conditions; the matron should always be provided with a report of the findings.

The points which a pharmacist, assisted where appropriate by a technician, might check on a routine inspection of ward cupboards are:

1. That the condition of cupboards themselves, including locks, is satisfactory.
2. That the cupboards are used for the correct types of pharmaceutical preparation.
3. That internal and external use preparations are physically separated.
4. That the contents correspond to the ward stocklist making amendments where necessary.
5. That patients whose individually dispensed medicines are stored in the cupboards are still inpatients.
6. That any drug samples on the ward were issued through the pharmacy.
7. That products with an expiry date are still within their shelf-life.
8. That undated products have not deteriorated to an unacceptable degree.
9. That the temperature in the refrigerator is maintained within acceptable limits.
10. That containers are, as far as possible, uniform in appearance with complete labels.

This checklist can be incorporated into a form to give a permanent record of the inspection, a copy, if necessary, being sent to the appropriate senior nursing officer. Some of the points may be checked more frequently than every three months, in which case it becomes more important to ensure that the other items are not forgotten.

DRUG ADMINISTRATION BY PHARMACY STAFF

Although administration of the medicine is the final component of the hospital drug distribution system, this activity is generally regarded and accepted as being a nursing function. However, if the clinical pharmacist accompanies the nurse on some of the medicine rounds he may be able to detect, for example, potential sources of medication error or problems in administration which can be solved by alternative forms of drug presentation.

In several American hospitals, medicines are administered by a team of nurses or technicians under the direction of the pharmacy department. Advantages claimed include absolute pharmaceutical control of the medicines from purchase to administration, fewer interdepartmental procedures and more effective use of professional time.

The use of specialised medication nurses is said to work well for medicines to be administered at regular intervals, although it is less satisfactory for those to be given 'as required'. These nurses are able to gain a wider knowledge of drugs (including their potential adverse reactions) than would otherwise be the case, which should improve patient safety, but it is likely to be more difficult for them to be aware of all aspects of the patient's treatment. The system is said to reduce the opportunities for pilfering of drugs and to free ward nurses for greater flexibility in patient care.

Medication technicians, trained to assist in the unit dose drug distribution system and to administer drugs to patients under the supervision of a pharmacist, have been introduced into a few American hospitals because of dissatisfaction with the existing system of administration and because of a shortage and high rate of turnover of nursing staff. The technicians may generally administer all medicines except where these form part of another procedure (e.g. wound dressing), intravenous injections by bolus, enemas, bladder irrigations, intradermal tests and blood or blood substitutes. Rubin and Harrison (1975) gave a job description for such a post and described a training programme of 9 weeks duration, 6 weeks being spent on observation of medicine rounds, lectures and private study and the final 3 weeks on the ward administering of drugs under the supervision of a pharmacist; the ability of trainees to administer drugs in a satisfactory manner is evaluated and examinations must be passed before a certificate is awarded. A minimum of seventeen technicians are required, according to Rubin and Harrison, to provide drug administration, unit dose and i.v. admixture services to 120 beds, all critically ill patients. Resistance to change on the part of nursing staff, legal complications and additional pharmacy costs are some of the reasons given for the general lack of support for the concept in other hospitals.

Pharmacists themselves have been involved in the administration of methadone in drug abuse treatment centres. At Brooke Army Medical Center in America a pharmacist sets up intravenous injections of chemotherapeutic agents for outpatients, although a doctor is within easy call if required; this service was initiated because of a shortage of nursing staff and a reluctance on their part to work with these agents. All other medicines for both inpatients and outpatients at the Center are administered by medical and nursing staff.

Participation of pharmacists in the administration of drugs requires special training and raises ethical, legal and economic problems, which must militate strongly against its increase.

USE OF A COMPUTER IN MEDICINE DISTRIBUTION SYSTEMS

The prescription, supply and administration of a medicine for a patient, together with the subsequent monitoring of its effect, involves the handling of a large amount of data and generation of further potentially useful information. Electronic data processing (EDP) (i.e. data processing performed largely by electronic equipment such as a computer) should therefore have considerable potential in this field. In properly designed systems, the data should be handled rapidly, efficiently and relatively economically, releasing trained staff for other activities, and also providing information which was not previously readily available because manual processing was impracticable.

Access to a computer for these applications is often only possible in hospitals where EDP is used for other purposes. This may be of considerable advantage, allowing linkage of prescription data with, for example, other patient information (name, age, diagnosis etc), or laboratory results (for renal function, effect of drugs on tests etc). Where a hospital-based computer is not available, it may be possible, for example, to use a Regional Health Authority installation for certain aspects.

It is intended to give here only a general indication of the type of computer applications which are possible. Further details of actual applications, including the methods used to enter data into the computer, are given in the references cited by Knight and Conrad (1975). Although described here as a fully comprehensive system, it must be stressed that the individual components would normally be developed in a stepwise manner after very careful planning, wide consultation, detailed training of staff, and suitable pilot studies. The subsystems, such as pharmacy stock control, may in any case be developed without any overall plan for an eventual total system; in these cases the amount and method of data input may be different from that used in a comprehensive system (e.g. patient details may be omitted). It is advisable to commence with simple systems which will have a higher chance of success and can be subsequently expanded; long delays in implementation or total abandonment have resulted from a number of the very ambitious projects. In the design of programs the pharmacist should be closely involved with other disciplines in deciding the data required and how it should be recorded, displayed or transmitted. Accurate communication with the systems analyst and computer programmer are essential.

When the computer system is online and realtime the data enters the system as soon as it occurs and the computer responds in time to affect the real-life situation. The doctor may prescribe for his patient in such a system by using a terminal such as a teletypewriter or visual display unit to transmit his requirements to the computer. This process usually takes longer than conventional writing but the computer can be programmed to assist the physician by providing him with additional information such as contraindications and dosage regimes; the dose may be calculated by the computer using such factors as the patient's age, weight, and creatinine clearance (e.g. Hull & Baker 1974). The computer assists further by checking whether the medicine may interact with other drugs already prescribed and, from the patient details file, whether there is, for example, a known drug sensitivity, giving warning messages where necessary. If the doctor decides for any reason to ignore this warning it may be arranged that the computer accepts the prescription but informs the clinical pharmacist who can, if he considers it necessary, discuss the problem with the physician concerned. This could result in more effective use of the clinical pharmacist; he should be able to take action on prescriptions as soon as they are entered, with perhaps only one pharmacist required to do this at night. Clearly pharmacists would be closely involved in providing the basic information required to be stored in the computer before this type of check can be carried out. Prescriptions may be automatically cancelled after a set period, a reminder being raised the day before to indicate that represcribing may be necessary.

As an alternative to the above, or perhaps in an emergency or after a breakdown, the medical officer may prescribe on a conventional form and either a pharmacist or nurse may then be responsible for the input of details to the computer and the transmission to him of any subsequent warning messages. Errors due to misinterpretation of the handwitten prescription may, however, then be possible. Some systems have been criticised because a nurse has been required to interpret the prescription without subsequent checks by a pharmacist, or even the more limited range of checks through the computer. Nurses or pharmacy technicians may alternatively enter the details into the computer but it is arranged that these are not acted upon until the pharmacist has verified that they are correct.

A complete drug record is therefore produced in the computer, including both current and cancelled medicines. In conventional prescribing systems this record is often distributed over the main prescription sheet and supplementary forms, such as the diabetic, anticoagulant, fluid prescription or variable dose sheets.

The computer can be programmed to compare the drug prescribed with the ward stocks and provide the pharmacy with written details for those patients who will require individually dispensed medicines or need the issue of 'temporary' stock. If criteria can be set the computer could also show when a drug was used sufficiently to be included in the 'permanent' ward stock, and then produce an updated listing.

In a similar manner, outpatient prescriptions or those for inpatients being discharged from hospital can be transmitted through the computer to the pharmacy. The computer check of the doctor's personal confidential number, entered before he commences prescribing, may be sufficient for a 'signature', or alternatively the print-out may be personally signed and dated. It is possible to arrange for the computer to print the label for the dispensed medicine, as well as providing the pharmacist with full details of current and previous drug treatment in the form of a drug profile. The quantities of medicines issued on each occasion can be reviewed to ensure that the patient has sufficient, is taking them correctly, and does not receive excessive supplies. The pharmacist may himself enter conventionally written outpatient prescriptions into the computer to obtain a printed label, incompatibility warnings and, subsequently, drug usage data; the computer may be programmed to include special instructions on the label (e.g. 'shake the bottle') depending on the medicine prescribed (Seibert *et al* 1967). Only minimal details are required to be entered for repeat prescriptions.

The computer could, in the future, be interfaced with a mechanical dispensing device such as the 'Brewer system' described earlier; thus, for example, the computer may produce a medication card to activate the machine. For inpatients the dose could be ejected into a patient tray at the appropriate time for administration, or for outpatients a suitably labelled bottle of the appropriate medicine could be automatically provided.

The computer can be programmed to print out, for each medicine round, a list of the patients for whom drug treatment is required, together with the details of the medicine, dose and route taking account of new prescriptions and cancellations, etc. It can be arranged that the drug name used is compatible with the pharmacy labelling system, avoiding confusion between approved and proprietary names. After the round, details of missed doses etc, with explanations if necessary, may be entered into the computer to give a complete record of the patient's treatment. The computer may print reminder notices at regular intervals until it has been informed that the administration of the drug has been carried out; alternatively, details for the next medicine round may not be obtainable until action on the previous one has been notified.

Theoretically, pharmacy issues of ward stock containers could be compared with these nursing drug administration records to automatically show when further supplies are needed. Problems are likely to arise, however, if broken ampoules or dropped tablets are not recorded. In systems where prescription data is not entered into the computer the pharmacy may enter details of stock issues so that subsequent information can be obtained from the computer on ward and pharmacy stock levels and usage patterns. Preprinted requisitions or cards, especially if already partially coded for speeding computer input, can be of considerable assistance in this. The computer may itself provide preprinted requisitions for approved stock items. Control over drugs liable to misuse (e.g. antidepressants) can be considerably improved in computer systems.

Where a unit dose system is in operation, the computer may be programmed to inform the technician of doses required to be dispensed to cover a given time interval (as described, for example, by Evans & Howe 1971). This can be achieved in a complex system, where prescription data is entered at ward level, without the risk of transcription errors or prescriptions being absent from wards, potential disadvantages in unit dose systems which were described earlier. A system has been developed where the computer automatically prints envelopes for sending each of the doses to be administered at a particular time to the ward; these envelopes are used by the nurse to document administration of the drug.

Means et al (1975) showed that the medication error rate associated with their unit dose system 'compared favorably with most other (noncomputerized) unit dose systems' but that 'no particular benefit in terms of the medication error rate was attributed to the computer element'. Clearly this type of finding is dependent on the efficiency of the system used before introduction of the computer. Flaws in the original system may in any case be identified in the systems analysis necessary before programming and these can be improved or eliminated whether or not computerisation does finally take place.

Where an intravenous additive service is in operation the computer can, after input of sufficient information, be programmed to print lists of solutions to be prepared at specific times for named patients, where possible, grouping together orders for the same drug and intravenous solution, thus facilitating preparation (Nielson 1973). The computer may also screen for incompatibilities, print the required labels and supply nursing staff with administration details at the appropriate time.

Details entered into the computer of issues of medicines from the pharmacy may form part of the overall stock control system. Details of all receipts are also necessary; the computer can then maintain a continuous record of the stock balance for each item, automatically generating purchase orders when the programmed reorder level is reached, taking account where necessary of supplier's minimum order quantities or of outstanding orders. A less sophisticated system may produce a list of all items at or below the minimum stock level, arranged in alphabetical order of manufacturer and giving the reorder quantity. Lists for stocktaking purposes can also be produced, together with estimated usage for contract purposes. The accuracy of the stock control system and contract estimates can be considerably improved if the pattern and trends of drug usage (as opposed to ward issues, or hospital purchases) are known; information on this may be possible from complex computer systems.

When details of expiry dates and batch numbers of medicines issued to wards are entered, the computer may assist in routine recall of dated material or in the urgent withdrawal of that found to be defective. The possibility of 'unofficial' transfer between wards must, however, be recognised.

Charging of patients for the drugs received is an important computer application in American hospitals and has often provided an initial incentive to further pharmacy developments. Management information on, for example, patterns of drug usage and costs, related to individual wards, hospitals, consultant, patient diagnosis and length of stay in hospital or medical specialty, may, however, be very useful in United Kingdom Hospitals also. For example, the clinical pharmacist may be able to identify certain therapeutic trends, whether good or bad, and pass on this information to the physician. Drug usage data can help in efforts to rationalise prescribing and reduce the range of medicines stocked; it may be shown, for example, that optimal dosage regimes are not being used. The data may also be useful in monitoring the use of controlled drugs.

Other retrospective uses for the data recorded and stored could include provision of bulletins to nursing staff on aspects of their recording of drug administration. Thus, for example, histograms may be drawn to show, for each ward, the recorded administered doses as a percentage of those prescribed. The data may also be used to monitor adverse drug reactions and the investigation of drug efficacy.

In the United States many hospitals have their own formulary, drawn up by a pharmacy and therapeutics committee, to indicate to the medical staff those drugs which have been approved for use in that institution. The computer can be used in the updating of this by programming it to print out the lists of drug names in the desired sequence (e.g. pharmacologically), incorporating an index and details of costs or contraindications where necessary. It has been suggested that a list of drugs stocked in the pharmacy could be provided for ward use. This may enable a physician to prescribe a readily available preparation, minimising delays in the patient receiving his treatment and reducing the range of drugs stocked. However, unless other useful information is also provided as an incentive to refer to it, the list would probably be so cumbersome as to be of little practical benefit.

When a computer system is 'offline' the peripheral equipment such as terminals are not in direct communication with the computer. The extent to which some or all of the above applications are possible will then depend upon the delay before input to the computer is effected, but a loss in flexibility is inevitable. Realtime systems are, however, much more costly to develop and should only be used when the need has been clearly defined.

The potential for computer applications is enormous but it must be stressed that these should be realistically developed and that even introduction of rela-tively simple subsystems involves a great deal of effort from many disciplines. Specific controls are necessary to ensure the continuing accuracy of data and to avoid massive proliferation of unnecessary reports which could consume more staff time in reading than is saved by the system. Care must also be taken that the time taken to input data into the computer is not excessive, especially where staff in the clinical area are involved. Cost savings resulting from com-puter applications are often difficult to define and may depend upon minimis-ing future increases in expenditure rather than effecting immediate reductions.

Although not a panacea, increased use of the computer in the type of appli-cation described may, nevertheless, lead in the future to greater involvement of the hospital pharmacist in a clinical role which is less concerned with the more routine aspects of the supply of medicines.

APPENDIX: PACKAGING OF PHARMACEUTICALS

C. Hetherington

Ward pharmacy has many elements and fundamental to any scheme is a good drug distribution system. Interest in drug distribution systems continues to hold a premiere position in the thoughts of many hospital pharmacists and it is now generally accepted that any system must be supported by a packaging programme to provide the medicines most commonly in use pre-packaged in a form ready for issue to the user. Such prepackaging requirements almost invariably are being met by hospital-based facilities due to the lack of interest from the pharmaceutical industry to meet the varied packaging requirements of different hospital pharmacists.

Prepackaging

Baker and Barrett (1967) suggested that there was a case for the provision of small unit packs to standard specifications suitable for use in hospitals and that these, provided from the pharmaceutical industry, would improve safety and reduce the need for repackaging to be undertaken in pharmacies.

The Hospital Pharmacists Consultative Committee of the Department of Health and Social Security set up a working party to advise on a specification for 'Hospital Standard Packs' and, when prepared in 1969, discussions took place with the industry. Nothing of any consequence in respect of solid oral dose forms emerged from these discussions, primarily because hospital phar-macists wished to use screw-capped glass bottles of rectangular section as their standard container. Such containers are not easy to handle on high speed filling machines and also the industry was well advanced in moving away from glass containers. The only recommendation which was generally accepted and which over the years has been followed, was concerned with presenting ampoules in containers of ten instead of the previous practice of supplying large boxes of 50 or 100 ampoules which required further division at the time of supply.

The Guild of Hospital Pharmacists established a working party in 1970 to investigate the requirements of the profession and the manufacturers with a view to formulating guidelines for hospital packages of solid oral dose forms. These were published in 1971 and are reproduced for reference on pp. 339–342. As the demand from hospital pharmacy is only approximately 2% of the output of the industry, any packages for hospital use only are not likely to receive great support. The Guild working party, in formulating guidelines, recognised this problem and suggested a standard blister pack format which could be utilised by general practice pharmacists. Such packages are commonplace in North America where unit dose drug distribution systems are widely used.

Advantages of packaging standardisation

In hospital pharmacy advantages are primarily associated with the standardisation of shape, size and labelling. The hospital pharmacist is forced into a situation where he must standardise containers for ward use because of the constraints in the system which exist in the form of ward medicine cupboards and trolleys. Hospital wards may store considerable quantities of medicines for the use of their patients and therefore any packaging system which permits logical tidy storage is to be preferred to one which presents the nurse with a large range of containers all varying in size and shape, leaving her with the task of trying to fit these into a standard hospital drug cupboard. The advantages of standardisation can be seen in the pharmacy where the maximum use can be made of shelving when the containers are all of the same dimension. These arguments are particularly true when considering strip and blister packs, for both these methods of presentation require more space than the glass bottle or extruded aluminium tin of bulk tablets. However, blister packs compare very favourably with small (25s and 50s) packs in bottles or tins but strip packs still require 2–3 times the volume of space. The advantages of package standardisation are:

1. Efficient use of storage space in pharmacy or ward.
2. Less confusion and consequently reduced errors with standard labelling.
3. Limited range of cartons or boxes needed for dispensing larger quantities to outpatients.
4. Inventory control of packaging components made easier.
5. Fewer change parts required on packaging machinery.
6. Reduced time of product dispensing.
7. Dispensary stocktaking simplified.
8. Patient compliance more readily checked.

9.   Patient confidence increased.
10.   Prescribing quantities rationalised.

Recent developments

In psychiatric hospitals many patients are often permitted to stay with relatives or friends at weekends. Such absences from hospital require the provision of small amounts of medication to accompany the patient during these leave periods. As the absence is short, in many cases only 1 or 2 days and as it may well occur every weekend, an enormous strain is placed on pharmacies in psychiatric hospitals in dispensing such 'leave' prescriptions. Chatfield (1971) has reported on the use of strip packaged solid oral dose forms as a satisfactory answer to this problem. Individually packaged and labelled dose forms were found to reduce the time involved in dispensing leave prescriptions. The operation of a unit dose drug distribution system in Leeds also requires the packaging of a wide range of materials to be undertaken, often in small quantities and consequently a versatile system has had to be evolved. Using preformed blisters, obtained from commercial sources, it has been possible to use relatively inexpensive platen sealing machines to produce either push through packs sealed with hard tempered, vinyl lacquered aluminium foil, or peelable blister packs sealed with laminates composed of paper, aluminium foil and vinyl lacquer.

Other developments in hospitals have been concerned with the unit dose packaging of oral liquid preparations. Compact machines are available that are easy to operate and with a reasonable output that can satisfy the needs of hospital pharmacies for unit packs. Using either polystyrene or polypropylene containers with a sealing flange, the machine applies a peelable laminate lid material. This is cut to shape, leaving a peel flap for easy opening.

The advantages of unit dose liquid presentations are immediately apparent and include: direct administration to the patient from the container; accuracy of dosage; labelling of medication until actual administration; and saving in nursing time.

Like all 'unit of use' packaging, whether for foods, sterile supplies or pharmaceuticals, the benefits must be offset against greater bulk to be stored and possibly some increase in unit cost, at least initially.

The 'unit of use' packaging of eyedrops in single use packs has evolved in Britain for some years. The 'minims' unit (Smith & Nephew Ltd.), a small plastic tube containing unit dose eyedrops contained in an overwrap, has several advantages. There is no need to include bactericides as in multidose containers, thereby reducing the possibility of sensitivity reactions. The outer surface of the tube is sterile and therefore can be handled by the surgeon during operations. The solutions are of assured sterility.

Interest in prefilled syringes where the injection solution is packaged in syringe units has prompted discussions with industry as to the availability of components which could be handled in hospital pharmacy facilities. No system of British manufacture is available although several are used in North America The possible advantages of such packages was investigated in a unit dose study

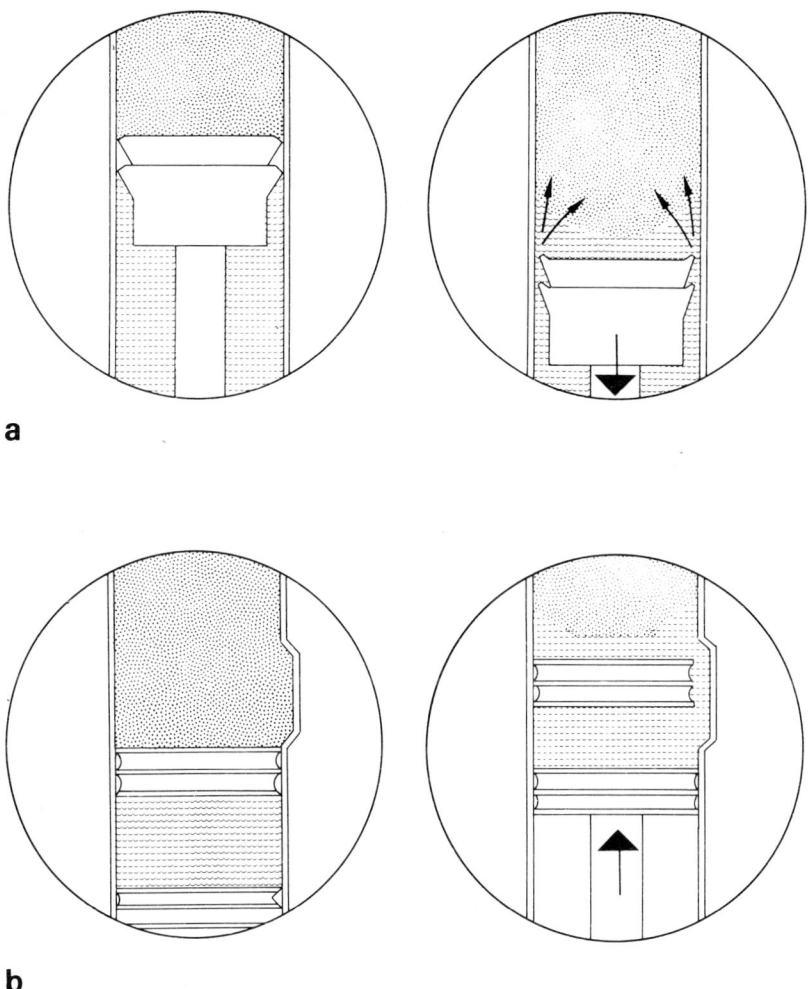

Fig. 10.8   Two designs of 'double chamber' syringes.

in Leeds by Ellis *et al* (1973) and the results suggested that where such units are used they must be simple to operate with the minimum of assembly manipulations required by the user. The claimed advantages of prefilled syringes in North America include less risk of microbiological contamination of parenterals; reduced possibility of dosage errors due to poor measurement of volume; better stock control; and reduced time of administration.

As many parenteral products are presented as lyopholised powders to ensure long shelf-life, the designers of syringes have produced double chamber syringes where the dry powder is held in one part of the syringe and separated from the diluent by a diaphragm. The action at the time of use to assemble the unit allows the diluent to mix with the powder and therefore presents a fresh solution for administration. The added advantage to this system is that it eliminates the risk of rubber particles being introduced into the solution, which is a constant hazard where rubber capped vials are involved (Fig. 10.8).

Packaging design

The design of packaging is most important and any new developments must ensure that the ease with which people can manipulate new style packs is not reduced. Reference has already been made to the design of prefilled syringe units being such that they are easily used by nursing staff; a multiplicity of styles of pack for any group of products can be misleading and even present a hazard to the patient. Packages for parenteral solutions are a good example of this problem. When all solutions were packaged in the MRC style 'blood bottle', the nurse could be trained in its use. With the introduction of vacuum packed bottles, rigid and flexible plastic containers and the multiplicity of administration devices, the nurse can easily be confused when handling such equipment. It is important to remember that progress in one field must not lead to deterioration of performance in another.

Materials

The purpose of a package is to protect the product up to the time that it is needed. This protection requires the maintenance of purity, stability, sterility (for some products) and efficacy of the preparation. The shelf-life of many products is affected by the materials of the package and is often a compromise between an acceptable shelf-life and the cost of the package. Deterioration may be caused by natural ageing, moisture, gas, vapour or contaminant penetration, and light. The packaging material itself must also be considered for factors such as permeation, extraction, sorption and modification on storage. The latter are particularly true where plastic materials are involved.

Glass

Glass has proved itself to be an excellent material for packaging pharmaceuticals. It is largely inert, stable, can protect from light, rarely contaminates the product, gives good physical protection and is relatively inexpensive. Glass is still used almost exclusively for prefilled syringes but has now been displaced from its leading position for almost all other dosage forms.

Aluminium foil

Aluminium foil is extensively used for both strip and blister packaging of solid oral dose forms. It is usually employed as a lacquered foil for push through blister packs or as a laminate material composed of foil and polythene or paper, foil and polythene when used for strip packs. These laminates have exceptionally good barrier properties and are excellent for giving moisture protection to very susceptible products, (e.g. effervescent tablets). The grade commonly used for blister packs is 0.020 mm foil with heat lacquer whereas 0.030 mm foil with 30 g/m² polythene is that used for strip packaging. Foil is fairly expensive and is therefore used only where maximum moisture protection is required.

Plastics

Strip packaging

One of the earliest strip packs employed waxed paper but since then plastic materials have been widely used either as films or as laminates incorporating various combinations of materials. Regenerated cellulose alone or laminated to polyethylene are both improved in moisture protection when coated with a heat seal lacquer. These are cheap and ideal for short-life packaged materials, such as those processed by hospitals for their own immediate use. More complex laminates have been developed to give longer shelf-life. These usually incorporate aluminium foil although good protection can be achieved with fluorocarbon-containing laminates.

Blister packaging

Thermoformable materials for blister packaging vary in their protective qualities against moisture, good quality foil or peelable laminate lid for sealing to the base materials are generally impermeable to water vapour. A number of materials have been used, as seen in Table 10.1.

Liquid preparations

Where rigid containers can be used, polystyrene has advantages, since it is cheap and perfectly clear, like glass. Polypropylene is a more stable material and compatible with a wider range of medicaments. For unit dose liquid preparations it is common practice in North America to use either glass vials or a lacquered aluminium container sealed with a peelable laminate lid material. PVC and foil sachets have been suggested as possible containers but again 'unit of use' design suggested that for the present nothing has been found superior in style to the shape of the traditional medicine glass bottle.

Table 10.1   Moisture protection properties of thermo-formable materials

Materials	Shelf-life comparisons	Increasing moisture protection
PVC 250 mm	1	
PVC/PVdC (polyvinylidine chloride) 200 mm with 48 g/m²	3½–6	
PVC/Aclar* 22A 187½ mm 37½ mm	8–12	
PVC/Aclar* 33C 187½ mm 18¾ mm		

*Aclar is the trade name for polymonochlorotrifluro ethylene copolymer film of Allied Chemicals Corporation, USA. Aclar type 33C is twice as moisture protective as Aclar 22A for a given thickness, but requires special equipment such as plug assist for blister forming.

Large volume sterile fluids are packaged in PVC polyethylene, polypropylene and nylon-melinex laminate containers.

Modern packaging machines often utilise the 'form-fill-seal' sequence of operation where the product is fed into newly formed containers produced in the machine from plastic granules and sealed before contamination can gain access. Such systems can utilise the thermoforming materials polyethylene and polypropylene. These systems of packaging are likely to be used increasingly for parenterals, oral liquids, ophthalmics and antiseptic lotions.

Equipment for packaging

Solid oral dose forms

The prepackaging of tablets and capsules into rigid containers of glass or plastic is conveniently undertaken using an electronic counting machine (Fig. 10.9). These work on the principle that as dose forms bisect a light beam, it is registered by an electronic device, and when a predetermined number have passed the beam, the flow of material is diverted and the cycle started again.

Strip packaging of solids is achieved by sandwiching the dose form inside a layer of one material (Fig. 10.10a) or between layers of two materials (Fig. 10.10b).

Blister or bubble packaging is achieved by locating the product in a pocket formed from thermolabile material and heat sealing a further backing into place so closing the pockets. The actual pockets can be made either by vacuum forming, pressure forming with male dies or a mixture of both. Vacuum form-

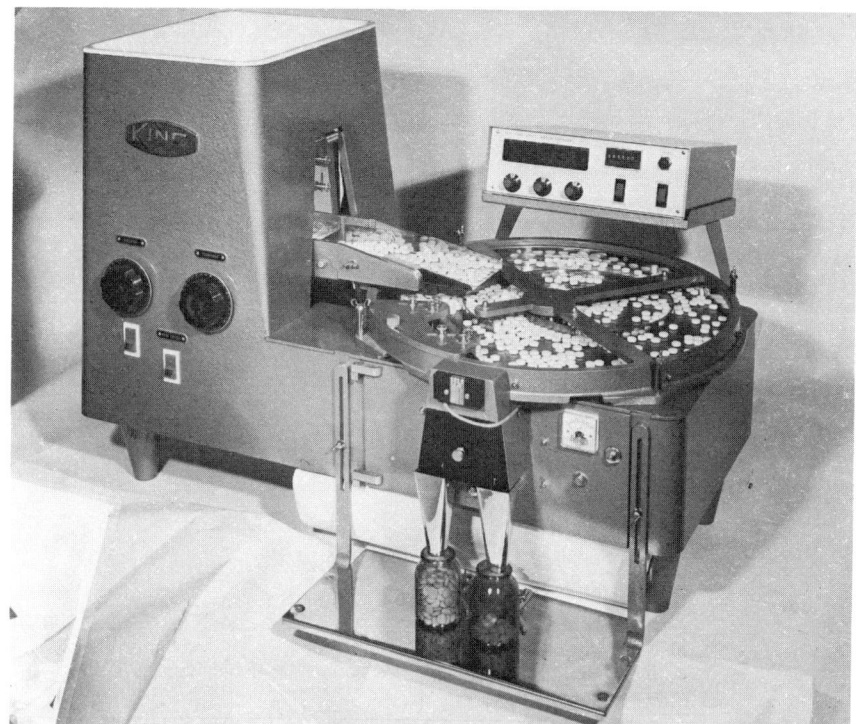

Fig. 10.9 Model TB4A Electronic Tablet Counter (C. E. King Ltd., Chertsey, Surrey).

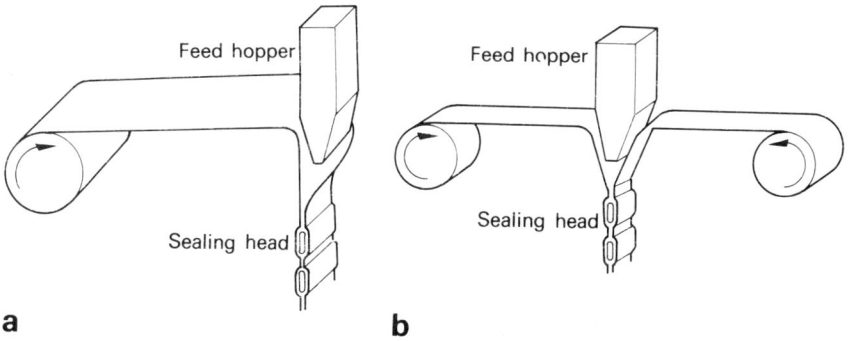

Fig. 10.10 (a) A 'form-fill seal' machine capable of producing sachets or pouches from one reel of laminate. (b) A strip-packing machine using two reels of laminate.

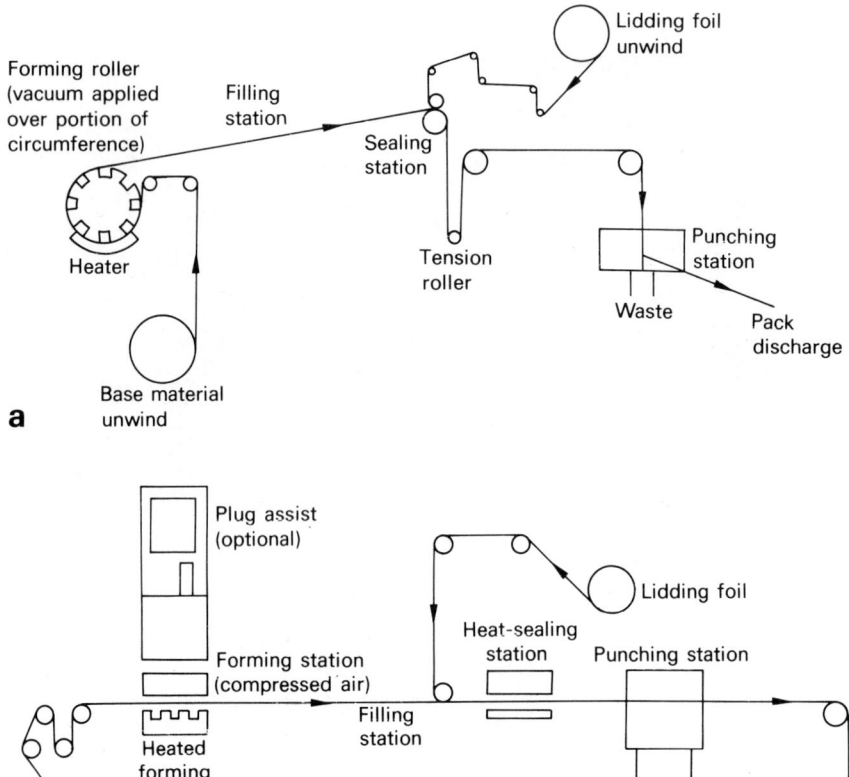

Fig. 10.11   (a) A vacuum-forming machine for blister packs. (b) Pressure forming with optional plug assist for blister packs.

ing is the simplest system (Fig. 10.11a) but care must be taken to ensure that the protective properties of the materials are not too markedly reduced due to the 'thinning' which takes place when it is drawn into the bubble shape. The pressure forming method using male moulds (plug assist) can largely overcome this problem (Fig. 10.11b).

Safety packaging

A considerable amount of discussion has been generated by the possibility of packaging pharmaceutical products in 'safety containers'. Several such containers are already in use in North America which require a precise series of actions to be performed before they can be opened. The hope for such containers centred on the prevention of accidental poisoning among young children by medicinal products. A working group of the Medicines Commission reported to the Secretary of State for Social Services in May 1974. This report recommended among other things that: 'a wider use should be made as soon as possible of unit packaging of all solid dose medicines which are known to present a hazard to children'. This group considered that unit packaged materials had advantages since even if available to a child each individual pocket had to be opened before the medicinal product was available to the child to consume. Such added restriction on the ease of taking medicines was thought to offer some child resistance and possible safety of such packaging. The need for monitoring of any change in presentation was highlighted by the committee. In March 1976 the Department of Health and Social Security issued HN(76)35 (*Health Services Management: use of reclosable child-resistant containers for dispensed medicines*). This notice asked health authorities to arrange for hospital outpatient prescriptions for solid dose preparations containing aspirin or paracetamol to be dispensed in reclosable child-resistant containers, unless otherwise suitably packaged, and the arrangements to take effect from 1 April 1976. The notice specifically asked that such containers should not be used for other prescribed medicines. 'Suitably packaged' in the Health Notice referred to 'unit packaged products'.

Guidelines for hospital packaging of drugs (Guild of Hospital Pharmacists 1971)

These proposals have been formulated with the hope that they will enable the pharmaceutical industry to design packaging for pharmaceuticals which will meet the requirements of the hospital service. It is hoped that they will form a basis for utilising modern packaging technology to the greatest advantage both for the supplier and all the various people who handle drugs as well as the ultimate user, be this nurse or patient.

A Single Unit Package is one which contains one discrete pharmaceutical dose form, properly labelled and presented so that the contents can be administered directly from the package.

A Multi Unit Package is one which contains a number of pharmaceutical dose forms, individually protected, properly labelled and presented so that the contents can be administered directly from the package.

Pharmaceutical manufacturers can package drugs more efficiently and economically than can hospitals; however standardisation of packaging would provide even greater efficiency and economy for hospitals. Every effort must be made to have all pharmaceuticals for hospital use packaged in a standardised form as soon as possible.

General Considerations

Packaging materials

The characteristics of the material necessary for product protection should be the responsibility of the manufacturer of the drug to determine and provide for each product. Comparable packaging material and equipment should be commercially available to enable the hospital pharmacist to achieve complete uniformity of the hospital packaging programme.

Shape and form

By definition the design of the package is such that the contents can be administered directly to the patient without transfer to any other container or device. In performing this function the package should be easy to open, easy to use, requiring little education or experience, and be easily destroyed.

Labelling

Each package label must carry the essential information detailed below; labels on outer cartons may have further details included where this is considered necessary or desirable by the manufacturer. Any information required only by the pharmacist should be capable of being removed before issue to the nurse or patient.

The desired format of label print to be as follows:

> Approved name.
> (Proprietary name, if shown.)
> Dosage form, if special.
> Strength.
> Batch number.
> Expiry date, where applicable.
> Special notes (e.g. below 4°C).

Approved name. To be the most prominent name on the package label. It is not considered necessary to have the proprietary name on labels. The style of type should be chosen to provide maximum legibility, contrast and permanence.

Special dosage forms. Reference to these should be incorporated (e.g. enteric coating, delayed release). For products other than for oral use, reference to the route of administration should appear on the label (e.g. topical use, i.m. etc).

Strength. Should be stated in metric units and whole numbers.

Batch number. Should appear on the label and the manufacturer's name and address.

Expiry date. For preparations of limited life should appear on the label.

Special notes. Such as storage conditions (e.g. store below 4°C); preparation requirements (e.g. shake before use); administration notes (e.g. not to be chewed).

The construction of packages should be such that their integrity can readily be checked at the point of use.

Package requirements: solid oral dose forms

Single unit packages

Bubble packages with pealable laminated closure which also serves as the label.
Size 40 mm × 20 mm.

Preferably perforated on the long edge and presented in strips of 10 units (i.e. 200 mm long).

The immediate carton to hold 10 strips of 10 bubbles (i.e. 100 units), and labelled on the narrow edge.

The bubble should be transparent material, thus allowing inspection of the contents for possible gross deterioration or damage. The laminate should be easily peelable and the adhesive such that it cannot be replaced. Provision should be made for it to be peelable from two corners and this indicated on the label.

Multi unit packages

Bubble package with push-through aluminium foil packing. Size 105 mm × 85 mm incorporating a label area 105 mm × 20 mm.

Contents

1. Tablets up to 11 mm diameter packaged as 4 rows of 7 dose forms=28.
2. Tablets above 11 mm diameter packaged as 3 rows of 7 dose forms. The centre row to have the central area blank to give a module content of 14 dose forms.
3. Small capsules, packaged as 3 rows of 10. The central section of the middle row to be blank to give a module content of 28.

4.   Large capsules packaged as 2 rows of 7.

These 105 mm × 85 mm modules to be packaged, in one row only, in outer cartons of 20 providing a pack size of 280 or 560 and labelled on the front edge.

REFERENCES

AMERICAN SOCIETY OF HOSPITAL PHARMACISTS (1972) *Unit Dose Drug Distribution Systems.* ASHP, Washington DC.

AMERICAN SOCIETY OF HOSPITAL PHARMACISTS (1974) *American Journal of Hospital Pharmacy* **31,** 1198.

ANDERSON P. O. & Taryle D.A. (1974) *American Journal of Hospital Pharmacy* **31,** 254.

ANON (1973) *Pharmaceutical Journal* **211,** 49.

ASHWIN J. & Lynn B. (1975) *Pharmaceutical Journal* **214,** 487.

AUSTIN, L. H. (1973) *Hospital Pharmacy* **8,** 351.

BAKER, J. A. (1967) *Journal of Hospital Pharmacy* **24,** 400.

BAKER, J. A. & BARRETT C. R. (1967) *Pharmaceutical Journal* **199,** 405.

BARKER K., KIMBROUGH W & HELLER W. (1966) *Hospital Formulary Management* **1,** 29.

BARKER K. N. & McCONNELL W. E. (1962) *American Journal of Hospital Pharmacy* **19,** 361.

BARNETT J. W. & CALDER G. (1969) *Journal of Hospital Pharmacy* **27,** 258.

BIRCH P., GEE N. & TALLETT, E. R., (1974) *Journal of Hospital Pharmacy* **32,** 94.

BOOTH T. G. & ELLIS S., (1973) *Pharmaceutical Journal* **210,** 248.

BRODLIE P., HENNEY C. & WOOD A. J. J. (1974) *British Medical Journal* **1,** 383.

BUTH J. A., COBERLY R. W. & ECKEL, F. M. (1973) *Drug Intelligence and Clinical Pharmacy* **7,** 276.

CALDER G. & BARNETT J. W. (1967) *Pharmaceutical Journal* **198,** 584.

CALDER G. & BARNETT J. W. (1971) *Pharmaceutical Journal* **207,** 562.

CARLIN H. S. & PERKINS A. J. (1968) *American Journal of Hospital Pharmacy* **25,** 271.

CHATFIELD R. F. (1971) *Pharmaceutical Journal* **211,** 276.

CROOKS J., CLARK C. G., CAIE H. B. & MAWSON W. B. (1965) *Lancet* i, 373.

D'ARCY P. F. (1976) In *Microbiological Hazards of Infusion Therapy,* eds. I. Phillips, P. D. Meers & P. F. D'Arcy. MTP, Lancaster.

D'ARCY P. F. & THOMPSON K. M. (1974) *Pharmaceutical Journal* **213,** 172.

DEPARTMENT OF HEALTH AND SOCIAL SECURITY (1958) *Report on Control of Dangerous Drugs and Poisons in Hospitals by a Joint Sub-Committee of the Standing Medical, Nursing and Pharmaceutical Advisory Committees, Central Health Services Council.* The Aitken Report. HMSO, London.

DEPARTMENT OF HEALTH AND SOCIAL SECURITY (1970a) *Security of Drugs Liable to Misuse.* HM (70)1. HMSO, London.

DEPARTMENT OF HEALTH AND SOCIAL SECURITY (1970b) *Report on Measures for Controlling Drugs on the Wards by the Joint Sub-Committee of the Standing Medical, Nursing and Pharmaceutical Advisory Committees of the Central Health Services Council.* HM(70)36. HMSO, London.

DEPARTMENT OF HEALTH AND SOCIAL SECURITY (1974) *Report on the Prevention of Medicine in Relation to Child Safety.* HMSO, London.

DEPARTMENT OF HEALTH AND SOCIAL SECURITY (1976) *Report of the Working Party on the Addition of Drugs to Intravenous Infusion Fluids.* HC(76)9. HMSO, London.

DURANT W. J. & HERRICK J. D. (1970) *American Journal of Hospital Pharmacy* **27,** 127.

Eling R. F. & Brissie, E. O. (1974) *American Journal of Hospital Pharmacy* **31,** 740.
Ellis S., (1972) *Control of Drugs in Small Hospitals: the West Cornwall System.* King Edward's Hospital Fund London.
Ellis S., Ford P. M., Hetherington C. & Watts G. E. (1973) *Pharmaceutical Journal* **211,** 276.
Ellis S. & Ford P. (1972) *Pharmaceutical Journal* **209,** 368.
Ellis S. (1973) Nicholas International Award Paper presented to meeting of Guild of Hospital Pharmacists, School of Pharmacy, London, 9 November 1973.
Evans S. J. & Howe D. J. (1971) *American Journal of Hospital Pharmacy* **28,** 500.
Gaunt M. S., & Riley B. B., (1971) *Journal of Hospital Pharmacy* **29,** 69.
Goldberg L. A. (1974) *Nursing Times* **70,** 998.
Grayson J. E. (1971) *Pharmaceutical Journal* **206, 64.**
Guild of Hospital Pharmacists (1971) Guidelines for hospital packaging of drugs. Report of a working party. *Journal of Hospital Pharmacy* **29,** 195.
Hassan W. E. Jr. (1960) *American Journal of Hospital Pharmacy* **17,** 490.
Hassan W. E. (1974) *Hospital Pharmacy.* 3rd edn. Lea & Febiger, Philadelphia.
Hetherington C. (1971) *Pharmaceutical Journal* **206,** 267.
Hetherington C. (1972) *Pharmaceutical Journal* **208,** 73.
Ho N. F. H. (1972) In *Perspectives in Clinical Pharmacy*, eds. D. E. Franke & H. A. K. Whitney Jr. Drug Intelligence Publications, Hamilton, Ill.
Horan V. (1973) *Journal of Hospital Pharmacy* **31,** 135.
Hull J. H. & Baker J. A. (1973) *Journal of Clinical Computing* **3,** 295.
Jacobs J. (1970) *Pharmaceutical Journal* **205,** 437.
Knight J. R. & Conrad W. F., (1975) *American Journal of Hospital Pharmacy* **32,** 165.
Kramer W. R., Inglott A. S. & Cluxton R. J. Jr., (1972) In *Perspectives in Clinical Pharmacy*, eds. D. E. Franke & H. A. K. Whitney Jr. Drug Intelligence Publications, Hamilton, Ill.
Lee E. V., Trice A. E. & Barrett C. W. (1971) *Pharmaceutical Journal* **206,** 195.
Lidgate R. A. (1970) *Journal of Hospital Pharmacy* **28,** 145.
Lockwood J. C. & Williams A., (1974) *Journal of Hospital Pharmacy* **32,** 111.
Lucarotti A. L., Prisco H. M., Hafner P.E., & Shoup, L. K. (1973) *American Journal of Hospital Pharmacy* **30,** 1147.
MacPherson D., Brown T. R. & Northern R. E. (1973) *Anerican Journal of Hospital Pharmacy* **30,** 1034.
Manzelli T. A., (1961) *American Journal of Hospital Pharmacy* **18,** 561.
Mathieson D. R. & Rawlings, J. L. (1971) *American Journal of Hospital Pharmacy* **28,** 254.
Mattei T. J. (1974) *American Journal of Hospital Pharmacy* **31,** 1053.
McLeod D. C., Ray D. V., Riddle J. I. & Eckel, F. M. (1971) *American Journal of Hospital Pharmacy* **28,** 568.
McMullan P. (1975) *Journal of Hospital Pharmacy* **33,** 9.
Means B. J., Derewicz H. J. & Lamy P. P. (1975) *American Journal of Hospital Pharmacy* **32,** 186.
Mehl B. (1968) *American Journal of Hospital Pharmacy* **25,** 71.
Moeys W. A. (1968) Report of Meeting of General Assembly of Hospital Pharmacists' section, Federation Internationale Pharmaceutique, Hamburg, 3–4 September 1968.
Moody P. M., Kisch R. M., Van Wey J., Hunniman C. E. & Parker P. F. (1970) *American Journal of Hospital Pharmacy* **27,** 473.
National Coordinating Committee on Large Volume Parenterals (1975) *American Journal of Hospital Pharmacy* **32,** 261.
Neill J. M. (1977) *The Prescribing and Administration of i.v. additives to infusion fluids.* Travenol Labs., Thetford, Norfolk.

NIELSON C. B. (1973) *Journal of Clinical Computing* **3,** 249.

PANG F. J. (1973) *Hospital Pharmacy* **8,** 10.

PAXINES J. & SAMUELS T. M. (1975) *American Journal of Hospital Pharmacy* **32,** 892.

PINCKNEY M. B. Jr., LUZZI L. A. & NEEDHAM T. E. Jr. (1973) *Journal of Pharmaceutical Sciences* **62,** 80.

PRITCHARD D. (1970) *Pharmaceutical Journal* **204,** 693.

REPORT OF SCOTTISH HOSPITAL PHARMACISTS' CONFERENCE (1966) *Pharmaceutical Journal* **196,** 241.

ROSS A. J. (1966) *Lancet* ii, 333.

ROSS A. J. (1967) *Journal of Hospital Pharmacy* **24,** 194.

RUBIN H. & HARRISON W. L. (1975) *American Journal of Hospital Pharmacy* **32,** 809.

SCOTTISH HOME AND HEALTH DEPARTMENT (1972) *Report on Control of Medicines in hospital wards and departments by a Joint Group appointed by the Standing Pharmaceutical, Medical and Nursing and Midwifery Advisory Committees of the Scottish Health Services Council.* HMSO, Edinburgh.

SCOTTISH HOME AND HEALTH DEPARTMENT (1973) *Standardisation of Hospital Medical Records. Report of the working group.* HMSO, Edinburgh.

SIEBERT S., BRUNJES S., SOUTTER J. C. & MARONDE R. F. (1967) *Drug Intelligence and Clinical Pharmacy* **1,** 342.

SILVERMAN H. M., GAMMARANO P. V., SIMON G. I. & SUHM, R. (1974) *American Journal of Hospital Pharmacy* **31,** 574.

SMITH W. E. & MACKEWICZ D. W. (1972) In *Perspectives in Clinical Pharmacy*, eds. D. E. Franke & H. A. K. Whitney Jr. Drug Intelligence Publications, Hamilton, Ill.

TYRELL P. J. S., DAVIES D. M., FRAZER E. S., LIDGATE R. A., LAWTHER A. & JOHNSON F. K., (1970) *Lancet* i, 408.

VERE D. W. (1965) *Lancet* i, 370.

VICTORINE M. (1958) *American Journal of Hospital Pharmacy* **15,** 973.

WALSH C. (1969) *Journal of Hospital Pharmacy* **27,** 318.

WARREN D. E. (1975) *American Journal of Hospital Pharmacy* **32,** 1127.

11

Ward and clinical pharmacy services

C. FEETAM

In recent years hospital pharmacists in Great Britain have been reassessing their role within the National Health Service. This has come about as a result of pressures arising within the profession from the Noel Hall Report (DHSS 1970a) and the desire of new graduates for more patient contact, as well as external influences such as changes in the law (Medicines Act 1968) and more government control over hospital pharmacy practice (e.g. *Guide to Good Pharmaceutical Manufacturing Practice;* DHSS 1977). In conjunction with this, the ever-increasing range and toxicity of drugs available to the prescriber has encouraged both medical and nursing staff to look to the pharmacist as a fellow professional whose main contribution to patient care is an expert knowledge of drugs and the safe supply of medicines to the patient.

The practice of hospital pharmacy in the past has been chiefly concerned with the acquisition, preparation, manufacture, distribution and control of medicinal products as well as, in some cases the purchasing and supply of various instruments and dressings. The increased contribution made by the pharmaceutical industry, however, as well as a general rationalisation and centralisation of supply services within the hospital service, have reduced the role of many dispensing pharmacists to little more than one of purchasing, counting, pouring and labelling. Recently, therefore, the emergence of a more patient-oriented approach, in addition to the traditional product-oriented approach, has become apparent. It is now acknowledged that the practice of pharmacy should evolve from the discovery, formulation and dispensing of compounds with potential medicinal properties to a study of their effects, both therapeutic and adverse, in man. Clinical pharmacy, although not a new concept, has yet to achieve a universally accepted definition. In its widest sense it is the term currently used to describe the steady movement of pharmacy away from the drug product in isolation, towards the patient. It is this trend in fact that has been suggested as being the most significant development in hospital pharmacy in the United Kingdom over the past decade (Whittet 1977).

Ward pharmacy was originally motivated by the need to prevent errors in drug therapy. Its introduction coincided with efforts in 1965 directed towards improvement of ward ordering procedures, stock control and recording practices as well as elimination of the transcription of prescriptions by nursing staff. Like clinical pharmacy, ward pharmacy is also without a universally accepted definition. Services currently in operation differ enormously; one thing common to all of them, however, is frequent, regular visits to the wards by pharmacists. Ward pharmacy can be regarded as a natural extension of an efficient drug distribution system which frees the pharmacist from much of the day-to-day routine supply function and enables him to visit the wards more frequently or to develop skills in one of the essential support services of a good ward or clinical pharmacy system such as drug information. The Noel Hall Working Party (DHSS 1970a) commented that the implementation of ward pharmacy services and related systems was to be commended and would be a major factor in the future development of the hospital service.

Before 'Noel Hall' the work of hospital pharmacists was organised on a relatively small scale which often resulted in duplication of effort and inflexibility in the deployment of resources. Insufficient use was made of supporting staff and pharmacists were often found doing work that could have been carried out by technicians or even unqualified assistants, who can and should assume many of the purely technical and repetitive functions in the dispensing, distribution and control of drugs. In considering the organisation of the hospital pharmaceutical service a distinction can be made between procedures which bring the pharmacist into close contact with medical and nursing staff as well as the patient and those which are usually carried out in relative isolation in the pharmacy department. The Noel Hall Working Party observed that there was a greater need than ever before for regular discussion between prescribers and pharmacists. One of the most effective ways that this may be encouraged is the active participation of pharmacists in the day-to-day management of patients at ward level. This obviously involves pharmacists making themselves available for discussion with medical and nursing staff. Once an effective ward pharmacy service has been established and a potential clinical role for the pharmacist identified, clinical pharmacy can then develop. In its evidence to the Royal Commission on the National Health Service in 1977, the Pharmaceutical Society of Great Britain suggested that the development of clinical pharmacy would assist in the improvement of drug therapy in hospitals and should therefore be encouraged by the Department of Health. It said that when pharmacists visited wards their advice on the actions and uses of drugs was frequently sought by physicians and nurses. The pharmacist should be able to give an unbiased assessment of the value of drugs which are used in a particular condition or in the circumstances of a particular patient. Ward visits by pharmacists to see prescriptions and to offer advice on appropriate drug treatment were also seen as valuable contributions to patient welfare in 1976 by a committee of the Central Health Services Council which considered the organisation of the hospital inpatient's day. This committee observed that professional skills within the National Health Service may not always be used in a way which provides the best service to patients. It commented that highly trained staff were wasted if their skills were not used to full advantage. This can certainly be true of pharmacists in the hospital service. Evidence was presented to the committee suggesting how pharmaceutical skills may be put to better use and a recommendation was made that an understanding of the skills available amongst all the paramedical professions should be encouraged by interprofessional discussion and the inclusion of relevant personnel on medical ward rounds. The Pharmaceutical Society, in its evidence to this committee, said that as the concept of ward pharmacy develops, the involvement of pharmacists at ward level was becoming apparent. Despite this new role currently being suggested for the hospital pharmacist, he must not abdicate his traditional skills as an expert on drugs with particular reference to their preparation and formulation. The clinical pharmacist can best define his own role by appreciating the problems he is equipped to solve. He must not try to step outside the area of his expertise—that of drugs, drug use and drug information. He should extend his original horizons to include an influence on prescribing and a knowledge of the clinical use of drugs, not forgetting the collation and dissemination of advice and information about drugs. His main efforts must be directed towards promoting the safe and efficacious use of drugs and to correcting deficiencies in their use by both patients and prescribers. It is clear that unless pharmacists are prepared to generate a clinical interest within their departments and to use their skills more for the direct benefit of the patient, their role and function within the hospital service may diminish. Many departments are unable to meet the stringent requirements of the Medicines Act (1968) which demands that hospital manufacturing departments match the highest standards of the pharmaceutical industry. As a result, bulk manufacture of both sterile and non-sterile items may be severely restricted unless major improvements are carried out. Consequently, in time, quality control within such departments could also diminish. Equipment and expertise which might otherwise become idle could perhaps be usefully redeployed in the measurement of drugs in body fluids and the development of a pharmacokinetic service. This would then link the pharmacy department directly with the bedside and so provide an excellent back-up service for the clinical pharmacist.

PHILOSOPHY

It has been said that a ward pharmacist by definition is committed to the care of patients on a ward or group of wards within a hospital (Bass 1973). For this to be true there must be recognition by pharmacists, physicians and nurses that the responsibility for health care can be effectively shared and that, in fact, optimal patient care can only be achieved through cooperative efforts (Fig. 11.1). The pharmacist's contribution should neither begin nor end when drugs are dispensed. He must have a knowledge and an understanding of the patient as a whole and be able to consider present or future drug therapy in terms of the patient's current status, his behaviour, the objectives of therapy and his prognosis. He should also understand and be able to communicate on the appropriateness of drug therapy, benefit-to-risk ratios and be able to suggest alternative regimes. A complex relationship links the patient, his disease and its treatment. The process of making drug therapy decisions and ultimately providing the patient with drugs is complex. It can be expressed diagramatically; outlining each stage sequentially and identifying the likely causes of treatment failure as well as highlighting possible areas of involvement by the clinical pharmacist (Fig. 11.2).

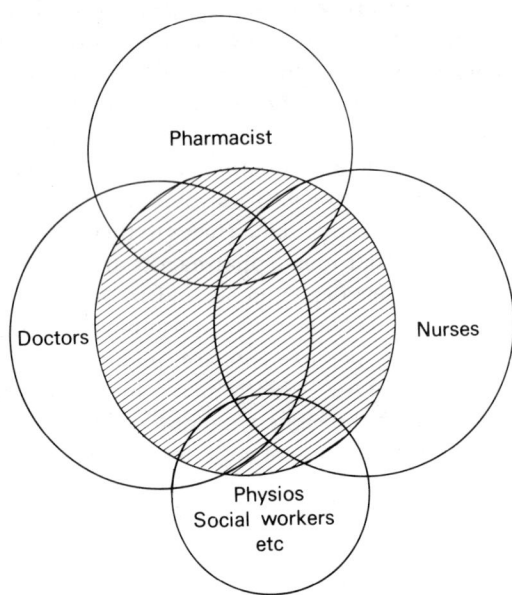

Fig. 11.1   The health care team. The shaded central area represents the patient.

Drugs often induce illness. They may also complicate disease. Medical and drug histories are usually recorded for each patient shortly after their admission to a hospital. It has been suggested that unwanted drug effects have occurred in as many as 28% of patients in the USA and are responsible for 3–4% of all hospital admissions to medical beds in the USA (Miller 1973; Caranasos et al 1974). The prior use of certain drugs may even predispose a patient to ill effects during either present or future therapy. Because of pharmacists' specialised knowledge, drug histories taken by them can be more informative than those obtained by medically trained personnel, especially where self medication with 'over-the-counter' medicines is concerned (Covington & Pfieffer 1972; McHale & Canada 1969; Wilson 1971). Pharmacists also frequently find it easier to clarify confusion regarding the strength or brand of particular dosage forms than their medical colleagues.

The hospital pharmacist has traditionally advised medical staff on drugs for general use within a hospital. He usually decides upon the source of supply and frequently works with medical and nursing colleagues to eliminate the use of duplicate or highly toxic drugs and to rationalise the range of drugs kept and supplied by his department. The pharmacist on the ward, however, is in a good position to advise on drug therapy before or at the time the prescription is written. In doing so he should evaluate all factors which may modify

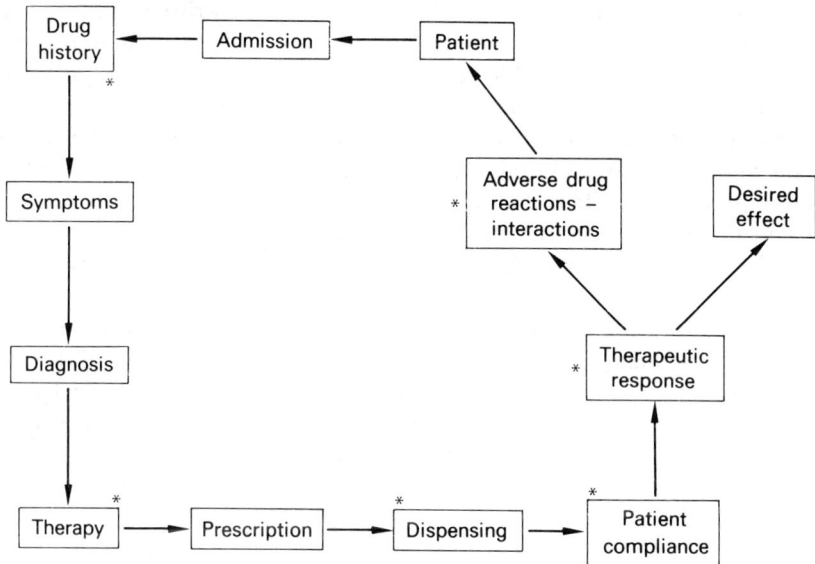

Fig. 11.2 The process of making drug therapy decisions. *Areas of involvement of the clinical or ward pharmacist. After Katcher (1972).

or preclude drug selection and he should have some idea of the efficacy and safety of treatment considered in terms of the incidence of side effects and possible adverse reactions. Various authors in the USA have documented the impact of the pharmacist as a drug therapy advisor in the ward situation (Bell 1970; 1973; Hill & Eckel 1973).

In hospitals that operate a stock system of drug distribution to the wards without a comprehensive ward pharmacy service, prescriptions are frequently interpreted by nurses, who may only question the prescriber or perhaps other nursing colleagues when the dose appears to them to be unusual or where there is a problem with its administration. This provides very few safeguards for the patient against inadvertent errors in prescribing and there is little attempt to detect inappropriate concurrent prescribing or potential drug interactions. In his capacity as therapeutic advisor, the pharmacist is able to provide information to both medical and nursing staff on the optimum dosage, dosing frequency, dosage form, as well as the times and routes of administration. Drugs are sometimes used inappropriately due to a lack of knowledge of formulation on the part of the prescriber. Having all the relevant information to hand on the ward, the clinical pharmacist is able to advise on the best formulation to suit a particular patient's needs. Likewise unnecessary or excessive drug use can be discouraged far more effectively whilst on the ward than from a distance, where the relevant background information is not usually available.

Once the diagnosis has been made, the prescriptions written and the drugs dispensed, the pharmacist has an important role to play in monitoring the effects of drug therapy. Problems concerning drug therapy in hospitals are not only related to poor systems of drug distribution, drug administration and record keeping, but also include lack of application of product information to the preparation and administration of drugs, inadequate drug information on the part of prescribers and a poor appreciation of the need to recognise and document adverse drug effects. The pharmacist, however, can only begin to make a significant contribution in this area when he is able to appreciate certain clinical chemistry and haematological data with respect to past, present and future drug therapy together with those parameters which commonly serve as therapeutic endpoints, and the organisation of medical records. He should be thoroughly familiar with the physical and pharmacological properties of the drugs prescribed, the normal dose range for the condition being treated, the pharmacokinetics involved, any possible adverse effects that might be expected, significant potential drug interactions and any factors which modify drug activity. It is therefore essential that the pharmacist develops and extends his knowledge of the clinical use of drugs. In view of the vast range of drugs currently available, this is perhaps best achieved if in the first instance attention is focussed on those drugs known to have narrow therapeutic indices where careful dosage adjustments are necessary in the event of certain predisposing factors such as old age, renal impairment or other concurrent medication. By monitoring drug use in this way and by attempting to detect and decrease adverse drug reactions and interactions, and by reducing unnecessary drug use and suboptimal or excessive dosing, the clinical pharmacist can then hope to improve drug therapy and so contribute significantly to direct patient care.

The pharmacist's contribution, however, need not end there. Having achieved a desired therapeutic response, patients usually leave hospital and return home. It is often necessary to continue drug treatment after discharge and it is now well recognised that education of the patient in the use of drugs thus supplied to him is the weakest link in the therapeutic chain. Treatment carefully worked out in the sheltered environment of the hospital often fails quite simply because of non-compliance or inability of the patient to take drugs according to directions when he gets home. In an attempt to improve upon this situation it is essential that the dosage form, time and frequency of administration as well as other concurrent drug therapy are all tailored to help the patient. The pharmacist both on the ward and in the pharmacy department from where he may hand over a supply of drugs directly to the patient, is in a good position to ensure that all instructions and precautions are understood, and that the patient can actually cope physically with his medication in the way that it is presented to him. Pharmacists should also see that patients are provided with as much knowledge as is necessary for them to make the best use of the drugs supplied. Consequently, in cooperation with medical staff, they should be able to tell the patient, either verbally or in writing, ideally just before he is discharged, why he should continue to take his drugs, which selected side-effects he might expect to experience, how, if necessary, to obtain further supplies and when to revisit his doctor. Other aspects of patient education by the hospital pharmacist should include information on the safety and storage of medicines and poisons in the home as well as promotion of a good relationship between the general public and pharmacists working in the community who can provide a useful link between the patient and secondary health care by collaboration and communication with hospital-based colleagues.

Education and training by the clinical pharmacist should also extend to medical and nursing staff as well as to fellow pharmacists. This can be in the form of lectures, informal discussion groups and bulletins produced at regular intervals by the pharmacy drug information service. The clinical pharmacist should actively participate in the education of student nurses, and, where geographically possible, undergraduate pharmacy students. He also has a valuable part to play in the in-service training of qualified staff. Nurses fully occupied with their day-to-day nursing duties, welcome help, advice and information concerning drug use specifically tailored to their needs. A clinical pharmacist has the advantage of ward experience and is therefore able to appreciate some of the problems frequently encountered by nursing staff and is able to pass on some of his knowledge of the use of drugs in the clinical situation. This is yet another way in which the pharmacist can promote safer and possibly more economic drug use both in terms of administration to the patient and stock control at ward level.

In order to achieve some of the objectives outlined, various obstacles have first to be overcome, not least of which being the attitudes and aspirations of many pharmacists currently within service. The movement for change has to come from within. The enthusiasm of young graduates opting for hospital pharmacy as a career may be lost if direction and leadership is not forthcoming. Whilst a great deal can be done on a personal basis by individual pharmacists, official recognition of the need for clinical pharmacy services is essential. Such recognition will bring with it the resources necessary in terms of funding for extra staff, expensive equipment and essential training programmes, all of which are required before such services can be fully developed. Quite naturally there has been and will be opposition, scepticism and cynicism from certain members of the medical profession, some of whom quite erroneously feel their position to be threatened. No pharmacist would question the ability of a physician to make diagnostic decisions or would suggest that all he does is not in the best interests of his patient; however, in recent years, with the ever expanding range and toxicity of drugs, it is the physician's ability to make appropriate decisions about drug therapy that has been questioned. Such doubts have been highlighted by the incidence of drug-induced disease and adverse reactions as well as the high cost of prescribing. It has been suggested that the concept of clinical pharmacy will be seen as a threat to physicians although some argue that pharmacists are unable to participate in drug treatment decisions since they have insufficient knowledge of medical terminology and are therefore unable to communicate effectively. A traditional task of a pharmacist has been to perform a safety check on prescriptions and whilst on the wards he is also able to monitor drug administration. This may give the appearance of evaluating the performance of medical and nursing colleagues. The motives and interests of clinical pharmacists must therefore be made clear. Their aim is to reduce drug errors, to encourage rational drug therapy and consequently to benefit the patient. They must not operate as new members of the health care team who can only function within the incompetence of other members of that team, but as professionals, trained to complement the services already provided by fellow professionals, who are expert in their own field. To maintain credibility, pharmacists must not play on the mistakes and bad prescribing habits of some physicians but develop a more constructive approach in which they monitor drug therapy for the benefit of the patient and offer advice, not just information, to the prescriber (Parish 1976).

CLINICAL PHARMACY IN AMERICA

Clinical pharmacy in the USA has evolved over the last decade. In this relatively short time the extent of such services has increased and developed rapidly and, although clinical pharmacists have not abdicated their traditional role concerned with the manufacture and distribution of drugs, they have nevertheless expanded their outlook to include a knowledge of the clinical use of drugs and attempts to influence prescribing. The report of the Millis Commission entitled *Pharmacists for the Future* was published in 1976. This study commission on pharmacy in the United States spent more than 2 years examining the practice of pharmacy as an integral part of the health service and also of the process of pharmacy education (Parish 1976). The report acknowledged that the primary aim of clinical pharmacists is to attempt to enhance the benefits of drug therapy and to reduce or correct deficiencies in drug use. The Commission began its examination on the assumption that judgements about the expected benefits and risks of various drug treatments in the individual are necessary, that pharmacists should be involved in drug-related decisions and that the organisation of pharmacy education with regard to the future of pharmaceutical services must be based on an understanding of the extent of services possible. The Commission acknowledged the traditional definition of pharmacy as the 'art and science of compounding and dispensing drugs' but at the same time recognised the possible extension of that definition which suggests that pharmacists should now be concerned with increasing their knowledge of the clinical use of drugs and their effects in man. Although this official recognition came as late as the mid 1970s, Brodie made an accurate forecast in 1965. He wrote in his report that 'the ultimate goal of the services of pharmacy must be the safe use of drugs by the public. In this context the mainstream function of pharmacy is clinical in nature. One that may be defined accurately as drug-use control' (Brodie 1965). He goes on to define drug-use control as 'the sum total of knowledge, understanding, judgement, procedures, skills, controls and ethics that assures optimal safety in the distribution and use of medication'. He continues: 'in the future, pharmacists will have increasing opportunities to participate in the distribution of drugs in a clinical situation. Emerging patterns of drug distribution in hospitals place the pharmacist on the floor, interpreting chart orders for medication, preparing medication for nursing staff and providing consultative drug information when required.' He does not restrict this context to the hospital environment: 'if drug use control is the mainstream component of pharmacy service it should apply to community pharmacy as well.' In this comment he highlights another area of importance. This is the role in clinical terms of the general practice pharmacist. This group of professionals has the scope for more day-to-day patient contact than many of their hospital-based colleagues. It is often the retail pharmacist who is the first source of advice and information concerning drugs for the general public. In fact, it is sometimes argued that this branch of the profession has always practised clinical pharmacy.

The Millis Report was not alone in directing the way for clinical pharmacy in the United States, the American Society of Hospital Pharmacists has also played a leading part in encouraging its development (Oddis 1976). In 1957 it urged hospital pharmacists to extend their responsibilities and actively promote the safe handling of drugs in hospitals. In 1970, a statement on clinical pharmacy and its relationship to the hospital urged hospitals to support the concept of clinical pharmacy and to make their facilities available to schools of pharmacy for the clinical preparation of future pharmacy practitioners. However, it was not words alone which stimulated the emergence of a more ward-based pharmacy service in the USA. Concern about the extent of medication errors also played an important part. A report published in 1962 (Barker & McConnell 1962) suggested that approximately 18% of all doses administered to a group of hospital patients were in error. In an attempt to rectify this alarming situation, hospital pharmacists introduced unit dose distribution methods (Chapter 10) which are recognised as the safest distribution systems, despite their high cost in terms of both time and money. They also required for the first time a pharmacist at ward level to coordinate the system. Decentralised or satellite pharmacy units subsequently emerged which also introduced the pharmacist to the clinical areas of the hospital. The potential contribution of the hospital pharmacist to direct patient care was then soon realised. Alongside these events, the appearance of drug information centres in several American hospitals demonstrated that physicians needed assistance in assimilating and evaluating the wealth of drug literature available to them as well as advice on the application of such information to the clinical situation. Such events, coupled with the recognition by both medical and nursing staff themselves that they needed help in making drug-related decisions and in drug therapy monitoring, all provided the initial stimulus for the growth of clinical pharmacy in America.

It must be borne in mind that most of the relevant literature concerning the services currently provided by clinical pharmacists in the USA is of a qualitative rather than a quantitative nature. There are obviously some centres of excellence but these appear to be concentrated in the larger teaching centres. There is very little quantitative information concerning the extent to which clinical pharmacy services are being provided in terms of both geography and patient number.

The activities of clinical pharmacists in the USA have been extensively reviewed. They can, according to McLeod (1976) be divided into three groups, those that are broad functions within the drug-use process, those that are specific tasks rather limited in scope, and those which involve specialisation of clinical pharmacy practice. In some hospitals in the USA, pharmacists routinely take drug histories from patients on admission. Their findings are recorded subsequently in the patient's notes. Other activities which fall into the first classification include advising on drug therapy during physicians' rounds and clinical conferences. Attendance at such meetings provides a means of keeping up to date with patients' progress as well as offering a pharmacist's perspective on drug treatment. Drug therapy monitoring is another such service. In some cases the pharmacist makes daily rounds independent of a physician. He visits patients and provides recommendations in writing on a special pharmacy communication sheet in the patient's notes (Beaman 1974). Patient counselling is yet another important service classified within the drug-use process. It is an attempt to reduce drug defaulting and so improve overall benefit to the patient. Retrospective drug usage review is also frequently carried out by pharmacists in conjunction with medical colleagues. Such studies are often of benefit to future patients since publication of results frequently leads to correction of inappropriate drug use.

Specific clinical activities include adverse drug reaction and drug–drug interaction detection and prevention, as well as antibiotic use control and cardiopulmonary resuscitation. According to McLeod (1976) pharmacists participate in the latter service in a number of ways from preparing and recording the drugs used during a cardiac arrest to even recommending appropriate drug therapy and helping to establish therapeutic endpoints. Total parenteral nutrition is another specific therapeutic area calling for widespread pharmaceutical involvement. It requires precise formulation with strict aseptic technique as well as careful assessment of the patient. Pharmacists also actively participate in monitoring the effects of anticoagulation and chemotherapy. Outpatient counselling has proved successful in terms of improved compliance and understanding by the patient (Chubb & Winship 1974; Linkewich *et al* 1974), particularly in those specialities concerned with cardiac, hypertensive and diabetic patients as well as those on narcotic withdrawal treatment with methadone. Specialisation towards clinical pharmacy has naturally led to specialisation within clinical pharmacy itself. Many general services depend for their success upon more narrow areas of interest which often correspond to well-recognised medical specialties. Examples of these include paediatric, psychiatric and geriatric pharmacy, clinical toxicology, pharmacokinetics and drug information. The reader is referred to McLeod's extensive review for further information on any of these services.

The increased involvement of the American hospital pharmacist in direct patient care has resulted in recognition of the need for a different, more specialised form of training. The stimulus for a change in direction of pharmaceutical services has come from both practitioners and educators and, as a result, there has been a proliferation of clinical pharmacists (Oddis 1976). One of the greatest problems, however, which hindered would-be practitioners has been the total lack of role models. Consequently young graduates have been left to define their own roles and in many cases have undertaken anything they consider appropriate which will help the patient. This however may include encroaching upon the areas of other health professionals. A pharmacist who has studied drugs and their effects extensively for several years both at undergraduate and postgraduate level should not be content to become merely an assistant to a physician or to undertake tasks that no one else sees fit or is able to find the time to do.

In 1972 Calder reported on the way in which pharmacy students in America were prepared for their potential new role. Certain objectives for instruction in clinical pharmacy had been put forward as early as 1968 (McCarron 1975). These included an acquaintance with general clinical pharmacological and pharmaceutical principles and an awareness of the general methods of diagnosis and patient-care specifically related to drug therapy. Students should be capable of effective interaction with patients as well as their fellow health care professionals and must also develop a patient awareness in the provision of a pharmaceutical service. Students should be helped to integrate their basic knowledge within the clinical situation and to develop an understanding of their responsibilities in the areas of drug therapy monitoring and drug usage. By 1972 most courses in clinical pharmacy included visits, clerkships and/or teaching seminars on wards and in clinics within hospitals. Many even made provision for some teaching within the community. Certain questions however still needed to be answered. Was there a need for separate, clearly defined preclinical and clinical programmes? Should all pharmacy undergraduates go through the same clinical pharmacy course or should options be made available at various levels? How should teachers of clinical pharmacy be qualified? Should they all hold joint appointments between the academic institutions and the hospitals? Should all instruction in clinical pharmacy be conducted in a 'real' situation—on the ward or in the clinic?

Many academics in England are currently concerned about the apparent desire to swing away from basic science subjects in the curriculum and Calder was similarly concerned to observe that some colleges in the United States were producing graduates who would not be capable of working for a higher degree in the fundamental pharmaceutical sciences. His view was that educators in America had failed to reach a satisfactory compromise between increased clinical input and either an extension in the total length of the course or at the expense of reducing its traditional pharmaceutical content. He was concerned at the lack of basic pharmaceutical ability evident in many of the practitioners he observed but at the same time their obvious enthusiasm and clinical knowledge was impressive. It seems that the Americans have succeeded in changing the attitude of pharmacists, but has this been at the expense of the pharmaceutical science content of their basic undergraduate course?

For several years, pharmaceutical education in the United States has been gradually moving towards its goal of meeting all the needs of the practising profession. The impact of clinical pharmacy on the curriculum and its educational development have been extensively reviewed (Rodowskas 1976). Currently the 5-year Bachelor of Pharmacy degree is the standard professional qualification. Its syllabus, although including a strong clinical emphasis, is basically tailored to suit the needs of the general practice pharmacist. This is not surprising, since only 12% of pharmacy graduates opt for hospital pharmacy as a career while at least 75% practice in the community. Related clinical subjects covered in the course include biopharmaceutics, pharmacokinetics, applied pharmaceutics and clinical clerkships. It is however the Pharm.D. which has rapidly become the degree programme associated with the advanced clinical training necessary for practice as a clinical pharmacist. This qualification is considered to be equivalent to a doctorate of medicine or dental surgery and, to obtain it, it is necessary to study for a further 1–3 years. This period is variable because several colleges offer a residency programme as part of the course. It is in such hospitals, which are in general closely associated with a college of pharmacy, that the practice of clinical pharmacy is most highly developed (Franke & Witney 1976). In these institutions a number of professors of clinical pharmacy hold joint appointments between hospitals and the academic institutions which thus allows them to be teacher-practitioners. Most colleges will only accept students for the Pharm.D. course who have already attained the Bachelor of Pharmacy degree. A total of 24 approved colleges of pharmacy in America offer courses leading to either a Bachelor degree or a Pharm.D. Of these, three institutions offer instruction exclusively to Pharm.D. level. Residency programmes in American hospitals are now well established and are highly regarded as part of the overall postgraduate pharmacy education. In 1975 there were 72 such approved residency programmes and the figure increased to 100 by 1977.

CLINICAL PHARMACY IN GREAT BRITAIN

Pharmacists in the United States appear to be nearer the goal of a more patient oriented approach to their work both in terms of education and practice than their counterparts in Europe. For many years pharmacists in Great Britain have been concerned that they should be exerting a greater influence in the correct use of drugs both by prescribers and patients. At the same time neither the medical and nursing professions nor the general public have been aware of the contribution pharmacists could make to health care. The level and depth of pharmaceutical education in Great Britain has gradually increased while the extent to which pharmacists have been able to make use of their knowledge has decreased. Clinical pharmacy is considered to be an outlet for some of this knowledge. When clinical pharmacy is the subject for discussion in Great Britain it is important to distinguish between rhetoric and practice. Baker (1976) has defined clinical pharmacy as 'pharmacist involvement in monitoring patients' therapy and giving advice which directly influences decisions concerning drug therapy and the way in which it is administered'. Unfortunately, there are few, if any, hospital pharmacy departments in Great Britain where this can be seen to be in operation on a large scale. Some of the aims of clinical pharmacy further defined by Baker (1976) as 'closer pharmacist involvement with clinical staff and patients to secure efficacy, safety and cost effectiveness in the use of drugs' are achieved by individual pharmacists committed to the ideal but who depend upon a particularly favourable local environment for much of their success. Pharmaceutical education as well as services will have to develop further before pharmacists in Great Britain are either adequately prepared to practice clinical pharmacy or before it is accepted nationally as the standard level of service.

Ward pharmacy in Great Britain

Ward pharmacy in its various forms is well established in many hospitals throughout Great Britain. It has become recognised as a valuable contribution to patient care since it was first introduced by the Westminster Group of hospitals between 1965 and 1966. In general terms, ward pharmacy can be considered to be a means of controlling the use of drugs at ward level and it was recommended as such in 1970 to Regional Hospital Boards, Boards of Governors and Hospital Management Committees by the DHSS circular HM (70) 36. This document, after outlining the problems associated with drug administration and advising on the correct way in which prescriptions should be written, suggested that regular ward visits by pharmacists should be introduced as soon as possible. This was to 'enable the pharmacist to check the pharmaceutical aspects of and draw attention to pharmacological anomalies of prescriptions, to be available for consultation by doctors and nurses and to examine and review ward stocks and stocklists' (DHSS 1970b). Calder (1975) has described the basic role of a pharmacist in 'patient services' as that of 'reading and interpreting every prescription and ensuring that the patient receives the correct medication of the proper quality, in the right dose and at the right time'. He said 'the pharmacist should also advise the prescriber of any known or anticipated untoward response to the medication'. This definition can be used to describe the activities of a ward pharmacist.

Drug distribution

Ward pharmacy cannot be entirely separated from the distribution function of a department. A complete stock system is both expensive in terms of the amount of stock necessarily carried by each ward and inadvisable in terms of patient safety unless a pharmacist regularly visits the ward at frequent intervals to monitor all prescriptions and to check stock levels. When all drugs are issued as stock and a pharmacist does not visit the ward, drugs may be selected from ward stock for administration to patients without nursing staff being aware of all the possibilities in terms of strength, formulation, dosage form etc. This is particularly hazardous when specific dosages are not prescribed. Similarly a distribution system in which every item is individually dispensed for each patient is often uneconomic and inefficient. Consequently many hospitals have adopted a compromise system of drug distribution backed up by ward pharmacy. This involves the wards keeping as stock only those items which are most frequently prescribed. Drugs used infrequently, those which require closer monitoring because of possible interactions with either other drugs or food, those which require specific dosage adjustments in the event of renal or hepatic impairment as well as new or particularly expensive items are all usually dispensed individually for each patient. It is important however that in the eyes of both medical and nursing staff, a ward pharmacy service is seen as an expansion of the role of the pharmacist and not as an extension to the existing distribution process (see Chapter 10 for a description of different drug distribution systems).

Ward stocks

One of the first duties of a ward pharmacist when establishing a new service is to rationalise and possibly reduce the number of drugs kept as stock at ward level. Regular supervision by a ward pharmacist who should maintain comprehensive up to date stock lists for each of his wards is of paramount importance in reducing wastage and ensuring that only drugs in good condition are used. Bradley and Griffiths (1977) have highlighted the cost benefits of ward pharmacy in this area. Prior to the implementation of a ward pharmacy service in a hospital, excessive stocks of drugs, some of which are rarely used, are frequently found in ward drug cupboards. This can result in patients receiving medication which is below standard due to age or inappropriate storage conditions. The ward pharmacist should come to an agreement with the ward sister as to which items are to be held as stock on her ward. This should be done bearing in mind the conditions treated on the ward and also possible emergency admissions which could occur especially when the pharmacy department is closed. Such stock levels should be flexible, it must be possible to change them at short notice when either medical staff or fashions in prescribing change.

Frequency of visits

The time and frequency of visits to a ward by the pharmacist are also decided jointly by the pharmacist and ward sister. The frequency depends upon the average length of stay per patient as well as the 'type' of patient and disease state dealt with on the ward in question. An acute medical, surgical or admission ward warrants a daily, or even twice daily visit while long stay units where changes in drug treatment occur infrequently could be adequately covered by a weekly or even monthly visit depending upon geographical location and the staff available. The time at which the pharmacist visits should ideally always be the same each day and should enable adequate contact with medical and nursing staff. A most convenient time to all concerned is often just after or even during the main prescribing round.

Tasks

The tasks performed by a ward pharmacist during a ward visit vary. Basically, the main objective is to ensure that all prescriptions are clear, unambiguous, appropriate and safe, and that nursing staff have clear and complete instructions for administering drugs in such a way that the best use is made of them. It is vital for a nurse to be able to relate a particular prescription to a name that appears on the label of a container. Since it is the practice of most hospital pharmacy departments to use approved names for labelling drugs the ward pharmacist often annotates the prescriptions with the approved name and also the strength of particular dosage forms where necessary. At the same time it is also common practice to indicate on the drug chart for the benefit of the nursing staff whether or not a particular item is to be found as stock on that ward. A supply or distributive function may also be part of the ward pharmacist's role. Where this is the case he usually initiates the supply of a newly prescribed non-stock drug and in doing so helps to ensure that prescriptions remain on the ward at all times. The details of such new prescriptions which are signed and dated by the pharmacist are usually recorded either in a notebook or on a preprinted form. Alternatively the labels may be written on the ward and taken back to the pharmacy department for dispensing. The drugs are eventually transported to the ward by the normal portering service. Further supplies of such individually dispensed items are obtained when necessary by sending the empty containers to the pharmacy where their contents are replaced according to the details on the labels. By regular monitoring of all prescriptions the pharmacist is able to ensure that prescriptions are still valid and that drugs supplied in this way are still appropriate. This supply function is often considered by medical and nursing staff to be one of the biggest advantages of ward pharmacy services which operate in this way. When new prescriptions for non-stock drugs are sent to the pharmacy for dispensing they may remain away from the ward for several hours. This can lead to dangerous situations whereby duplicate prescriptions may be written possibly from memory to enable drug administration to take place, or new items may be prescribed on fresh charts, resulting in the patient ending up with more than one treatment chart. It is obviously both tiresome and inconvenient to medical and nursing staff, as well as dangerous to the patient, if prescriptions are absent from the ward at any time. It must be remembered however that such a supply function on the part of the ward pharmacist is only possible when frequent ward pharmacy visits are made such as to an acute or admission ward. To wait for the ward pharmacist's visit before newly prescribed drugs are supplied to patients in a long stay unit could result in unnecessary and possibly hazardous delays in treating those patients.

As the ward pharmacist reads the prescription he is alerted to the possibility of drug interactions, possible adverse reactions, incompatibilities and contraindications. The importance of this is emphasised by the fact that prescribing for inpatients is frequently delegated to junior and relatively inexperienced medical staff with a varying amount of supervision from their superiors. Similarly, drug administration is often the responsibility of relatively inexperienced nurses whose only guidance is the written prescription and the label on the container. Ward pharmacy evolved from investigations into the frequency with which errors occurred when drugs were administered in hospitals. It was apparent at the time that many sources of error would be eliminated by devising safer methods of prescribing and administering drugs. Although this was done, a chronic shortage of nursing and junior medical staff did not help to improve the situation. Pharmacists have been welcomed on to the wards to help fill the gap created by such inadequacies. Ward pharmacists must not however exist merely to make good the deficiencies in other areas. They must be seen as experts in their own field, capable of giving advice which is clinically useful and participating in the day-to-day management of the patient.

In some hospitals, much of the pressure to introduce ward pharmacy came from outside the profession. Senior medical and nursing staff are often involved in preliminary discussions before such services are implemented. The concept of ward pharmacy should have widespread approval within a hospital before it can be considered to be truly successful. It must be seen as an integral part of an existing service which places less demand on, and more closely meets the needs of, both medical and nursing staff. At the same time it is important that ward pharmacy should not be regarded as an expensive messenger or portering service.

'Take home' drugs

Drugs prescribed for patients to take home are also often dealt with by the ward pharmacists. Perhaps the least satisfactory way in which this is done is for the pharmacist to take the prescription back to the pharmacy for dispensing. Once again this means that the chart is missing from the ward. The use of special carbon backed prescription pads for 'take home' drugs is therefore preferable. When the prescription is written, two copies are made automatically. After he has checked that the drugs prescribed for a patient to take home correspond to his inpatient treatment, one copy is taken to the pharmacy department by the pharmacist for dispensing, after which it remains there as a record. The main prescription stays on the ward with the patient until he is discharged, after which it is stored in the patient's notes. The second copy often serves as a communication between the hospital team and the patient's general practitioner. This avoids the obvious danger and inconvenience of transcription from the original prescription and enables the general practitioner to see exactly which drugs the patient was sent home with.

One of the prime requisites of a ward pharmacy service is continuity. It is essential that a particular pharmacist remains with a group of wards, if not 'permanently', then for a period of at least 12 months. Only in this way can the right relationships be formed with medical and nursing staff. An experienced ward pharmacist with a sound knowledge of the range of drugs used on his wards and a commitment to keeping himself well informed and up to date, as well as with the ability to communicate adequately and establish good relationships, can as a ward pharmacist contribute significantly to the improved efficacy and safety of drug therapy. With frequent changes of junior medical and nursing staff the ward pharmacist is increasingly relied upon for information and advice on drug therapy. Such continuity enables him to build up a relatively specialised knowledge of the drugs used on the wards he covers. Provision of information to all grades of staff is one of the most important duties of a ward pharmacist. As he becomes more experienced such information should be advisory as much as factual. He should always be ready to admit uncertainty or ignorance of a particular topic but, at the same time, express his intention of looking into the problem and providing an answer either verbally or in writing at a later date. Obviously therefore an effective ward pharmacy system can only operate in conjunction with an efficient and comprehensive drug information service.

Ward rounds

In some hospitals recognition of the role of the ward pharmacist has occurred to the extent that they regularly attend clinical ward rounds. This can be very time consuming and in general the time spent is often only of an educational benefit to the pharmacist concerned with very little contribution possible on his part. A more satisfactory arrangement is for the ward pharmacist to be available during or immediately after a clinical round whilst he performs his routine ward pharmacy tasks. When this is so his advice is regularly sought by clinicians and he is often invited to take part in discussions involving problems of particular interest to him. Conversely in this way doctors are equally available to the pharmacist should he wish to bring anything to their attention. Since the routine attendance of pharmacists on medical ward rounds is considered by many to be of questionable value to any one other than the pharmacist, such participation is usually limited to educational programmes intended to equip pharmacists for a future clinical role. There are of course exceptions. Grant (1976) has described a clinical pharmacy programme involving the regular participation of six pharmacists in medical ward rounds in a district general hospital. The premise on which such a programme is based is a definition suggested by Lipman (1974). He describes clinical pharmacy as 'the provision of both solicited and unsolicited clinical drug information in the patient area on a regularly scheduled basis at the time that drug therapy decisions are being made'. In practice this can be interpreted as being possible only if a pharmacist is routinely present on clinical rounds and is free to participate in patient conference sessions. Pharmacists initially attended ward rounds in the hospital in question in a learning capacity. In fact the programme evolved from the clinical involvement of students undertaking study for a master's degree. It was noticeable at first that pharmacists present were often accredited with a greater background knowledge of disease and therapeutics than they possessed and it is admitted that in the beginning the contribution to patient care was small. This increased however as the clinical experience of the pharmacists widened. Six consultants currently have pharmacists as members of their team. The principle aim of this programme is to ensure that the patient receives maximum benefit from drug therapy. Involvement of the pharmacist also includes patient monitoring, compilation of drug histories, participation in adverse drug reaction screening, documentation of new therapies and the provision of advice on the clinical use of drugs. Although the programme appears to be costly in terms of time, the benefits are considered by all concerned to outweigh the disadvantages.

History taking

Further extensions to the role of the ward pharmacist are the taking of drug histories, patient counselling and adverse drug reaction monitoring. The specialised training and knowledge of a pharmacist enables him to obtain a comprehensive medication history involving both prescribed drugs and self medication. The detection of side-effects, iatrogenic disease or other consequences of therapy are also important considerations when such activities are undertaken. In a study conducted over a 4-month period on a gynaecological ward in a district general hospital it was observed that significantly more items were reported by a pharmacist than by the doctor when medication histories were taken from the same patients in admission by both parties (L. G. Dodds, pers. commun. 1976). It was noted that the doctor frequently failed to report self medication even when it was being taken in fairly large quantities. The pharmacists' report also contained more information about the adverse effects of therapy such as nausea, vomiting, dizziness, diarrhoea and constipation. Recognition and possible avoidance of such effects in the future could significantly improve patient compliance with subsequently prescribed medication.

Patient non-compliance

Non-compliance in the taking of prescribed medicines is currently an area of great concern. It is also one where the pharmacist's potential contribution goes unchallenged by researchers and is welcomed by clinicians. A considerable amount of time and expertise go into deciding upon and finally providing suitable drug therapy for a patient. All of this is wasted if, on discharge, a patient fails for whatever reason to take his prescribed medication correctly. One study of 130 patients discharged from four hospital wards dealing mainly with acute medical cases showed that 66 deviated from the drug regime prescribed on discharge. Of these, 46 did not have a clear understanding of the regime and 20 understood the instructions but did not follow them (Parkin *et al* 1976). Non-compliance is not only wasteful; it can also be harmful to the patient. Particular groups of patients, despite the fact that they depend upon regular medication for a symptom-free existence, have been identified as the worst defaulters. Such patients include those suffering from tuberculosis, hypertension and schizophrenia. Very little can be done to persuade deliberate defaulters to comply but much can be achieved in helping other patients to understand and to cope with their medicines more effectively.

In the past it has usually been a nurse who hands over discharge drugs to a patient, often at the very last moment just as he leaves the ward. The transition from the sheltered environment of a hospital ward back to the home can be a difficult one, particularly for a patient who has suddenly to cope with a number of different kinds of medicines. The ward pharmacist is ideally placed to try to help a patient with this transition. Elderly people in particular may experience difficulties. Because of their age they are likely to suffer from more than one disease and consequently they may be prescribed a number of different drugs. A survey has recently shown that 25% of elderly patients could not manage to take more than three preparations correctly during any one period (Dass *et al* 1977) and in 1976 a general practice survey showed that 24% of elderly patients were on more than three drugs regularly (Law & Chalmers 1976). Studies have also shown that the level of compliance in the general population falls off with an increase in the frequency and number of different preparations prescribed. In 1972 in the United Kingdom people who were taking prescribed medicines were taking an average of 2.2 different items (Dunnell & Cartwright 1972), and it is quite conceivable that patients in the high risk elderly age group are probably on at least twice as many. The first task of a ward pharmacist in promoting compliance is to work in conjunction with prescribers to ensure that a patient is discharged on as few drugs as possible and also that those that are prescribed are convenient for the patient wherever possible in terms of dosage form and frequency. The total number of items can often be reduced by careful consideration of the real need for such drugs as hypnotics and also by the use of various combined preparations which have recently gained considerable favour with prescribers concerned about the problems of non-compliance amongst their patients.

Elderly patients in particular may suffer from poor eyesight. It is then important that instructions on containers as to how medicines should be taken are made legible for them. This may necessitate containers which enable the use of larger labels with bolder print. Separate information sheets may even be necessary in some instances. Patients with arthritic hands also deserve special consideration. They are often unable to cope with bubble or blister packs and welcome their drugs supplied in containers that are somewhat larger than usual. The ward pharmacist should be aware of such difficulties likely to be experienced by his patients. He should be able to help overcome them and so hope to promote compliance.

Another way of overcoming some of the problems of drug defaulting, particularly in the confused or elderly patient who may be taking a number of different items regularly, is by the use of containers such as the 'Dosette'. This is a container invented in Sweden. It holds a weeks supply of drugs and has a transparent plastic cover which slides open to uncover one at a time, four separate compartments for each day of the week. Into each compartment can be placed all doses to be taken at either breakfast, dinner, tea or bedtime. It is coloured bright red and all letters and figures, as well as being raised, are shown in braille. A window on the back of the container holds a card on which details of the drugs prescribed may be written. Although such aids are too expensive and inappropriate for routine use by all patients, the savings incurred if they are used by otherwise non-compliant patients carefully selected by the ward pharmacist and prescriber, could be considerable.

It is quite clear from the various studies carried out in both America and Great Britain that comprehension and recall of prescription directions are necessary if drugs are to be taken correctly. There is a need for the ward pharmacist and prescriber to take an active part in educating the patient. This must be seen as a joint responsibility but care must be taken to see that verbal and written instructions from both parties are consistent. Very often little effort is made to explain to patients that as a result of hospital contract buying, tablets and capsules obtained subsequently from a retail chemist via a prescription from their general practitioner may differ in size, colour or markings from those they were taking whilst in hospital and were discharged with. They are also often confused by the apparent discrepancy between trade names and approved names. All of these are relatively minor problems when considered individually. However, they may all contribute to the major problem of non-compliance. In an attempt to overcome the source of these difficulties some hospitals have introduced training programmes whereby the patient is counselled by a ward pharmacist several days before he is due to be discharged. At the same time he is supplied with the drugs that he will eventually take home and is encouraged to administer them to himself during the last few days of his stay on the ward. He does this under a certain amount of supervision from both the ward pharmacist and the nursing staff. In this way his potential degree of compliance can be assessed. If necessary his prescribed therapy can be reviewed and possibly changed before discharge should the circumstances demand it. Verbal instructions and counselling can be reinforced by the use of written instructions, calendars and cards on which the patient can tick off doses taken. It has been shown that, particularly in the elderly, compliance can be improved by giving patients written as well as verbal instructions (Wandless & Davie 1977).

Adverse drug reaction monitoring

Drug therapy monitoring is also an important function of many pharmacists working in the clinical field. One aspect of this is participation in schemes devised to monitor for adverse drug reactions, the objectives being to diminish the time interval between the general release of a new drug and the full recognition of any undesirable effects it might produce. This is particularly important in the case of side effects occurring either infrequently or only after prolonged administration. Such effects are unlikely to be detected during premarketing trials. It is also important to investigate fully those adverse reactions already identified in order to ascertain their frequency and distribution and to disseminate such information to the medical, nursing and pharmaceutical professions. In recent years national registers have been established in several countries with the main aim of providing an early warning that a drug is capable of causing a serious adverse effect. These registers in general depend upon the voluntary spontaneous reporting of suspected adverse reactions by doctors.

An adverse reaction is an unwanted and unexpected effect of a particular drug. It may occur as a result of a drug–drug or drug–food interaction or it may involve interference with a laboratory test. Some adverse reactions are self evident, others may closely simulate natural disease states. Reactions observed may be so bizarre that a familiar drug may escape suspicion or alternatively the appearance of an adverse effect may be long delayed or the clinical situation may be so complex that a drug-related effect may pass unnoticed. Also doctors may be reluctant to admit that a patient may have been harmed by their treatment.

The British Register of Adverse Reactions was established in 1964. Doctors are asked to report unexpected and severe reactions to all drugs and all re-actions, including mild ones, which occurred as a result of the administration of new drugs. Despite wide publicity the response has been disappointing. This is attributed to a number of factors. Doctors may fear exposure to criticism or charges of negligence. There appears to be no immediate or direct benefit of submitting such reports and so consequently doctors are poorly motivated. A high work load and the shared responsibility of the hospital team are other excuses put forward. It is often extremely difficult to establish a causal relation-ship between the observed effect and drug responsible, especially in patients who may be suffering from more than one disease and who are being treated with more than one drug. The main aim therefore of a pharmacist involved in adverse drug reaction monitoring is one of encouragement and promotion in an attempt to improve the situation.

Any system of monitoring adverse drug reactions must set out to answer a number of questions. It is important to have some idea of the incidence of such reactions. Do the beneficial effects of treatment outweigh any risk or dis-advantage? What specific populations are most at risk and which adverse effects observed are related to interactions with food or other drugs? Two forms of monitoring are possible; spontaneous voluntary reporting by medical prac-titioners or intensive drug monitoring programmes. The first has the advan-tage of cheapness and allows an enormous population of patients and a wide range of drugs to be covered. It potentially involves all prescribers. Its major disadvantages have already been outlined, the main ones being under report-ing and the submission of incomplete information. Intensive drug surveillance involves a more defined population, subjected to drug therapy, which is monitored continuously to determine the frequency with which certain events are associated with drug administration or whether a causal relationship between drug and effect is probable. It also allows the identification of sub-populations at greatest risk. Such systems, although costly and time consum-ing, are more effective than those which depend upon voluntary spontaneous efforts. A number of such intensive monitoring programmes set up in America have involved pharmacists as monitors (Allen & Greenblatt 1975). In Great Britain the ward pharmacist is taking on more and more responsibility in this area. It is interesting to note that in hospitals where monitoring systems are established or where ward pharmacists show a particular interest there is a significant rise in the level of reporting of adverse drug reactions.

Extended hours service

One criticism of many of the activities outlined is how can they be carried out effectively on a 'part-time' basis. This somewhat harsh comment is a reflection of the fact that hospital pharmaceutical services, with notable exceptions, generally operate according to a nine-to-five working day. Most hospitals however do perform some unofficial on call or out-of-hours service but nothing as yet is officially recognised in terms of pay and conditions of service. Until pharmacists can be seen to be working on an equal footing with medical, nursing and other paramedical staff with regard to hours and on-call duties, they cannot expect to assume a truly clinical role.

Specialised units

In general, ward pharmacy appears to be well established in Great Britain and is accepted as a useful extension of the pharmaceutical service. The way in which ward pharmacy is organised varies according to the type of hospital, staffing levels and geographical location. An acute district general hospital will operate a very different system from that found in a geriatric or psychiatric unit. Each specialty has its own problems and calls for different levels of involvement. A geriatric unit may provide more opportunities to participate in patient counselling; psychiatric hospitals may require particular involvement of the pharmacist with day patients and those likely to take overdoses, while a paediatric hospital has special problems with regard to formulation and particular dosage forms. Similarly, the widely differing grades and abilities of nursing and medical staff found in various units also demands different aspects of a particular service. To be successful, therefore, a ward pharmacy service must suit the requirements of its recipients. It is impossible to describe a stereotype, only to indicate different areas of possible involvement and opportunity to fulfil some of the basic aims.

Increasing specialisation within medicine has led to the realisation that health care depends upon the coordinated activities of a large team of people all with different training and skills. The role of the pharmacist in the health team as described is an important one and clinicians will come to depend more and more upon specialist knowledge in areas such as bioavailability, formulation and drug interactions. The ward pharmacist therefore has a definite and expanding role in patient management, especially since the ever increasing range and toxicity of drugs available to the prescriber has resulted in therapeutics being handled less efficiently than diagnosis. There are many, however, who would dispute this. Eaton (1977) has said that clinical pharmacy in particular might be seen as a threat to physicians, with regard to both their clinical freedom and their authority. It has also been said that pharmacists are not competent to participate in drug treatment decisions since they have insufficient knowledge of diagnosis and medical terminology. In reply it is often pointed out that the time devoted to therapeutics and pharmacology in the medical school curriculum is generally less than the time allocated to other subjects. Like ward or clinical pharmacists in not directly challenging a physician's responsibility towards his patient, another group, the clinical pharmacologists, has emerged in recent years which also claims considerable expertise in drug use and whose declared aim is also to improve patient care and safety by promoting a more rational approach to prescribing.

Clinical pharmacology

The scope of clinical pharmacology was outlined in 1972 by a study group of the World Health Organisation as promoting the safer and more effective use of drugs in man, research, teaching and providing services such as analysis, drug information and advice on experimental design. In 1977 a working group of the World Health Organisation on clinical pharmacology services suggested that clinical pharmacology has much to contribute to safe and effective drug therapy and should be integrated into medical practice. It acknowledged the increasing concern in many countries that drugs are not being used as efficiently and safely as they might be. It recommended that clinical pharmacology be introduced into regional and district hospitals in order to ensure safe and effective drug therapy and continuing education in drug use.

Clinical pharmacologists are in general confined to the teaching centres. They have the advantage of coming from within the medical profession. They are usually physicians who have a particular interest in drugs and whose specialty has shifted from diagnosis to therapeutics. They are often laboratory based and frequently conduct research on patients as well as fulfilling teaching commitments to both medical students and colleagues. It is clear that the ranks of clinical pharmacologists are too thin to carry out all the functions assigned to them by the World Health Organisation even in the major teaching centres. Properly trained clinical pharmacists could, however, augment their number and collaborate in many of the defined areas. In fact, hospital pharmacists are already performing many such functions effectively. The principal responsibility of the clinical pharmacologist lies in teaching and research. He does not have the time or necessarily the interest in the day-to-day service functions that usually comprise the activities of a ward or clinical pharmacist.

Education

Having outlined some of the aims, objectives and activities of ward and clinical pharmacists, it could be said that the distinction between ward and clinical pharmacy remains in dispute or unclear. It is however apparent that whatever role or title a hospital pharmacist in Great Britain chooses to assume it is likely that he will have been inadequately prepared for it. In the desire and enthusiasm to implement ward pharmacy it is important that such services do not involve pharmacists who lack the knowledge, experience and training necessary and who perhaps do not possess the right motives, or an appreciation of their own limitations. It is lack of the right calibre of staff that has held back the development of ward pharmacy in some hospitals while at the same time lack of success in others has been due to the use of inadequate or poorly motivated staff. Pharmacists should not be educated entirely by academics but in part by practitioners of their profession. In Britain, the first degree of a pharmacist trains him to be a scientist. With the movement for increased clinical involvement of the pharmacist has come pressure to increase the clinical content of the undergraduate course. This may be both a dangerous and difficult thing to do. Dangerous because it is vital, for the future of the profession, that pharmacists retain their basic scientific knowledge and the undergraduate syllabus leaves no room for expansion; difficult because practical considerations would result in clinical aspects being taught in isolation without patient contact.

The obvious place for training in clinical competence therefore is at postgraduate level. Any such course or training programme should aim to promote constructive interaction between pharmacists and other health care professionals and to provide an environment in which the student can apply his theoretical knowledge to the clinical situation. Clinical pharmacists should be encouraged to be patient-oriented rather than product-oriented and to develop and extend the role of the pharmacist within the hospital service. Students should develop an awareness of the pharmacist's potential role in the day-to-day management of patients. This involves not only a knowledge of pharmaceutics and pharmacology but also a knowledge of the sequence of drug use, the alternatives, the pitfalls of treatment and when to stop or change therapy. Any course in clinical pharmacy should therefore provide a basic knowledge of the clinical use of drugs in common disease states and an insight into the ways a clinician arrives at a diagnosis and selects a particular treatment. It should also provide an understanding of medical terminology to enable effective communication with other health care professionals. Students should have a basic knowledge of the interpretation of laboratory data and the relevance of such data to previous or subsequent drug therapy. Above all, however, it is vital that the student understands what he is being trained to do and is provided with the communication skills to enable him to go out and do it.

REFERENCES

ALLEN M. D. & GREENBLATT D. J. (1975) *Drug Intelligence and Clinical Pharmacy* **9,** 648.

BAKER J. A. (1976) *Pharmaceutical Journal* **216,** 272.

BARKER K. N. & McCONNELL W. E. (1962) *American Journal of Hospital Pharmacy* **19,** 360.

BASS B. H. (1973) *Pharmaceutical Journal* **212,** 255.

BEAMAN M. W. (1974) *The Role of the Clinical Pharmacist.* Geigy Travelling Fellowship presented to a meeting of the Guild of Hospital Pharmacists, University of Aston, Birmingham, 5 April 1975.

BELL J. E. (1970) *American Journal of Hospital Pharmacy* **27,** 29.

BELL J. E. (1973) *American Journal of Hospital Pharmacy* **30,** 300.

BRODIE D. C. (1966). *Report to the Commission on Pharmaceutical Services to Ambulant Patients by Hospital and Related Facilities.* American Pharmaceutical Association and American Society of Hospital Pharmacists, Washington DC.

BRADLEY T. G. & GRIFFITHS G. (1977) *Pharmaceutical Journal* **219,** 435.

CALDER G. (1972) *Pharmaceutical Journal* **207,** 287.

CALDER G. (1975) *British Journal of Hospital Medicine* November, 566.

CARANASOS G. J., STEWART R. B. & CLUFF L. E. (1974) *Journal of the American Medical Association* **6,** 713.

CHUBB J. M. & WINSHIP H. W. III (1974) *Drug Intelligence and Clinical Pharmacy* **8,** 431.

COVINGTON T. R. & PFIEFER F. G. (1972) *American Journal of Hospital Pharmacy* **28,** 692.

DASS B. C., MADDOCK S. G. & WITHINGHAM G. C. (1977) *Modern Geriatrics* **7,** 22.

DEPARTMENT OF HEALTH AND SOCIAL SECURITY (1970a) *Report of the Working Party on the Hospital Pharmaceutical Service.* The Noel Hall Report. HMSO, London.

DEPARTMENT OF HEALTH AND SOCIAL SECURITY (1970b) *Report on Measures for Controlling Drugs on the Wards by the Joint Sub-Committee of the Standing Medical, Nursing and Pharmaceutical Advisory Committees of the Central Health Services Council.* HM(70)36. HMSO, London.

DEPARTMENT OF HEALTH AND SOCIAL SECURITY (1977) *Guide to Good Pharmaceutical Manufacturing Practice.* HMSO, London.

DUNNELL K. & CARTWRIGHT A. (1972) *Medicine Takers, Prescribers and Hoarders.* Routledge & Kegan-Paul, London.

EATON G. (1977) *Health and Social Services Journal* 4 March, 380.

FRANKE D. E. & WHITNEY H. A. K. JR. (1976) *Drug Intelligence and Clinical Pharmacy* **10,** 511.

GRANT E. (1976) *Journal of Clinical Pharmacy* **1,** 5.

HILL J. H. & ECKEL F. M. (1973) *American Journal of Hospital Pharmacy* **30,** 687.

KATCHER B. (1972) *Failures in Drug Therapy: Continuing Education in Health Sciences University of California at San Francisco School of Pharmacy.* University Press, California.

LAW R. & CHALMERS C. (1976) *British Medical Journal* **1,** 565.

LINKEWICH J. A., CATALANO R. B. & FLACK H. L. (1974) *Drug Intelligence and Clinical Pharmacy* **8,** 10.

LIPMAN A. G. (1974) *Hospital Pharmacy* **9,** 257.

McCARRON M. (1975) *Drug Intelligence and Clinical Pharmacy* **19,** 12.

McHALE M. K. & CANADA A. T. (1969) *Drug Intelligence and Clinical Pharmacy* **3,** 115.

McLEOD D. C. (1976) *American Journal of Hospital Pharmacy* **33,** 904.

MILLER R. R. (1973) *American Journal of Hospital Pharmacy* **30,** 584.

MILLIS COMMISSION (1976) *American Journal of Hospital Pharmacy* **33,** 134.

ODDIS J. A. (1976) *Pharmaceutical Journal,* **216,** 271.

PARKIN D. M., HENNEY C. R., QUIRK J. & CROOKS J. (1976) *British Medical Journal*
2, 686.
PARISH P. (1976) *Pharmaceutical Journal*, **215,** 425.
RODOWSKAS C. A. JR. (1976) *Drug Intelligence and Clinical Pharmacy* **10,** 522.
WANDLESS I. & DAVIE J. W. (1977) *British Medical Journal* **1,** 359.
WHITTET T. D. (1977) *Pharmaceutical Journal* **218,** 196.
WILSON R. S. (1971) *American Journal of Hospital Pharmacy* **28,** 49.

FURTHER READING

FRANKE D. E. & WHITNEY H. A. K. JR. (1972) *Perspectives in Clinical Pharmacy*. Drug
Intelligence Publications, Hamilton, Ill.
HERFINDAL E. T. & HIRSCHMAN J. L. (1975) *Clinical Pharmacy and Therapeutics*. Williams
& Wilkins, Baltimore.
KNOBEN J. E., ANDERSON P. O. & WATABNE A. S. (1973) *Handbook of Clinical Data*.
3rd edn. Drug Intelligence Publications, Hamilton, Ill.
ROWLES B. & SCOTT E. A. (1975) *Clinical Pharmacy Handbook for Patient Counselling*. Drug
Intelligence Publications, Hamilton, Ill.
SWARBRICK J. (1970) *Current Concepts in the Pharmaceutical Sciences. Biopharmaceutics*. Lea
& Febiger, Philadelphia.

12

Clinical pharmacokinetics and concentration monitoring

E. VAN DER KLEIJN

CLINICAL PHARMACOKINETICS SURVEILLANCE SERVICE

The majority of patients visiting a physician will be prescribed one or more drugs to cure or relieve the disease symptoms. The logic of drug choice, choice of drug formulation, route of administration, dosage, frequency of administration and duration of treatment in relation to the disease symptoms and their severity together with requirements for onset, intensity and time course of activity is largely controlled by university training, literature from objective and sale-oriented sources and experience on an often epidemiologically small population. Unlike many infectious diseases where the discovery of drugs has led to an almost complete cure rate or even elimination of the disease from medical practice, the treatment of many other diseases has not benefited by drugs to the same extent. The success of drug treatment in medicine, although undoubtedly indispensable for the complete or partial control of symptoms or causes has, in many cases until now, not fully satisfied patients or physicians and scientists. Without pretending to understand the causes of diseases, it has become evident that the effectiveness of treatment could gain from individualised 'fine' adjustment of drug dosage regimens.

The idea of taking the individual as his own reference standard has changed the treatment routine of patients. This has created possibilities for prospective planning, in-process vigilance, retrospective monitoring and feedback procedures. Plasma concentration determinations have alerted physicians to their relatively unjustified trust that all prescribed regimens should lead to the intended effect. Retrospective statistical analyses have made it clear that, despite all good intentions, only a small fraction of a patient population reaches the concentration range accepted as therapeutic (Guelen & Van der Kleijn 1977) (Fig. 12.1). Many factors can be held responsible for this low figure. Some of them are susceptible for correction; some are still so little understood that the solution cannot yet be foreseen (Van der Kleijn *et al* 1975, 1977). Drugs, here defined as substances that are foreign to the body by nature or amount, often initiate a sequence of chemical and physiological processes. Body foreign

372

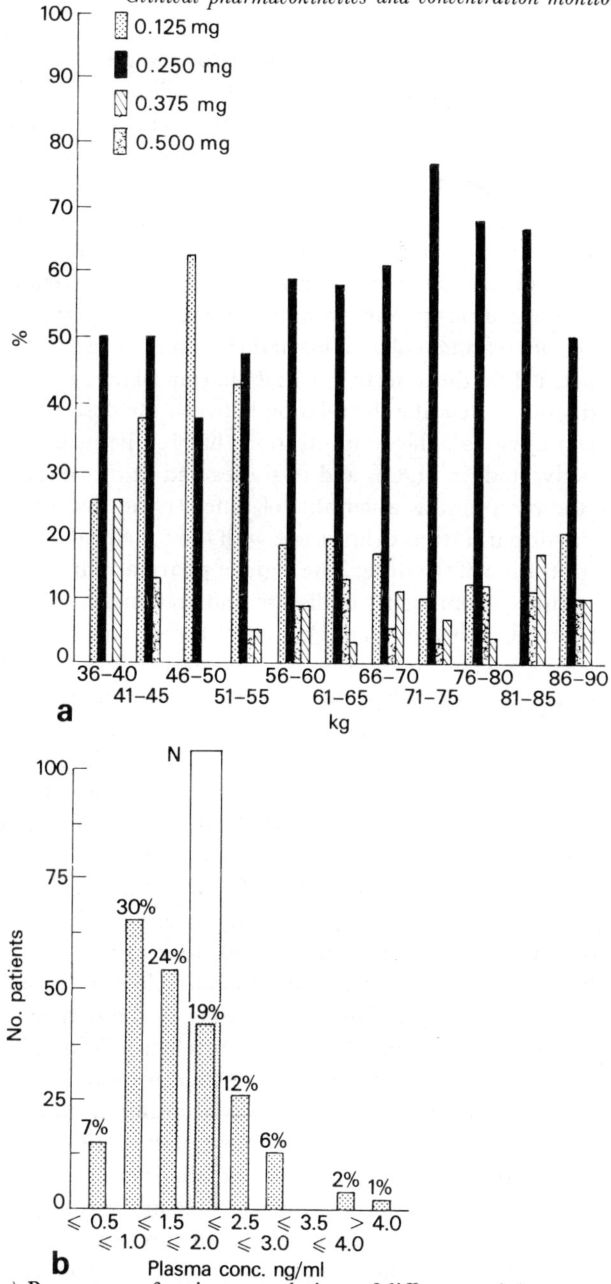

Fig. 12.1   (a) Percentage of patient populations of different weight groups receiving dosages of digoxin per day. Note that 50% or more of the patients of each weight group from 36 kg to 90 kg receive prescriptions for the commercially most common tablet strength of 0.25 mg. (b) Distribution of patients for which the plasma digoxin concentration has been determined. Note that only 19% of the patients investigated have a plasma concentration that is considered optimal. More than half of the patients are undermedicated, while almost 20% have an increased risk for toxicity. N=222 patients.

substances, semantically distinguished as food, luxury, therapeutic drug or toxoid, are absorbed, become distributed in and are eliminated from tissues and organs by a multitude of mechanisms. The rate at which these processes occur simultaneously are categorically characteristic for every drug with respect to a number of variables. These rates determine the onset, the time course and the intensity of the effect to the body. 'Pharmacokinetics' involves the studies of these rates of absorption from the various loci of administration, distribution in the body, metabolic and anabolic transformation and excretion. The application of the information obtained from theoretical and experimental pharmacokinetics for the treatment of patients in the various categories of health care is further specified by the adjective *clinical* pharmacokinetics. It is the aim of pharmacokinetics to describe the relation between the dose of a drug administered to an individual, the concentration that results in blood, plasma or any other body fluid, in organs and in tissues and in the so-called biophase near or on the receptors, as a variable of time. It tries by measurements of pharmacokinetic parameters to link these with the beneficial or adverse results of the administration of the drug. The logic of pharmacokinetics seems to bypass the descriptive approaches of disease and treatment. Pharmacokinetics is more concerned with the quantification of the driving forces than of the description of the phenomenon of the effect (pharmacodynamics). In principle pharmacokinetics is not restricted to drugs but also applies to biogenous compounds. It is well understood that the quantitative influence on or of enzyme systems, trace elements, hormones etc. is of the highest importance, but our knowledge about them appears to be lacking most often due to analytical problems. Confident analytical procedures may be still the primary and dominant problem in the usefulness of the determination of drugs in body fluids. Next to the ability to quantify the time course of a drug there appear to be many therapeutic and domestic variables that play a roll in the motivation to use 'plasma concentration determinations' and therefore clinical pharmacokinetics. The sequence initiated by the drug should ultimately lead to a change in condition and to a recognisable improvement in the patient. This change is often one of linear exponential precursor-product relationships.

The influence of even large temporal drug concentration changes may have a smaller and more delayed influence on the concentration changes of its metabolites and also on the intensity and time course of the anticipated effects (Fig. 12.2). For restoration and control of chronic abnormal physiological conditions, as in epilepsy, psychiatry, cardiology, diabetes, asthma and infectious diseases treated with bactericidal antibiotics, an agreed primary requirement of drug treatment is to maintain an adequate and as constant as possible amount of drug in the body during the course of the disease. This amount will result in various concentrations in different regions in the body depending on the nature of the drug and of the body regions. For instance some of these regions (compartments) are blood, plasma or other body fluids available for sampling like saliva, tears, urine, wound exudates etc.

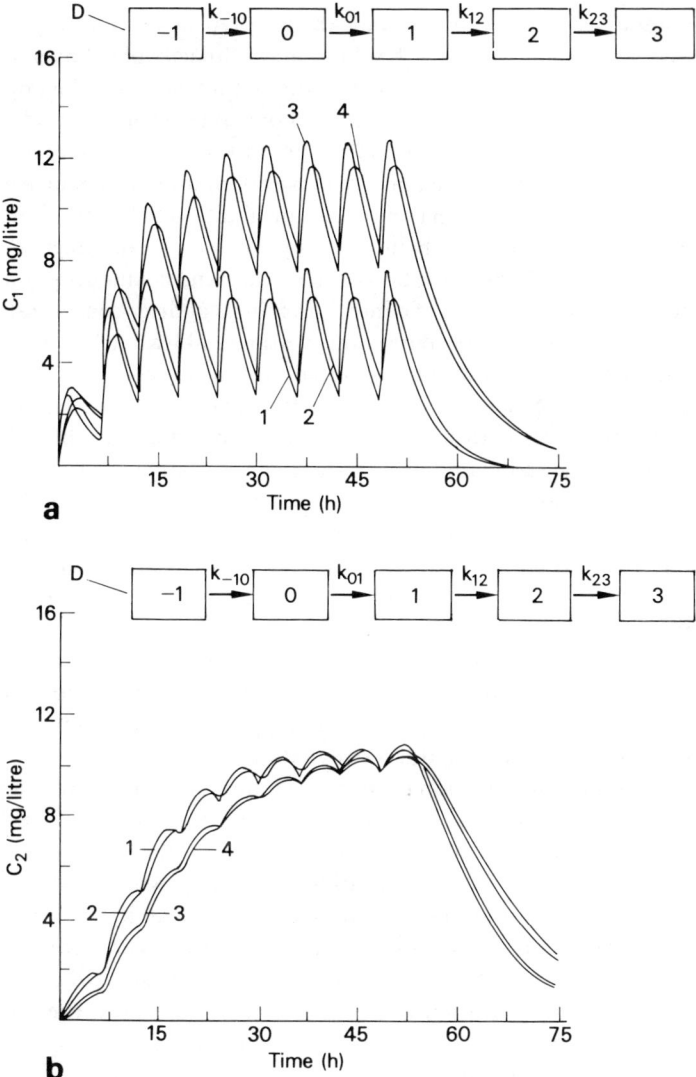

Fig. 12.2   (a) Concentration of procainamide in compartment 1. Comparison of two variations of the rate of release from a dosage form with two variations of the rate of metabolism: (1) rapid release, rapid metabolism; (2) slow release, rapid metabolism; (3) rapid release slow metabolism; (4) slow release, slow metabolism. In (b) the influence of these variations on the course of the metabolite is given. By decreasing the rate of release (k_{-10}) as is tried in sustained release formulations it appears that neither the rate of accumulation nor the amplitude of the concentration of the drug and of the metabolite are significantly influenced in this simulation. $\Delta t = 6$ hours. Dose = 1000 mg.

   (b) Course of the simulated plasma concentration of e.g. *N*-acetylprocamide as a metabolite of the parent compound procainamide in compartment 2. It is obvious that the level of accumulation is not influenced by the rate of metabolism of procainamide. Only the rate of accumulation is influenced. Sustaining the release of the active compound hardly influences the level of the pharmacologically active compounds. $\Delta t = 6$ hours. Dose = 1000 kg.

The amount adequate to maintain the restored or normal physiological functions is largely controlled by the elimination capacity of the liver and kidney, the apparent distribution volume at the output side and the amount of drug supplied to the body per time unit or at one time at the input side. When the metabolic capacity of the liver and/or the capacity of the excretory organs is in large excess, linear proportionality between input, maintenance amount and output can be expected. Within reasonable limits such linear relationships have been found for many drugs in carefully controlled experimental conditions, indicating confident constancy of the pharmacokinetic parameters. Nevertheless the entire subject of clinical usefulness of drug concentration determinations in plasma has become controversial or at least arbitrary particularly for some groups of drugs or individual substances, not the least because the relation between concentration and effect is generally not well understood.

This chapter deals with a number of conditions and variables that can influence the value and confidence of the pharmacokinetic parameters of a variety of drugs that can be assayed in clinical conditions. In patients one is bound to practical limitations (e.g. the number of samples and dosage schedules used in individuals). This does not allow the estimation of all possible parameters such as time constant or biological half-life time, apparent volume of distribution etc., but does allow calculation of at least the clearance.

In the sequence of events leading from drug administration to the ultimate effect, direct linear proportionalities are assumed. The proportionalities are often of a nature mathematically describable by one or by the sum of differential equations. When integrated, these equations can be solved to yield relations between the concentration or amount at any time and one or a sum of exponentials that can describe the time course of the drug in the body.

The rate of change in amount or concentration in the body appears proportional to the amount or concentration remaining, which means that an equal fraction of the dose applied is eliminated per time unit, or that an equal fraction accumulates per unit time during constant infusion. Chronic intermittent medication can often be considered pseudoinfusion when the time interval of drug administration is short enough in relation to the biological half time so that concentration oscillations are minimal.

Pharmacokinetic considerations are important in the choice of treatment when the clinical condition has been diagnosed. In principle, seven variables can be differentiated in the prescribing of a medicine:

1. The chemical, pharmacologically active substance.
2. The dose.
3. The dosage form.
4. The formulation.
5. The route of administration.
6. The time course of treatment.
7. The nature and the severity of the (changing) disease state.

Individually and combined, these variables control the onset, intensity and time course of the effect. All these variables have pharmacokinetic implications and have to be weighted and judged when plasma concentration determinations are requested. When these data are incomplete or unknown it is questionable whether the clinical judgement of the efficacy of drugs is satisfactorily adequate to justify prescription for a longer or shorter period of time. There are reasons to doubt the quality of the choices, assessments and audits of the above variables.

Comedication, age and body weight (or surface area) appear to be dominant in causing subsequent variations of clearance of drugs and the plasma concentration during chronic treatment. There appear to be great differences in the medical tradition of treating for example epilepsy, among physicians of different regions and countries. This is shown in epidemiological studies of the prescribing habits in various countries (Guelen & Johannesen 1977). The unpredictable influence of one drug on the clearance of another, forces one to adapt the dosage. Moreover, little is known of the dose-related nature, intensity and time course of the therapeutic, pharmacological or adverse effects of combinations of two or more apparently closely related compounds. The picture of treatment of many diseases is complicated by the subjective and non-statistical observations and apparent responses of patients to dosages that are generally considered subtherapeutic.

Pharmacokinetic logic

In abstract pharmacokinetic terms, it is considered that amounts of drug are homogeneously distributed in compartments of particular volumes. The resulting concentrations are subject to continuous change as a result of input and output of the materials. The dominant driving forces are haemodynamics, secretion and enzyme–substrate reactions. The analogies used are strongly simplified and have no direct relation to the anatomy and physical physiology of living individuals. It bears most resemblance to communicating vessels where the flow rates are controlled by taps.

Homogeneous distribution does not necessarily imply that the concentrations are equal in each part of the body. It does mean that absorption and distribution of the drug have no quantitative influence on the elimination process. A compartment is a volume of complete abstract entity.

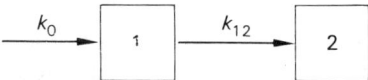

The amount of drug Q present at time $t=0$ diminishes in the body, here represented by compartment 1, as a result of metabolism, anabolism and/or excretion.

It is collected, as in a sink, represented by compartment 2.

When the amount or concentration in 1 is measured at subsequent time periods it appears that the course of values follows a curve asymptotically approaching zero when time approaches infinity. Because a similar pattern is observed for the course of the concentration of most drugs in human and animal subjects, the analogy with discharge of an electric condenser and a sink outlet is obvious. Mathematically this curve is described by the differential equation:

$$\frac{dQ_1}{dt} = -k_{12} Q_1 \qquad (1)$$

in which Q_1 is the amount of drug (mg), t the time (h), k_{12} the reciprocal time constant for elimination describing the convexity of the hyperbola (per hour).

$$Q = C.V \qquad (2)$$

in which C is the concentration (mg/litre) and V the apparent distribution volume of the compartment 1. When the amount of the drug administered is related to the resulting plasma concentration it may appear that this volume has anatomically and physiologically, an unrealistic high value, sometimes several times larger than the factual body volume. Due to preferential partitioning of the drug in tissues inaccessible for sampling and non-homogeneous distribution in regions outside the plasma, the value for the relative volume may be as large as 20–40 litres/kg (e.g. for antidepressant and neuroleptic drugs). This can be explained by the fact that the anatomical distribution is not homogeneous, but due to the physicochemical properties of the drug, much higher concentrations than in plasma exist in different regions of the body (Fig. 12.3).

Solving equation 1 by integration one obtains

$$C_1(t) = C_1(0) \, e^{-k_{12}t} = \frac{Q_1(0)}{V_1} . e^{-k_{12}t} \qquad (3)$$

Because of the nature of this equation, the terms first order or exponential elimination are used. Graphically, the course of the concentration can be represented in Fig. 12.4.

Mathematical conversion of this equation yields

$$\ln C_1(t) = \ln C_1(0) - k_{12}t \qquad (4)$$

or $$\log C_1(t) = \log C(0) - 0.434 k_{12}t \qquad (5)$$

Presentation on log-linear graph paper yields a straight line (Fig. 12.4).

The three most important parameters that determine the time course of a drug in the body are Q, k and V. All are mutually independent. A number of important parameters are deduced from these:

$$Cl = k \times V \qquad (6)$$

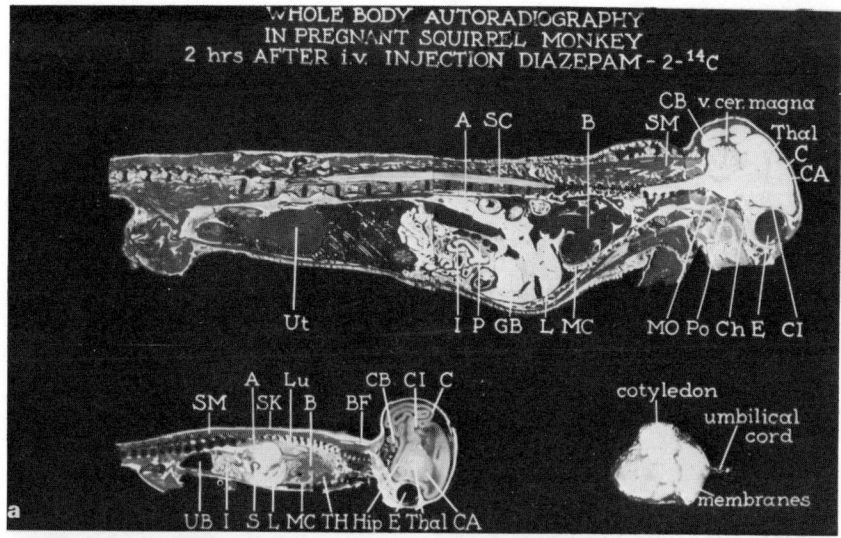

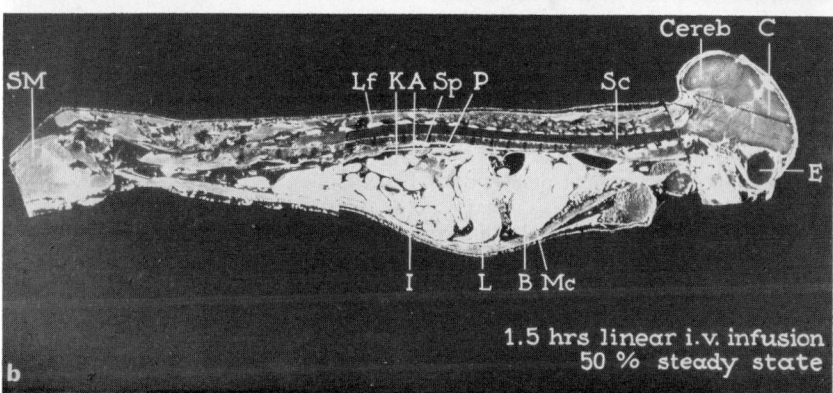

Fig. 12.3 (a) Whole body autoradiography of a pregnant squirrel monkey 2 hours after i.v. bolus injection of 2-^{14}C-diazepam. White areas indicate the presence of radioactive material. Note that while the blood concentration is low the brain concentration is high and shows various regional differences.

(b) Whole body autoradiography of a squirrel monkey 1 hour after i.v. infusion of ^{14}carboxy valproate. White areas indicate the presence of radioactive material. Note that although this drug is active as an antiepileptic drug only very low concentrations of radioactive material are present in the brain. The blood concentration is relatively high.

in which Cl is the clearance of the drug (per hour), and

$$t_{1/2} = \frac{0.693}{k} \tag{7}$$

in which $t_{1/2}$ is the biological half-life time (h). This parameter can be derived from $C(t_{1/2}) = 0.5C(0) = C(0)e^{-kt_{1/2}}$. The Dose Q, is often referred to body weight

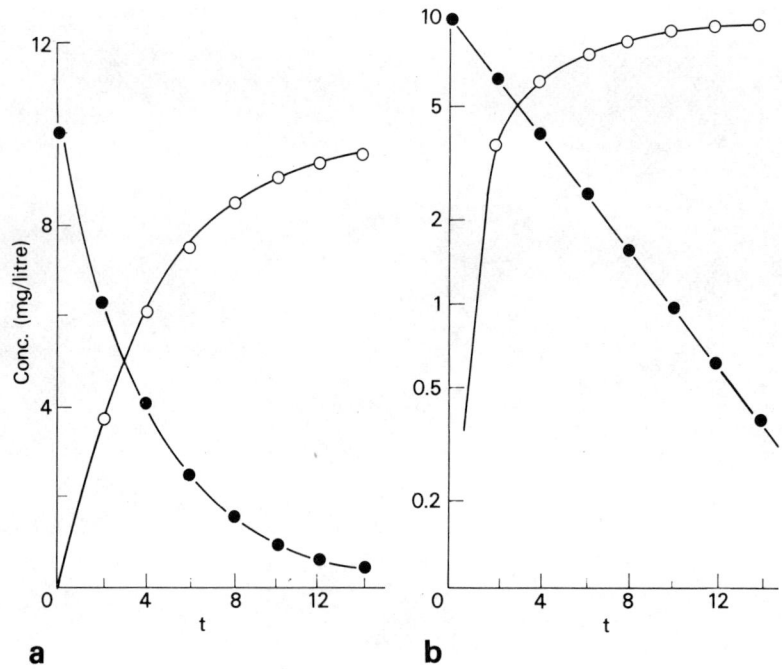

Fig. 12.4 Graphical presentation of the simulated course of the concentration of a drug in a one-compartment open model. Black circles, C_1; white circles, C_2. (a) Both ordinate and abscissa have a linear scale. The curve approaches zero as an asymptote. (b) The ordinate has a logarithmic scale while the abscissa has a linear scale. The curve is a straight line.

(kg) or body surface (m²). This reference is only justified when a confident statistical value has been established for the proportionality between dose and, for example, the resulting plasma concentration or, preferably, the effect in a wide range of body weights or body surfaces. The proportionality constant between dose and concentration in simple one-compartment steady state kinetics is called clearance. In other words, reference to body weight or body surface is only justified when the clearance parameter can be considered constant within reasonable confidence limits. In these cases use can be made of the symbols V^* and Cl^*, the relative volume of distribution and the relative clearance (Fig. 12.5). Many physiological, pathological and metabolic factors can influence the clearance value. Therefore individual determinations of this parameter can improve the dosage. Since elimination is an asymptotic process it is sometimes useful to use the concept of $t_{0.90}$, the time in which the drug is removed from the body to a residual value of 10%. The relation between $t_{0.9}$ and $t_{1/2}$ and other states of elimination is given in Table 12.1.

When agreement has been reached about the maximum oscillation in amount or concentration in the body during chronic medication (e.g. 10 or 20%), use can be made of the $t_{0.1}$ or $t_{0.2}$ values

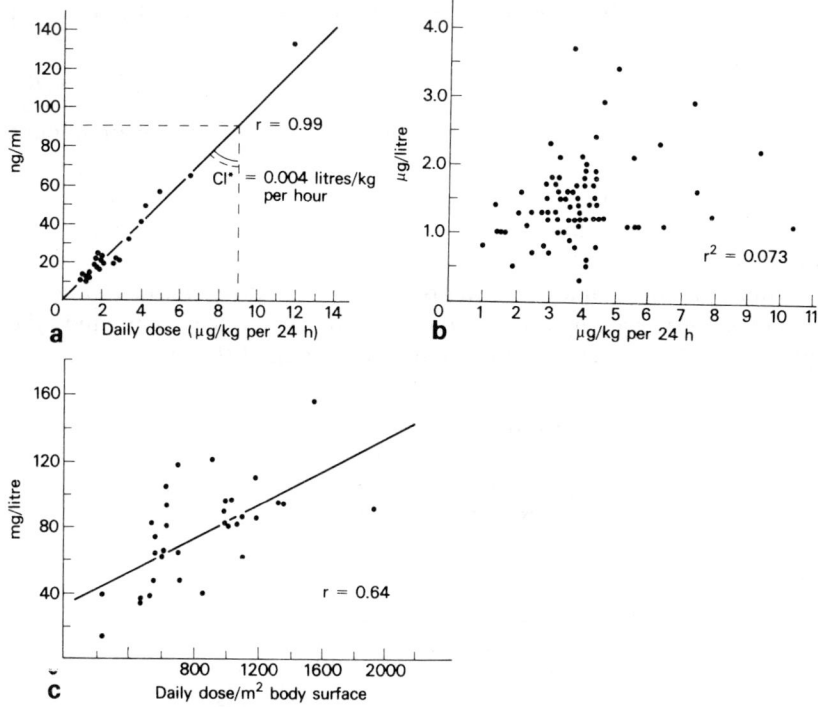

Fig. 12.5 (a) Relationship between the dose per time unit/kg body weight (pseudoinfusion rate on the abscissa) and the steady state plasma concentration C of digitoxin on the ordinate. When the conditions of a one-compartment infusion model are valid there is a confident proportionality between dose per time unit and C. Thanks to the long biological half-life the confidence of the proportionality or *clearance* factor is very high.

(b) Relationship between the dose per time unit/kg body weight (pseudoinfusion rate) on the abscissa and the steady state plasma concentration C of digoxin on the ordinate (no. patients=83). It is obvious that the confidence value of the proportionality clearance factor is very low. Reasons for this low figure can be the bioavailability problem, the relatively short half-life in relation to its dosage interval, sampling time, limited compliance, intercurrent diseases etc. Digoxin requires an intensive, individual monitoring for which both clinical, as well as concentrations and clearance, parameters can be useful.

(c) Relation between the dose per time unit/m² on the abscissa and the pseudosteady state plasma concentration on the ordinate of valproate. The confidence of this correlation was slightly better for surface area than for the body weight reference.

$$e^{-kt_{0.1}} = 0.9 \qquad t_{0.1} = \frac{0.1054}{k} \tag{8}$$

$$e^{-kt_{0.2}} = 0.8 \qquad t_{0.2} = \frac{0.2231}{k} \tag{9}$$

In order to calculate the dosage interval, Δt, the following rule of thumb can be applied:

$$\Delta t = t_{max} + t_{0.2} \tag{10}$$

in which t_{max} is the time taken to reach the maximum concentration or amount in the body.

Following intravenous injection t_{max} can be neglected. Following oral, intramuscular or rectal administration t_{max} will differ from 10 minutes to many hours depending on the substance and the formulation. As a mean, the maximum time of absorption for an oral preparation is in the order of 1–3 hours, although large variations are observed depending on the compound, the emptying of the stomach and the physical condition of the individual.

Table 12.1 The relationship between $t_{\frac{1}{2}}$ and other states of elimination

x	$x = y \times \dfrac{1}{k}$	$x = z \times t_{\frac{1}{2}}$
	y	z
$t_{0.1}$	0.1054	0.15
$t_{0.2}$	0.2231	0.32
$t_{0.5}$	0.6931	1
$t_{0.8}$	0.6094	2.32
$t_{0.9}$	0.3026	3.32
$t_{0.95}$	0.9957	4.32
$t_{0.99}$	0.6052	6.64

Determination of the pharmacokinetic parameters

Graphical method

The accuracy of the k and V values and thus the Cl values, is largely controlled by the number of assay points by which the curve is fitted. The quality of the analytical assay in the biological medium, especially near the limits of detectability, is of great importance for the final confidence of the parameters. In the graphical method, use is made of semilog paper in which the ordinate is calibrated in one, two or three decades in a logarithmic scale. Often, the most likely line is drawn through the data points and the intercept with the ordinate corresponds to the apparent concentration value at time $t=0$, as if distribution was complete and homogeneous. Because the dose Q is known, it is possible to calculate the apparent volume of distribution V. When body weight is also known V^* can be derived. From the slope of the regression line, $t_{1/2}$ and k can easily be found. Table 12.2 gives these parameters collected from the literature for a number of drugs.

Analog computer

The analog computer is an excellent instrument to simulate and to fit concentration or amount–time courses even for complex sums of exponentials and for non-linear equations. It can be used to estimate the parameters from the fitted curves. The rate of discharge of electronic condensers similar to flow in communicating vessels is controlled by resistors or potentiometers supplying relative values for the reciprocal time constants.

Digital computers

Most programmable digital computers (from pocket calculators to multicore CPUs) are able to transfer concentration–time data into parameters describing multiphasic curves including their confidence statistics and the most appropriate model (Metzler 1969). By combining graphical methods and digital computing it is possible to rapidly establish the most relevant parameters. More complex multiphasic linear models are resolved with slower computers, by a process of best fit through the last so-called terminal concentration data and a feathering or residual slopes technique by subtracting the concentration values from the curve at earlier times from this regression line (Wagner 1975). When more phases can be discriminated in multicompartment systems this will lead to the identification and estimation of the parameters.

Chain model of consecutive compartments

With first-order input (absorption) and first-order output (elimination):

Differential equation for compartment 1:

$$\frac{dQ}{dt} = k_{01}Q_0 - k_{12}Q_1 \tag{11}$$

Solution and conversion of integral

$$C_1(t) = \frac{F.Q_0}{V_1} \cdot \frac{k_{01}}{(k_{01}-k_{12})} \cdot (e^{-k_{01}t} - e^{-k_{12}t}) \tag{12}$$

F is the biological availability factor that has a maximum of $[(F.Q_0)/V_1] = C_0$ in cases of complete absorption.

When in a practical experiment, Fig. 12.6 has been constructed from enough data points, it is possible to estimate k_{01} by calculating the residuals of the ascending part of the curve from the extension of the elimination phase to the ordinate.

Table 12.2   List of drugs currently used and assayed for clinical accompaniment of pati●

Drug group Generic name	Sample time during chronic treatment hours after intake/route		Sample vol. ml blood	Assay method
Antiepileptics				
Phenobarbital	4–12	oral	0.5–2	GC-FID/EMIT
Phenytoin	2–5	oral	0.5–2	GC-methyl-FID/EMIT
Primidone	2–4	oral	0.5–2	GC-methyl-FID/EMIT
Ethosuximide	4	oral	0.5–1	GC-FID
Carbamazepine	4	oral	1–2	HPLC
Clonazepam	4	oral	2	GC-hydrol.
Valproate	2–8	oral	0.5–1	GC-FID
Nitrazepam	4	oral	2	HPLC
Diazepam	4	oral	2	GC-ECD/HPLC
Desmethy-diazepam	4	oral	2	GC-ECD/HPLC
Ataractics				
Diazepam	4	oral	2	GC-ECD
Desmethyldiazepam	4	oral	same sample	GC-ECD
Oxazepam	1–3	oral	0.5–1	GC/hydrol./ECD
Anaesthetic				
4-Hydroxybutyrate	protocol	i.v.	1–2	GC/FID
Hypnotics				
Hexobarbital	1	oral	2–4	GC/(A)/FID
Heptabarbital	2	oral	2–4	GC/(A)/FID
Cyclobarbital	2	oral	2–4	GC/(A)/FID
Vinylbarbital	4	oral	2–4	GC/(A)/FID
Butobarbital	4	oral	2–4	GC/(A)/FID
Secobarbital	4	oral	2–4	GC/(A)/FID
Phenobarbital	4	oral/i.v.	2–4	GC/(A)/FID
Nitrazepam	4	oral	5–10	HPLC
Analgesic				
Salicylate	1–3	oral	2–4	Sfp
Cardiacs				
Digoxin	5–12/prot.	oral/i.v.	0.5–1	RIA/EMIT
Digitoxin	5–12	oral	0.5–1	RIA
Lidocaine	protocol	i.v.	2	GC
Procainamide	protocol	oral/i.v.	2	GC
Antidepressant				
Li_2CO_3	1–2+8	oral	1	FSp
Antiasthmatics				
Theophylline	protocol	oral/i.m./ i.v./r.	2	GC/HPLC
Antineoplastics				
Methotrexate	protocol	oral/i.v.	3	HPLC/EMIT
Methotrexate children	protocol	i.v.	3	HPLC/EMIT

GC, gas chromatography; EMIT, enzyme multiplied immunoassay test; HPLC, high-pressure liquid chromatography; FSp, flame spectrophotography; RIA, radioimmunoassay; Sfp, spectrofluorophotometry; protocol, according to sample protocol;

Table 12.2 (*cont.*)

Saliva/plasma ratio	t_{ss} (days)	C_{therap} (mg/l)	Cl* (l/h/kg)	Δt practice (h)	$t_{\frac{1}{2}}$ (h)	Cl (l/kg)
0.32	20	30	0.004	12–24	130	0.7
0.10	3	12–15	0.018	6	20	0.7
0.97	1.5 (25)	8–10	0.060	8	8	1
0.88	6	60–80	0.018	8	40	0.65
0.25		6–8	0.150	6	15	1.2
—	4	0.03–0.06	0.100	8	30	3.3
0.06	5	60–80	0.012	6	8	0.25
—	3	0.08–0.12	0.080	8	20	1.8
—	5	0.4	0.030	8	30	1.8
—	7	0.3	0.020	12	50	1.8
—		0.400	0.030	8	30	1.8
—		0.300	0.020	12	50	1.8
—						
—		2–4	0.290		4.5	1.1
—		2–4	0.160		7–9	0.78
—		2–4	0.030		11.6	0.49
—		2–4	0.031		28–33	0.74
—		2–4	0.030		30–40	0.8
—		2–4	0.060		25–30	0.9–1.0
0.32		10	0.005		60–120	0.7–1.0
—		0.060	0.080		20–25	2.1
0.033	1.5	150	0.016	4–6	7	0.25
0.78	8	0.0015–0.0020	0.140	12	40	8
—	25	0.015 –0.030	0.0042	24	150	0.9
—		2–4	0.57	—	1.5	1.1
1.6		4–8	0.40	4	3.5	2
1.5–2.7	2–3	25–35 0.8–1.1 mmol	0.025–0.050	8	10–35	0.7
0.65–0.75	1–2	10–20	0.060	2–6	2–10	0.38
		$10^{-4}–10^{-8}\,\mathrm{M}$	0.150		6.9	0.32
		$10^{-4}–10^{-8}\,\mathrm{M}$	0.36		4.6	1.07

oral, after oral administration; i.v., after intravenous administration; i.m., after intramuscular administration; r., after rectal administration; TI, thymidine incorporation.

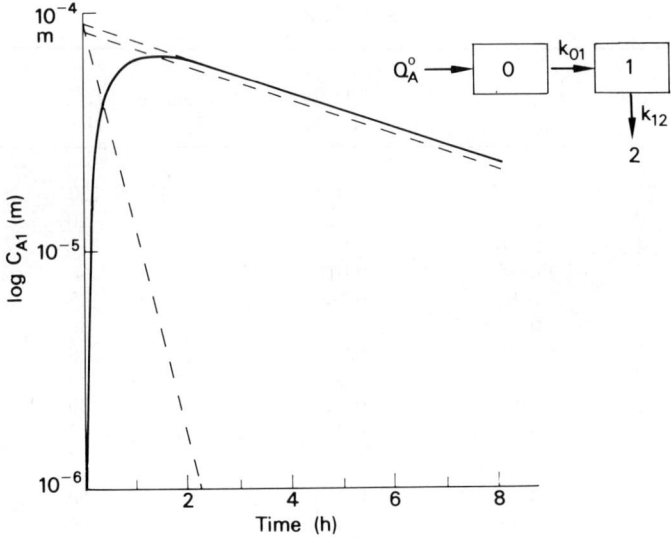

Fig. 12.6 Simulated concentration–time profile of a drug after e.g. oral absorption, according to a simple chain model. The rate of absorption can be deducted from the curve constructed by the residuals of the ascending curve and the extension of the descending curve.

When more intricate absorption processes take place and the number of samples allow more accurate analyses of the data, more sophisticated kinetics have to be applied.

When instead of first-order input (absorption) a zero-order input, such as an infusion of drug, is applied then the schematic model is:

$$k_0 \rightarrow \boxed{1} \xrightarrow{k_{12}} \boxed{2} \xrightarrow{k_{23}} \boxed{3}$$

and the differential equation reads:

$$\frac{dQ_1}{dt} = k_0 - k_{12} Q_1 \tag{13}$$

The integrated solution reads:

$$Q_1(t) = \frac{k_0}{k_{12}}(1 - e^{-k_{12}t}) \text{ or} \tag{14}$$

$$C_1(t) = \frac{k_0}{V_1 k_{12}}(1 - e^{-k_{12}t}) \tag{15}$$

The graphical representation is given in Fig. 12.7.

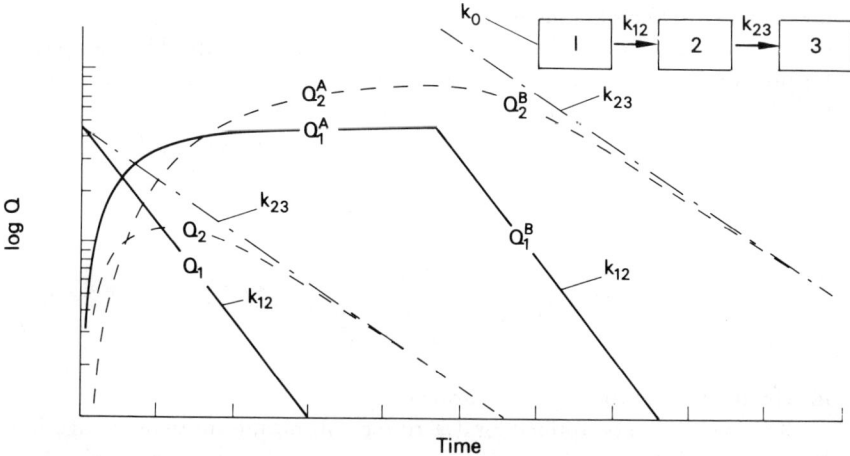

Fig. 12.7 Simulated concentration–time profile of a drug during and following intravenous infusion according to a simple chain model. The rate of elimination can be found from the residual curve of $Q_{max} - Q_1$ (t) during infusion and from the post-steady state profile. The profile of a metabolite is also given in this figure as Q_2.

The equation for a possible metabolite formed from the parent drug in this model reads:

$$C_2(t) = \frac{k_0}{k_{23} \cdot V_2} \cdot \frac{1 + (k_{23}\, e^{-k_{12}t} - k_{12}\, e^{-k_{23}t})}{k_{12} - k_{23}} \tag{16}$$

For many drugs with pharmacologically active metabolites, it appears necessary to include their kinetics in the clinical interpretation.

As in the foregoing model, it is possible to find the rate of elimination (k_{12}) from the residual curve of $C_{max} - C_1(t)$. This is especially useful when confident assays in the low concentration range are impossible. The rate of elimination can also be calculated from the elimination curve following the arrest of the infusion where the equations read:

$$C_1(t) = \frac{k_0}{k_{12} \cdot V_1} \cdot e^{-k_{12}t} \tag{17}$$

$$C_2(t) = \frac{k_0}{(k_{23} - k_{12}) \cdot V_2} \cdot (e^{-k_{12}t} - e^{-k_{23}t}) + \frac{k_0}{k_{23} \cdot V_2} \cdot e^{-k_{23}t} \tag{18}$$

In a biological process, in particular with neuroleptics, antidepressants and ataractics, the chain is not restricted to two compartments or one metabolite. As long as it is possible to determine the concentrations of these in a chain of linearly related exponentials for associated substances or their effects, it will be possible to determine the major pharmacokinetic parameters.

The further the intrinsic distance of these substances or effects in this chain from the parent compound, the more complex the relation will be. Because the oscillations in effect and/or concentration will be quenched, the more the metabolite or effects are alienated from the parent compound, the more the observations in steady state will be clearer and more accurate. This also pleads for precursor–product relations in drug design, (i.e. the prodrug), as a better tool for sustained release than pharmaceutical formulation.

When $t = \infty$ equations 15 and 16 can be simplified to:

$$C_1(t) = \frac{k_0}{k_{12} V_1} = \frac{k_0}{Cl_1} \tag{19}$$

and

$$C_2(t) = \frac{k_0}{k_{23} V_2} = \frac{k_0}{Cl_2} \tag{20}$$

in which Cl is the total body clearance.

This model can be applied for describing chronic intermittent medication. When drugs show a small k_{12} value (large $t_{\frac{1}{2}}$) and are given at a relative high frequency per day (small dosage interval) than

$$k_0 = \frac{Q}{\Delta t} \tag{21}$$

A more accurate notation is to include the biological availability factor F. Equation 20 then reads:

$$Q = \text{dose} = C \times Cl \times \Delta t \times \frac{1}{F} \tag{22}$$

Since F in most cases is equal to 1 or will otherwise be included in the clearance, this equation can generally be used for dosage calculation

$$\text{Dose} = C \times Cl^* \times \Delta t \times W \tag{23}$$

in which W is body weight and Cl^* is the relative clearance litre/kg per hour. The concentration in this equation is the mean plateau concentration and is generally referred to as the therapeutic concentration. When, in the course of chronic intermittent treatment, absorption and elimination are taking place, it is possible to derive the equations for the maximum plasma concentration C_{max} and the minimum concentration prior to the next administration C_{min}:

$$C_{max} = \frac{F.D.k_{01}}{V(k_{01} - k_{12})} \cdot \left[\frac{e^{-k_{12} max}}{1 - e^{-k_{12} \Delta t}} - \frac{e^{-k_{01} t max}}{1 - e^{-k_{01} \Delta t}} \right] \tag{24}$$

$$t_{max} = \frac{1}{k_{01} - k_{12}} \cdot \ln \left[\frac{k_{01} (1 - e^{-k_{12} \Delta t})}{k_{12} (1 - e^{-k_{01} \Delta t})} \right] \tag{25}$$

$$C_{min} = \frac{F.D.k_{01}}{V(k_{01} - k_{12})} \cdot \left[\frac{1}{1 - e^{-k_{12} \Delta t}} - \frac{1}{1 - e^{-k_{01} \Delta t}} \right] \tag{26}$$

where D = dose.

In these equations k_{01} is the rate constant for absorption and k_{12} the elimination rate constant, $C_{max} - C_{min}$ corresponding to the concentration amplitude or oscillation, is influenced primarily by the dosage interval Δt and to a smaller extent by k_{01}. Therefore, it is necessary to adapt Δt to the boundaries that one allows for optimal therapy. In chronic clinical conditions, oscillations of over 20% are often unacceptable and therefore Δt can be adapted accordingly using equations 24 and 26:

$$\frac{C_{max} - C_{min}}{C_{max}} \times 100 = 20\% \qquad (27)$$

Tables 12.3 and 12.4 summarise for a number of drugs that comply to this model how one can influence the theoretical plasma concentration oscillation by the choice of the dosage interval.

In addition, by influencing t_{max}, it is possible to influence the oscillation amplitude. Pharmaceutical techniques (e.g. acid-resistent coating), cogranulation with polymers, chemical derivative formation to a prodrug that first has to be transformed metabolically, are used to manipulate the release rate of the active principle. The chain model is then extended with a 'compartment' before the absorption takes place, assuming first-order release.

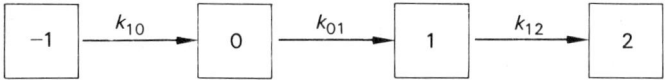

The implicit extension of the equation for compartment 1 by one term will have only a minor influence on the area under the curve of $C_1(t)$. The intrinsic rate of absorption is not changed by the presence of a biological disintegration and dissolution rate. This model can be used in judging the merits of, for example, sustained release formulations. In general, when drugs with short half-lives (large k_{12}) are pharmaceutically manipulated to sustain dissolution (k_{10} decreases without changing k_{01}), no sustained concentration profile will result (Fig. 12.2a). In these cases, decreasing the dose and the dosage interval Δt, will have a larger effect in reducing the plasma concentration fluctuations, than sustained release formulation, especially when first pass metabolism is involved in elimination of the drug. This then will result in more frequent administration which may create problems with patient compliance. Nevertheless with adequate explanation patients can be motivated to adhere to these instructions. When a pharmacologically active metabolite is generated, it appears that the influence of a decreased rate of dissolution does not influence the plasma concentration profile. The influence of the individual rate of metabolism is much more important and clinically more relevant (Fig. 12.2b).

A secondary problem with sustained release preparations at least *in vivo*, but often also *in vitro*, is the limited and unpredictable reproducibility of the release in consecutive administrations (Fig. 12.8). This results in a less reliable plasma concentration profile. In cases where the normal formulation may give

Table 12.3 Parameters for the calculation of concentration values and of concentration amplitude

Parameter	Phenobarbital	Valproate Depakine[R]	Carbamazepine Tegretol[R]	Nortriptyline Sensaval[R]	Digoxin Lanoxin[K]			Dimension
F	1	1	1	1	0.8	0.8	0.8	—
Cl	0.7	0.25	1.1	20	8.57	7.15	5.72	litre/kg
k_{01}	0.7	0.7	0.35	0.7	0.693	0.693	0.693	per hour
$t_{\frac{1}{2}}$ absorption	1	1	2	1	1	1	1	hours
k_{12}	0.005775	0.07	0.07	0.0231	0.0231	0.0173	0.0116	per hour
$t_{\frac{1}{2}}$ elimination	120	10	10	30	30	40	60	hours
Cl^*	0.004	0.028	0.077	0.462	0.198	0.124	0.050	litre/kg per hour
dose/day per kg	3	12.9	8.6	1.43	0.00357	0.00357	0.00357	mg (per 24 h)/kg
body weight	70	70	70	70	70	70	70	kg

Table 12.4 Mean C, maximum plateau C_{max} and minimum concentration C_{min} and the maximum oscillation of a number of model drugs in the usual dosage regimen

	Phenobarbital			Valproate Depakine[R]			Carbamazepine Tegretol[R]			Nortriptyline Sensaval[R]			Digoxin						Dimension
dose interval (Δt)	24*	12	8*	24	12	8*	24	12*	8	24	12*	8	24	12	24	12*	24*	12	hours
Dose/Δt per kg	3	1.5	1	12.9	6.4	4.3	8.6	4.3	2.9	1.43	0.71	0.48	0.00357	0.00178	0.00357	0.00178	0.00357	0.00178	mg/kg per Δt
C_{max}	32.4	31.5	31.2	50.1	37.05	33.4	6.71	5.3	5.0	0.154	0.138	0.134	1.10	0.96	1.40	1.30	1.97	1.86	mg/litre
C	31.3	31.3	31.3	30.6	30.6	30.6	4.6	4.6	4.6	0.129	0.128	0.128	0.89	0.88	1.20	1.22	1.80	1.80	mg/litre
C_{min}	29.1	30.1	30.5	13.1	21.7	27.2	0.26	3.6	4.1	0.050	0.116	0.121	0.72	0.80	1.01	1.14	1.58	1.70	mg/litre
$\dfrac{C_{max}-C_{min}}{C_{max}} \times 100$	10.2	4.3	2.4	73.9	42.7	18.6	96.1	31.1	16.6	67.6	16.1	9.2	35.1	16	27.6	12.3	19.4	8.4	%

* preference dosage interval

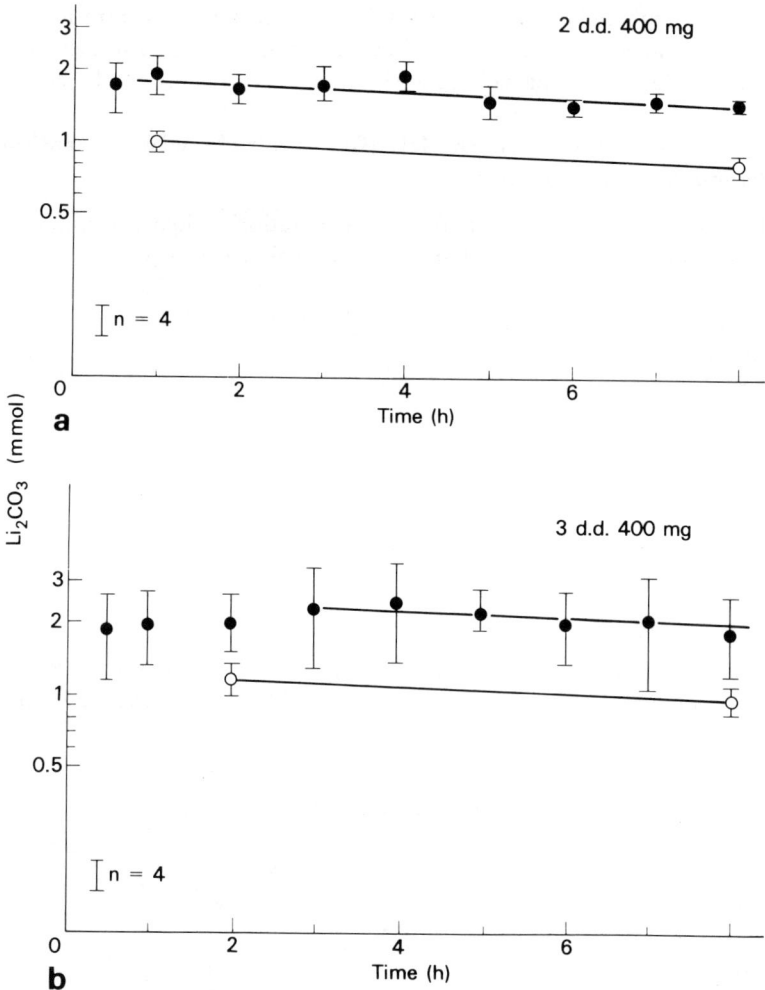

Fig. 12.8   (a) Concentration–time profile of lithium in saliva (black circles) and plasma (white circles) following the administration of regular Li_2CO_3 tablets during treatment. (b) Concentration–time profile of lithium in saliva (black circles) and plasma (white spheres) and plasma following the administration of sustained release tablets in the same patient as in (a). Note the differences in reproducibility of the concentration values and the limited influence of the sustained dissolution on the maximum of the concentration. (In this study the sustained release preparation was given to reduce gastrointestinal side-effects rather than sustain the plasma concentration, hence the dosages.)

gastrointestinal irritation, coating may be indicated as long as no sustained effect is expected.

When k_{10} as well as k_{01} are very small (e.g. with intramuscular implantation tablets and depot injections), a successful reduction of the concentration amplitude can be achieved. For oral preparations, this is unlikely to ever happen because of the limited passage time through the gastrointestinal tract.

Two-compartment open model after a single administration of intravenous bolus injection

Although the terminology is confusing, the notation of the two-compartment open model has become familiar in pharmacokinetics. Because many substances comply to this model after intravenous injection and subsequently can be characterised accordingly, this model and approach have gained great popularity.

Because differential equations and their integrated solutions have been published many times only a few examples will be given (Wagner 1975). Integrated equation:

$$C_1(t) = A\,e^{-\alpha t} + B\,e^{-\beta t} \tag{28}$$

$$Q_2(t) = P\,e^{-\beta t} - P\,e^{-\alpha t} \tag{29}$$

in which:

$$A = \frac{Q(\alpha - k_{21})}{V_1(\alpha - \beta)} \tag{30}$$

$$B = \frac{Q(k_{21} - \beta)}{V_1(\alpha - \beta)} \tag{31}$$

$$\alpha = \tfrac{1}{2}[(k_{12} + k_{21} + k_{13}) + \sqrt{(k_{12} + k_{21} + k_{13})^2 - 4k_{21}k_{13}}] \tag{32}$$

$$\beta = \tfrac{1}{2}[(k_{12} + k_{21} + k_{13}) - \sqrt{(k_{12} + k_{21} + k_{13})^2 - 4k_{21}k_{13}}] \tag{33}$$

$$P = \frac{Q \cdot k_{12}}{\alpha - \beta}$$

$$V_{dss} = \frac{\alpha + \beta - k_{13}}{k_{21}} \cdot V_1 = \frac{k_{12} + k_{21}}{k_{21}} \cdot V_1$$

V_{dss} is the apparent volume of distribution at steady state.

The mathematical solutions of the model enable predictions about the course of drug outside the body fluids accessible for sampling. Reference is made to central and peripheral or shallow and deep compartments. The real course of the concentration can only be traced when actual determinations are done in the body region or fluid that is considered relevant for the peripheral compartment or for the effect.

In some cases, parallelity of the course in the peripheral compartment with clinical effect has been established (Fig. 12.9). At times where the plasma concentration is almost negligible, the maximum effect can be measured. In other

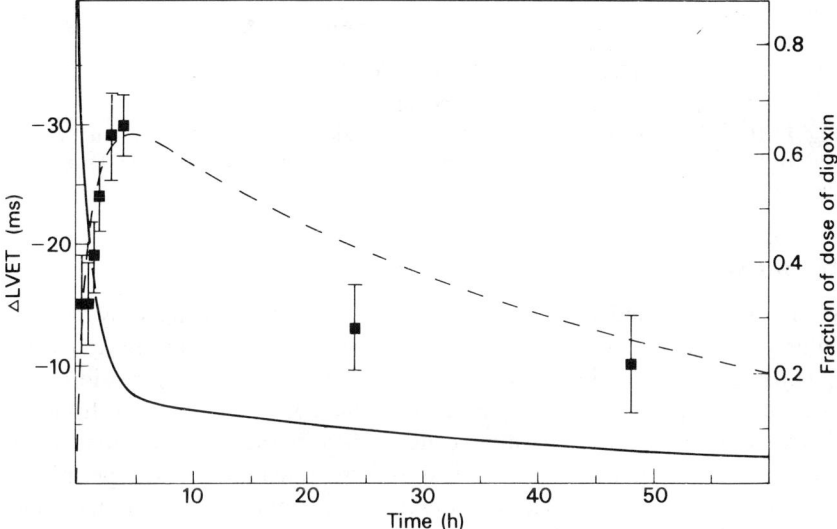

Fig. 12.9 Plasma concentration–time profile (solid line) of digoxin following a single bolus injection and the simulated course of the digoxin concentration in 'tissue' (dotted line). The tissue concentration course appears to follow the course of the pharmacological effect here expressed as ΔLVET index.

cases, the effect follows the plasma concentration more closely as in the case of the bronchodilating agent thiazinamine (Multergan[R]) that can best be measured by the heart rate (Jonkman 1977) (Fig. 12.10). For psychotropic drugs, a similar parallelity has not been adequately documented, largely due to the inaccessibility of the detailed locations for the effect, presumably the brain, and the lack of feasibility to sample and determine the pharmacological and therapeutic effect. Moreover, it is very likely that very poorly perfused regions of the brain, like the thick myelinated structures of the corpus callosum, lag behind in drug accumulation at a different rate and course than the second compartment, and accumulation to the therapeutically obvious effect only appears after prolonged administration.

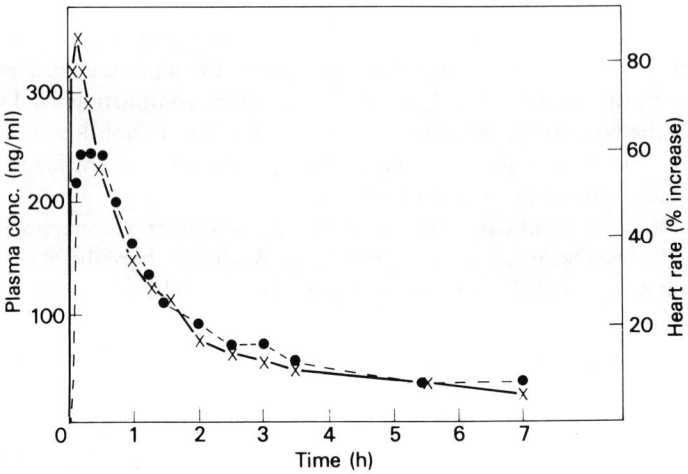

Fig. 12.10   Plasma concentration–time profile (solid line) and heart rate–time profile (dotted line) of thiazinamine (Multergan^R) after i.m. administration of 25.0 mg. Note the close correlation between the two profiles.

Open two-compartment model with first-order input

In principle, this model is very similar to the previous one. It has only didactic value to explain the course of the drug, unless the subjects are sampled frequently enough to allow confident pharmacokinetic interpretation. For example, at a point where 50% of the drug has still to be absorbed from the gastrointestinal tract the maximum concentration in the central compartment, the plasma, has already been reached and the maximum in the peripheral compartment is only reached when absorption is practically complete (Fig. 12.11a). After repetitive drug administration, the drug keeps accumulating in the peripheral compartment, whereas the accumulation in the central compartment is relatively small and will easily be overlooked and underestimated. The model also shows that a steady residue remains at the absorption side (Fig. 12.11b). In practice one has to watch variations in rate and extent of absorption, even in one individual, since position of the patient, upright or in bed, sitting or ambulant, can cause differences (Fig. 12.12).

Integrals:

$$C_1(t) = \frac{k_{01} \cdot F \cdot D}{V_1} \cdot \left[\frac{k_{21} - \alpha}{(k_{01} - \alpha)(\beta - \alpha)} \cdot e^{-\alpha t} + \right.$$

$$\frac{k_{21} - \beta}{(k_{01} - \beta)(\alpha - \beta)} \cdot e^{-\beta t} +$$

$$\left. \frac{k_{21} - k_{01}}{(\alpha - k_{01})(\beta - k_{01})} \cdot e^{-k_{01}t} \right] \tag{34}$$

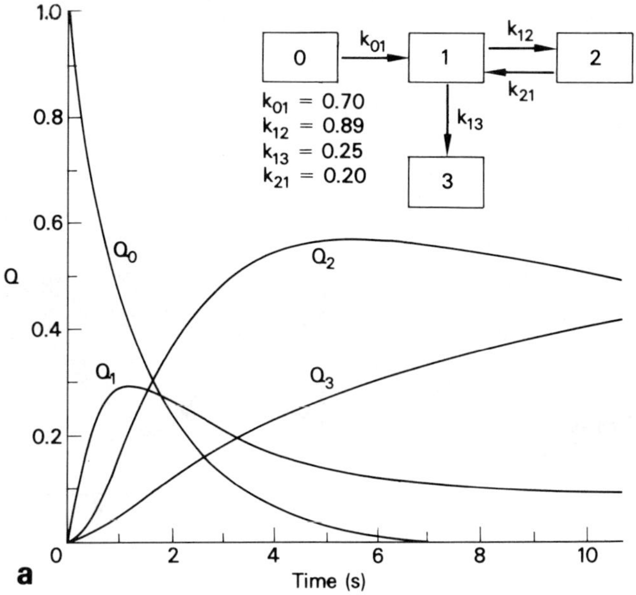

Fig. 12.11 (a) Simulated concentration or amount–time profiles when absorption in the body takes place. When still 50% of the drug has to be absorbed the maximum of the plasmaconcentration has already been reached. (b) Simulated concentration or amount–time profiles of a drug after six successive administrations. Note that a rather large fraction of the drug remains unabsorbed before the next administration takes place. Although the absolute accumulation of the drug in compartment 1 is of minor importance the drug keeps on accumulating in compartment 2.

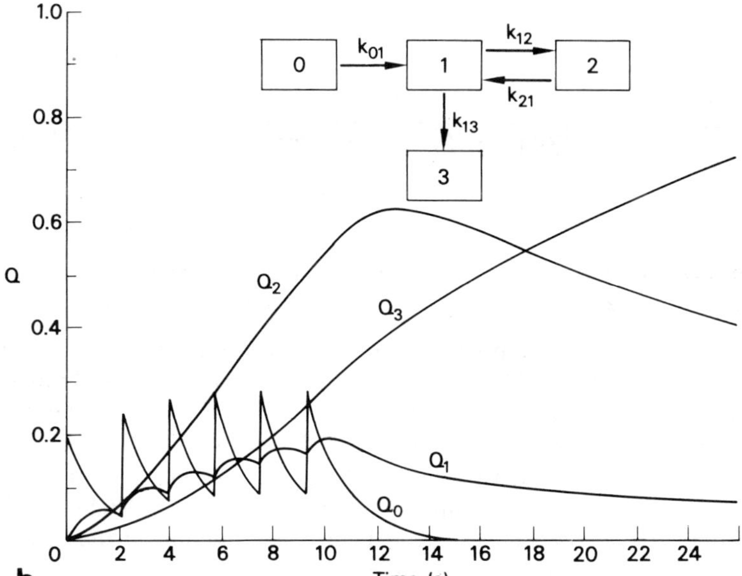

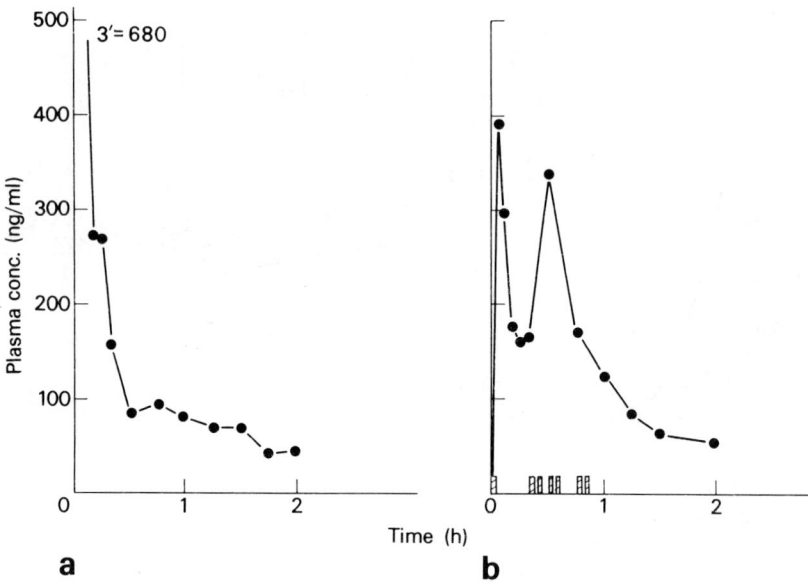

Fig. 12.12   Plasma concentration–time profile of thiazinamine (Multergan^R) after intramuscular injection of a dose of 25 mg to a subject (a) in resting position and (b) in resting position interrupted by small periods of walking as indicated by bars.

$$C_2(t) = \frac{k_{12} \cdot k_{01} \cdot F.D.}{V_2} \left[\frac{e^{-\alpha t}}{(k_{01}-\alpha)(\beta-\alpha)} + \frac{e^{-\beta t}}{(k_{01}-\beta)(\alpha-\beta)} + \frac{e^{-k_{01}t}}{(\alpha-k_{01})(\beta-k_{01})} \right]$$

$$(35)$$

One-compartment model with zero-order elimination
(non-linear or enzyme-capacity-limited elimination)

Ethanol is the classical example of a substance that, although 'effective' only in fairly high doses (10–20 g), can saturate the capacity of its eliminating enzyme, alcohol dehydrogenase (ADH). The result for the course of the plasma concentration, in contrast to all previous models with first-order kinetics (in which a constant fraction of the original amount is eliminated per time unit), is that a constant amount is eliminated per time unit. This model is valid for the period that the enzyme is saturated. At lower amounts in the body, the original first-order characteristics will regain dominance (Fig. 12.13).

The mathematical solution for this model has been given by Wagner (1973) and Van Ginneken *et al* (1974). The elimination rate appears to be dose and

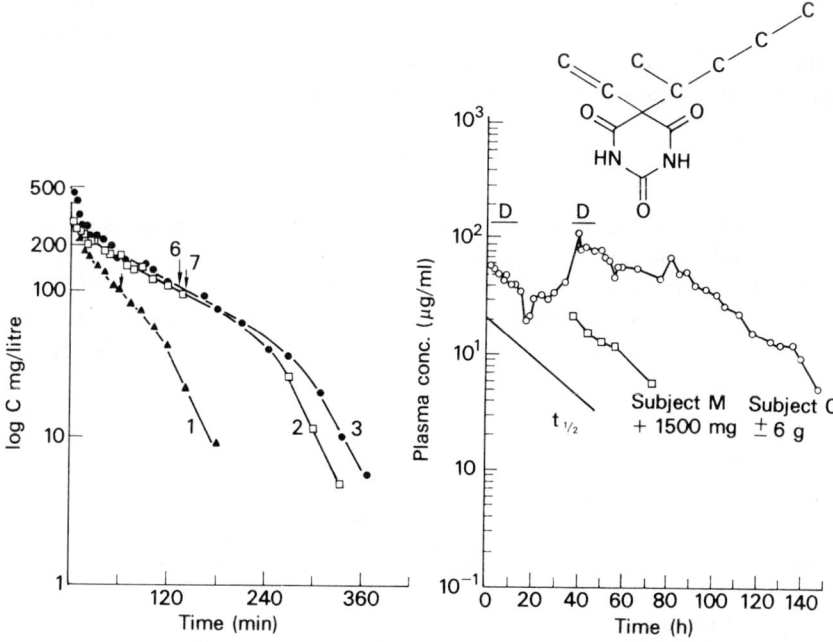

Fig. 12.13 (left)   Plasma concentration–time profile of 4-hydroxybutyrate after intravenous injection. Note the concave curve that can be explained by the capacity limitation of the enzyme lactate dehydrogenase that is responsible for the elimination of the compound. Triangles: patient no. 1, 50 mg/kg, squares: patient no. 2, 60 mg/kg; circles: patient no. 3, 60 mg/kg; arrows indicate mode of awareness.

Fig. 12.14 (right)   Log concentration–time profile of vinylbital (Bykonox[R]) after severe intoxications. Note the enzyme-capacity-limited elimination pattern of the drug at the high plasma concentrations. After the capacity has been restored the normal elimination pattern and rate can be demonstrated. D is the haemodialysis period.

thus concentration dependent, the higher the concentration the slower the elimination and the longer the sustaining of the effect. More recently the same phenomenon has been described for other drugs: salicylic acid (Levy *et al* 1972), phenytoin (Ritchens 1975) and 4-hydroxybutyric acid (Vree *et al* 1975). Barbiturates can show enzyme-capacity-limited elimination at high and toxic concentration (Vree *et al* 1976), which has clinical implications in the treatment of intoxication (Fig. 12.14).

Phenytoin

For diphenylhydantoin, non-linear kinetics have relevance for the calculation of the dosage regimen, because non-linearity appears at therapeutic concentrations. The parameters that describe enzyme saturation kinetics are common in biochemistry and show analogy with the Michaelis-Menten constants: K_m

and V_{max}. The K_m value represents the concentration (mg/litre) at which half of the amount of metabolising enzymes present are occupied by the drug . V_{max} is the maximum rate of metabolism (mg/hour). The clearance of a drug that appears concentration dependent can be expressed by:

$$Cl = \frac{V_{max}}{K_m + C} \qquad (36)$$

The apparent volume according to our current state of knowledge is not concentration dependent.

In the literature, K_m values for phenytoin ranging from 1.5 to 25.2 mg/litre have been reported (Ritchens 1975). The disproportionate increase of the concentration with proportional increase of the dose is shown in Fig. 12.15.

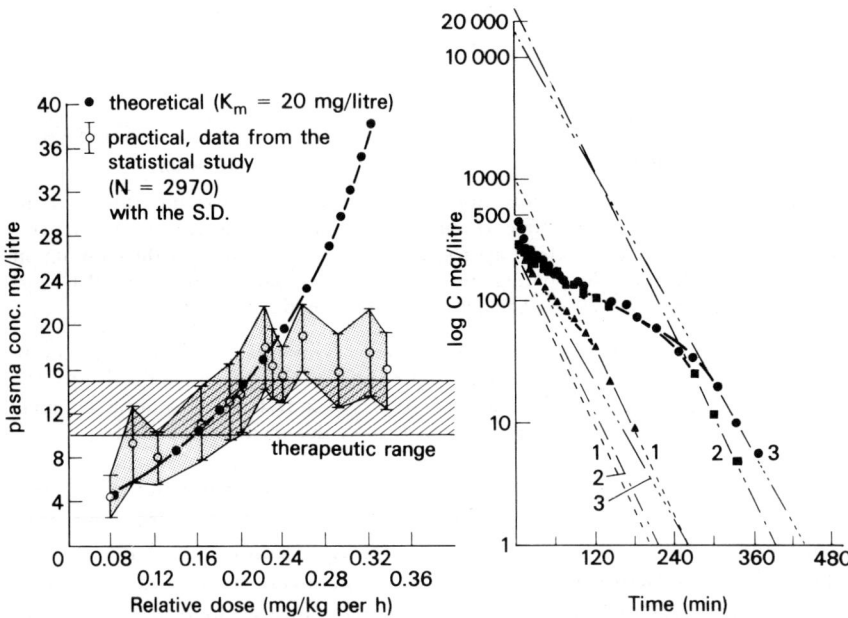

Fig.   12.15 (left)   Simulated concentration–dosage per time relation for phenytoin showing enzyme-capacity-limited elimination $K_m = 20$ mg/litre. $V_{max} = 0.68$ mg/kg per hour. In practice when, probably due to the limited patient compliance, toxic effects have a high occurence, this relationship is not followed.

Fig. 12.16 (right)   Plasma concentration–time profile of 4-hydroxybutyrate after i.v. bolus injection in order to induce anaesthesia. In the text the various methods are explained how to calculate K_m and V_{max} from the constructed intercepts with the ordinate and the first-order rate of elimination of the terminal phase of the curve. Triangles: patient no. 1, 50 mg/kg γOH; squares: patient no. 2, 60 mg/kg γOH; spheres: patient no. 3, 60 mg/kg γOH.

Calculation of K_m and V_{max}

When the plasma concentration profile after a single bolus injection has been constructed graphically with the aid of a sufficient number of samples, it is possible to determine the apparent Michaelis–Menten constants describing the concentration-dependent metabolism K_m and V_{max} (Fig. 12.16) (Ginneken *et al* 1974).

$$\ln C = \ln A + \frac{A-C}{K_m} - k \cdot t$$

(37)

or

$$C = A \cdot e^{(A-C)/K_m} \cdot e^{-kt}$$

(38)

in which k is the reciprocal time constant of the terminal part of the curve, A is the intercept of the curve with the ordinate, A^* is the intercept of the extrapolated terminal (linear) phase of the concentration curve with the ordinate. When $C < 0.1 K_m$

$$\ln C = \ln A^* - kt$$

(39)

$$\ln A^* = \ln A + \frac{A}{K_m}$$

(40)

K_m can be calculated by the difference between intercept A^* of the regression line with the ordinate slope described by k and the real intercept of the curve A

$$K_m = \frac{\ln A^* - \ln A}{A}$$

(41)

Another method to calculate K_m graphically is given by:

$$K_m = \frac{A}{k \cdot \Delta t}$$

(42)

in which Δt is the shift of the slope described by k and A^* parallel to a line described by k and A.

V_{max} can be calculated by:

$$V_{max} + k \cdot V \cdot K_m = \mathrm{Cl} \cdot K_m = \frac{\mathrm{Dose}}{A^*} \cdot k \cdot K_m$$

(43)

The Michaelis–Menten constants can also be derived from multiple dose regimens using dose increments during chronic medication when a patient is treated for a period of approximately five times the apparent (concentration-dependent) half-life. After steady state is achieved with one dose, the dosage is then increased. When plasma concentration values are monitored for three to five periods it is possible to graphically determine K_m and V_{max} (Ludden *et al* 1976). An algebraic solution for K_m is given by the following equation:

$$K_m = \frac{D_2 \times C_1 \times C_2 - D_1 \times C_1 \times C_2}{D_1 \times C_2 - D_2 \times C_1} \qquad (44)$$

In this equation D_1 is the initially instituted dose, D_2 the dose during the second period after steady state when D_1 has been established and clinical effect has not yet been achieved. C_1 and C_2 are the corresponding plasma concentration values determined at the end of each dosing period.

Structure and organisation of a clinical pharmacokinetics and toxicology laboratory

Because of the presence of know-how and expertise in the analysis of drugs in formulations and body fluids, it is most logical to integrate a clinical pharmacokinetics and toxicology laboratory with the functions and responsibilities for the preparation, dispensing, information, research and monitoring functions of a pharmacy department. The combination of accompaniment at admission, treatment and discharge of patients and research make it a valuable extension to the already existing service and developing components of a pharmacy department, as well as a source of inspiration for identifying patients' needs and their solution.

The major areas for the laboratory can be categorized as:

1. Clinical toxicology.
2. Pro- and retrospective monitoring of therapeutics.
3. Choice of drugs to be admitted to the hospital formulary.
4. Design of therapeutic guidelines.
5. Research, metabolite identification, drug interaction studies, placental transfer, adverse effects evaluation etc.

Clinical toxicology

Frequently, patients are admitted to the emergency service of the hospital on suspicion of overdoses of drugs. Anamnestic interviews with patients and/ or companion(s) are taken to identify the drug(s) or poisons. Clinical symptomatology also leads to group identification. Qualitative and quantitative data are meant to help this decision making and prediction of recovery.

Phenobarbitone intoxication

The monitoring of plasma concentrations has most often served in the diagnosis of intoxication of patients when clinical signs were ambiguous. Very often in cases of severe intoxication only circulation- and respiration-supporting measures can help to overcome the crisis. Phenobarbitone elimination appears to be increased by hemodialysis, but only at high concentrations. Phenytoin elimination is not influenced by this method (Van der Kleijn *et al* 1973).

Carbamazepine intoxication

Because of its slow absorption, gastrointestinal lavage is thought advantageous even after 24–48 hours following abnormal carbamazepine (Tegretol[R]) ingestion. A case report on a severely intoxicated patient who had been treated with sorbitol 40% and 10 g activated charcoal every 4 hours during 1 day with the intention of enhancing intestinal passage and reduced absorption of the yet unabsorbed drug appeared to result in the opposite: an increased absorption and a prolonged coma (Fig. 12.17) (de Zeeuw *et al* 1978).

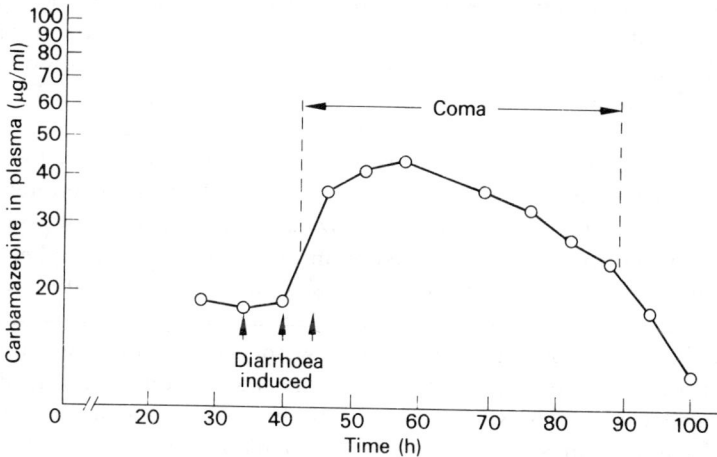

Fig. 12.17 Plasma concentration profile of carbamazepine (Tegretol[R]) following a massive overdose in an epileptic patient. After 48 hours when the patient has not yet recovered, the diminution of suspected unabsorbed drug was thought to be enhanced by induced diarrhoea by 40% sorbitol solution. In contrast an increased absorption could be observed.

Vinylbital intoxication

An instructive example of toxicity with enzyme-capacity-limited elimination for both effect and enzyme is obtained with an overdose of a barbiturate. Garrett *et al* (1974) showed with amobarbitone in dogs that when a plasma concentration of about 40 µg/ml is reached, the elimination process becomes zero order. In Fig. 12.14 the elimination curve of vinylbital of subject C is shown after taking 40 tablets of Bykonox (6 g). After admission to the hospital and estimation of the high plasma concentration of 60 µg/ml subject C underwent dialysis (D) with the initial success that the plasma concentration rapidly decreased. When dialysis was stopped the plasma concentration increased again due to the restoration of the equilibrium of vinylbitone between plasma and tissue and possibly, by absorption from the intestinal tract. A second period of dialysis did not result in the anticipated lower plasma concentrations. Eighty hours after admission, the plasma concentration started to decrease more rapidly and the half-life time of elimination could be estimated to be 18 hours. This half-life time of 18 hours was also reported by Breimer (1974) for healthy subjects.

A second subject (M), who had taken only 1.5 g of vinylbitone, did not reach the high plasma concentration of 30–40 µg/ml at which the mixed function oxydase, cytochrome P450, can be considered totally occupied. The elimination curve of subject M showed again the half-life time of 18 hours. The same behaviour (first-order elimination) was found with the compounds amobarbitone and secobarbitone. Up to concentrations of 16 µg/ml, a first-order elimination was found for both compounds with a half-life time of 18 hours for amobarbitone, and 30 hours for secobarbitone (in Vesparax^R). From the foregoing it can be concluded that the enzyme in subject C was totally occupied during 80 hours and the capacity for elimination was limited by its V_{max}. The phenomenon of capacity-limited elimination of barbiturates after an extremely high dose can be used to explain the elimination of vinylbitone in subject J after the intake of 40 tablets of Bykonox^R, 40 tablets of Seresta^R (oxazepam), ten tablets of Dalmodorm^R (flurazepam) and ten tablets of Tryptizol^R (amitriptyline). After a 3-day period of unconsciousness in a peripheral hospital, subject J was admitted to the intensive care and resuscitation ward of the University hospital. At the time of admission the plasma concentration of vinylbitone was only 11 µg/ml. This low concentration in comparison to that of subject C, indicated that the enzyme was no longer saturated. The prolonged sleeping time was concluded to be due to the oxazepam and flurazepam. In order to measure the half-life time, a blood sample was drawn every 4 hours over a period of 3 days. The half-life measured was 22.5 hours. Because the first part of the elimination curve was missing, it had to be proven that the enzyme cytochrome P450 was not damaged. For this reason, one tablet of vinylbitone was given at the very end of the elimination of the first toxic dose. The plasma concentration rose again and the compound was eliminated with the same half-life time of 22.5 hours, which could be considered typical for this individual. From the dose and blood concentration (1500 mg–12 µg/ml and 150 mg–1.2 µg/ml) the volume of distribution could be calculated as 125 litres. From Fig. 12.14 it can be derived that the K_m value of vinylbitone is about 25 µg/ml (1×10^{-4}M).

Pro- and retrospective monitoring of therapeutics

Determinations of plasma concentrations

The purpose of the determination of plasma concentrations still serves the predominantly diagnostic aims of identification and evaluation of toxic, therapeutic or subtherapeutic levels, patient compliance, disease states (e.g. impairment of renal or liver clearance), drug interactions, adaptation of dosage as a result of temporary disease conditions, diet or medication profile, incomplete or erratic absorption and elimination (e.g. linear or non-linear proportionality between dose, plasma concentration and effect) and variations in biological availability.

Therapeutic consequences can be: correction of the dosage regimen, enforcement of drug intake, treatment of the disease state, addition or withdrawal of one or more drugs and change to other formulations or route of administration.

Toxic, therapeutic or subtherapeutic levels

Very often clinical symptomatology is insufficient to distinguish states of overdosing and underdosing. For instance antiepileptic drugs may be epileptogenic at high levels and benzodiazepines may elicit excitatory states. When not identified, these symptoms may be treated by increasing dosage or addition of a related compound that may result in serious defects. Reliable therapeutic concentrations have been established for only a few drugs and again for a few clinical indications (Table 12.2).

Patient compliance

Compliance is a well-documented subject. It should be stressed that domestic organisation of drug use should be optimal before expensive assays are requested. Reduction of the number of drugs and administrations, instruction and encouragement of intake are indispensable. Packaging drugs in an instructive manner similar to the contraceptives is likely to improve this problem (Van der Kuy and Van der Kleijn 1972).

Disease states

Increased or decreased plasma levels and elimination kinetics may lead to the diagnosis of renal and hepatic dysfunctions. Breimer (1974) has successfully used hexobarbitone kinetics to discriminate between hepatic cirrhosis, acute hepatitis and normal subjects.

Drug interactions

It has been demonstrated in a number of cases that drugs may alter the kinetics of other drugs. This alteration may result in either decreased or increased plasma levels (Guelen *et al* 1972). Decreased plasma levels and consequently increased clearance values are found in the concomitant treatment of patients with phenobarbitone. Phenobarbitone, long time recognised as an enzyme inducer in rodents, is also thought to increase mixed functions oxidase metabolism in man (Guelen and Van der Kleijn, 1978). The reversed phenomenon of a drug causing an increase in the plasma concentration level of another drug has been demonstrated by Morselli *et al* (1971) and by Schobben *et al* (1975). Diphenylhydantoin and dipropylacetate appeared to cause an increase in the phenobarbitone concentration in patients maintained on the same regimen. Interactions with drugs may also occur with food. Concomitant drug intake with meals often results in a sustained absorption of the drugs. Depending on the therapeutic requirements for onset, intensity and time course of wanted and undesired effects, the drug intake may be rescheduled. Parenteral administration in different muscle areas may also result in different concentration profiles.

Incomplete or erratic absorption and elimination kinetics

Although it requires more frequent sampling to establish the absorption and elimination characteristics than would normally be feasible in clinical practice, absorption and elimination patterns differing between individuals can frequently be observed. Those drug formulations showing slow absorption when rapid onset of effect is required may be reformulated. When the absorption of a drug is influenced by decreased or increased motility or GI obstruction, concomitant drugs like anticholinergics and laxatives, or nutrition, it may be possible for the drug to be administered by another route or at other times. It may also be that the drug demonstrates a change to non-linear kinetics when dosages are increased. For phenytoin, this has been demonstrated even at therapeutic levels. At younger ages it has been demonstrated that drugs may be cleared at a much higher rate than can be compensated for by handrule calculated dosage.

Variations in biological availability

Bioavailability is a well-documented variable for drugs that is interesting to monitor. This and the variations in weight and content uniformity of the dosage forms should be kept as constant as possible during treatment.

Choice of drugs for formulary

The restriction of items with generic and/or therapeutic equivalence requires, as well as literature evidence, very often self-documented evidence and experience. *In vitro* and *in vivo* bioavailability testing has been proven necessary for a number of drugs in order to choose the optimal brand or formulation.

Digoxin and diphenylhydantoin are notorious examples of drugs with bio-availability problems. Also drug formulations for sustained release have to be watched carefully because the *in vitro* data do not always match the *in vivo* data. The design of the pharmaceutical formulation has to be closely in agreement with the current therapeutic aims.

Therapeutic guidelines

Very often it appears that the classical guidelines for drug therapy may lead to inadequate dosage regimens or, in other words, to too large fluctuations in amount of pharmacologically active substance in the body. Sometimes too large fluctuations are allowed in practice in the suggestion that too frequent drug administration is not feasible. For example for procainamide, a rather short time interval has to be prescribed in order to maintain adequate plasma levels of the drug and its *N*-acetyl metabolite. Due to the slightly longer half-life of the *N*-acetyl-procainamide metabolite, the fluctuations of the therapeutic substances are not as serious as for procainamide alone. Nevertheless, it requires intensive monitoring of plasma concentrations to check the maintenance of the therapeutic concentration. This is in particular necessary because the elimination rate shows a bimodal distribution pattern in epidemiological studies. Because it has its own pharmacological activity the sum of parent compound and product has to be considered in relation to activity. Therefore, it is an exemplary drug to monitor by plasma concentration profile in relation to well-observed antiarrhythmic effects. Other drugs that have a small safety margin and do require more rigid schedules and need to be monitored are theophylline, the toxic antibiotics gentamicin, kanamycin, rifampycin, and diuretics.

Establishment of therapeutically relevant plasma concentrations (C_{therap})

The therapeutically relevant plasma concentration has been determined for a number of drugs. These values have been obtained from careful clinical studies by closely monitoring predefined objective effects, adverse effects or lack of effect, in relation to a confident plasma concentration profile. Due to the difficulties in medical semantics and the multitude of experimental variables in patients, these values often show large variations.

Assuming reasonable control of the disease state in general practice, instructions through the daily self-control or monitoring by the accompanying nurses and doctors, therapeutic optimum values can also be obtained from epidemiological studies on plasma concentrations in large populations. There is little information on the therapeutic concentration values when combinations of drugs are given. Moreover, it has been observed in, for example, epilepsy, that extremely low concentrations of either one or more drugs are reported to be effective. Withdrawal of the drug has been reported to induce crises. This paradoxical phenomenon also needs further confirmation and investigation.

The quantitative dependence of C_{therap} on, for instance, the nature and severity of the disease state and also on technical factors like laboratory and assay quality, chemical stability of the sample and time of sampling, often still need clarification through interlaboratory, interdepartmental controls and standards.

In a similar manner to the established routine in clinical chemistry, standardisation is necessary to compare the results of different laboratories, methods, chemists, times of the day, week or month. The usefulness and necessities of such quality control has been proven (Ritchens 1975).

Research

Clinical pharmacokinetics still requires intensive research both at the fundamental level as well as under practical conditions. Within the framework of a good structure for the organisation of drug distribution and administration to patients, clinical pharmacokinetic data for drugs collected in the following tables may be considered fruitful. So-called routine determinations will only be applied for toxicology and for otherwise unprovable underdosing. In most other cases research will be applied to establish or improve guidelines for the treatment of patients with drugs in various pathological conditions. These efforts support decisions to be made in therapeutics committees and help those involved in the daily monitoring service of patients on wards. In this respect it appears to be necessary to reconsider old drugs that have been replaced. The emphasis of the research of a department of clinical pharmacy can be focussed on the following:

1.   Qualitative and quantitative investigation of the interactions of drugs.
2.   The quantitative adaptation of dosage regimens in pathological conditions.
3.   Comparison of drug substances and drug formulations within the same therapeutic group (biological availability).
4.   Testing and design of guidelines for treatment of patients suffering a pathological disease.
5.   Pharmacokinetics in the newborn child and infant, in cases of malnutrition as well as overnutrition and more generally in genetically differing populations and in the elderly.

Assuming participation of the major clinical departments in projects the following areas can be distinguished:

Antibiotics and chemotherapeutics. Monitoring is for research purposes, seldom for routine determinations. Research is carried out mainly to establish or improve feasibility and dosage regimen guidelines for the application of particular drugs in special conditions.

Cardiac glycosides and antiarrhythmics. These are routinely monitored mostly for inpatients and paediatrics.

Neuromuscular relaxants and anaesthetics. These are investigated for research on behalf of anaesthesiology.

Antineoplastic drugs. To improve protocols and to monitor patients in oncology units, in haematology, endocrinology, ENT, gynaecology and paediatrics.

Antihypertensives and diuretics. For improvement of therapeutic guidelines and for research purposes.

Theophylline. For monitoring and for research purposes in respiratory disease units.

Antidepressants and lithium. To monitor inpatients for compliance and research on guidelines.

Investigational drugs. To establish guidelines and efficacy and adverse reaction monitoring.

Laboratory facilities

A laboratory serving a large general or university hospital requires a floorspace of about $400\,m^2$ to be able to perform these duties. Instrumentation that is thought to be required consists, next to the standard laboratory equipment, of: gas chromatography; high-pressure liquid chromatography including UV, fluorophotometry and Coulombmetric detection; radioimmunossay involving beta and/or gamma counting; enzyme multiplied immunoassay technique; gas chromatography–mass spectrometry; computer equipment; time sharing, plotting, desk and hand calculator facilities.

Personnel requirements

Staff must be able to develop and carry out drug assay research and routine service. The job description of technicians should include the performing of assays, and assistance in their development, the execution of the calculations and interpretation of the acquired data. Preferably they should be able to communicate with the assay-requesting department about the therapeutic implications. Frequent participation in patients' conferences improves the quality and relevance of this work.

Assay requisition

In order to produce meaningful results from offered sample material, it is required that information on the individual drugs to be analysed, previous

SINT RADBOUDZIEKENHUIS NIJMEGEN Pharmacy Clinical Pharmacy tel: (080) 51 41 63 or 51 64 05	Pharmacochemical research in body fluids
INCOMPLETE FILLING OF FORMS WILL RESULT IN SERIOUS DELAYS	int. ext. 4162

	Reason for request ☐ Check (clinically well set up) ☐ Suspected underdose ☐ Suspected intoxication ☐

Requesting physician   Dept.   tel.

Patient: Weight: (kg)   Height: (cm)   Creatinine clearance

Diagnosis

Which drug do you wish examined?			**not to be completed**	
name of drug:	dose:	admin. times	conc. (mg/l)	rel. clear. (ml/h/kg)

Have other drugs been administered at the same time?		☐ yes ☐ no		
name of drug:	dose:	admin. times		

Has dosage changed in previous week?				
name of drug:	old dosage:	Date of change:		

Blood sample(s) date:	time taken:	time of last dose:		**not to be completed**

Remarks:

Advice:

	passed on:

Fig. 12.18 Requisition form for the assay of drug concentration in body fluids used in the department of Clinical Pharmacy, St Radboud Hospital, Nijmegen, the Netherlands. All pharmacokinetic information necessary for dosage regimen calculations such as clearance data etc. are reported on this form.

regimens, other drugs not to be analysed, diet (if relevant) special instructions for use as well as basic biometric and civil data, body weight, height and any additional clinical and laboratory data is supplied (Fig. 12.18). Without this information, it is useless to determine the concentration values because clearance values cannot be calculated and relevant information cannot be fed back. Since most assays are relatively expensive, great care should be paid to optimising their usefulness. The initial and. the feedback communication is often organised through a senior consultant who is informed about the details of time of sampling, sample processing, data interpretation and other pitfalls. Regular retrospective evaluation at patient conferences and prospective planning of newly admitted patients greatly improves the quality of the service. Depending on the position of the laboratory and its structural acceptance, more compulsory measures can be made to improve compliance to these instructions.

Because so many variables may influence the plasma concentration of drugs and subsequently the therapeutic adequacy of the dosage regimen of specifically active drugs, it is necessary to design a rather meticulous logistic procedure for the accompaniment of patients treated with one or more drugs. Before expensive and specialised procedures requiring drug analyses and kinetic consulting services are considered, domestic drug distribution procedures should be guaranteed. The practical clinical benefits of clearance parameters and plasma concentrations are not equal for every drug and condition. Lack of confidence in intra- and interindividual clearance and concentration parameters at subsequent times during treatment limits these values to the diagnosis of severe overdosing or underdosing when clinical signs are conflicting.

When an adequate number of samples are taken at well-considered time periods a concentration profile can be constructed allowing the calculation of the 'area under the curve' and the clearance values.

Sample material

Kinetic parameters are usually based on plasma or serum concentration determinations. When, however, invasive and painful blood sampling is not possible, it might be wise to make use of saliva. Next to that, cerebrospinal fluids, tears, urine and wound exudates are sometimes available. When the total plasma concentration is measured the protein concentration may play a considerable role, because the pharmacological activity is said to be determined by the free concentration. The protein-binding capacity is of great importance for psychotropic drugs. In general, because of their high lipophilicity, they show a high binding affinity for plasma protein. Therefore in some cases, it is necessary to take the albumin concentration of the sample material into account.

Saliva

With respect to protein binding, saliva may be a better reference for the free fraction (Fig. 12.19). For acidic and amphoteric drugs this supposition seems to be reasonable. For the basic drugs with a p*Ka* equal to or larger than 7 the partition between saliva and plasma appears to be in favour of saliva. A mechanism other than free diffusion of the undissociated fraction must play a role. Saliva sampling appears to be attractive when a large number of samples is indicated in cases of 'profile' determination. However, care should be taken for proper collection since the variation may depend on the moment

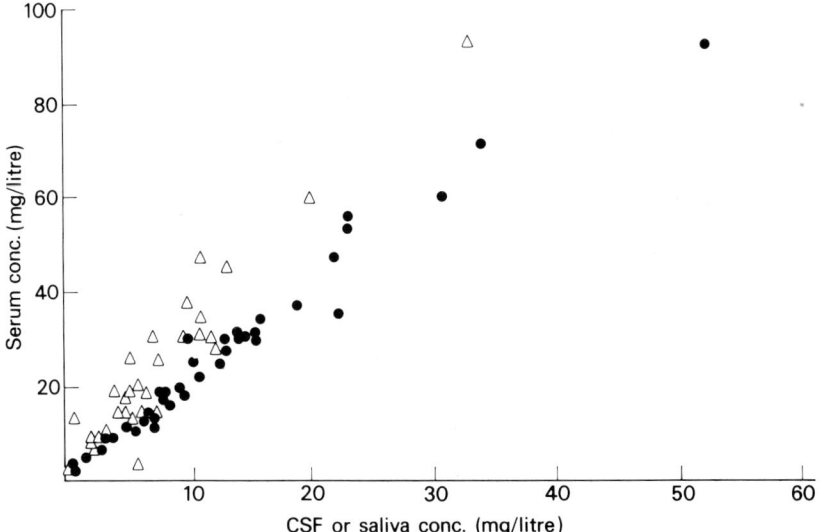

Fig. 12.19   Relationship between saliva (triangles), CSF (circles) and plasma concentration of phenobarbital in epileptic patients. Ratio saliva–serum = 0.32; ratio CSF–serum = 0.48.

of sampling in relation to intake of food and beverages. There may also be a difference in the excretions of the parotic and submandibular glands.

In cases of a rather high saliva–plasma ratio, the saliva concentration profile related to one or more plasma concentration values may be helpful. The conditions and variables for practical use of saliva data still remain to be investigated (Van der Kleijn *et al* 1975). So far clearance and concentration data for saliva have best been applied in the field of epilepsy and for lithium.

Urine

Urinary excretion rates could equally serve the purpose for monitoring patients. However, confident sampling is found difficult to comply with. In addition urine output and urinary pH may influence the renal excretion rate of the drug. Because an unknown ratio of metabolites may be present in the urine, the uncertainty of the relevance of the determination is great. Cumulative urinary excretion profiles have proved useful for the determination of bioavailability of various drug formulations.

Cerebrospinal fluid

For many lipophilic drugs, the uptake in CSF is negligible. It would not be practical to take CSF samples in routine monitoring but occasionally it may be indicated in suspected blood brain barrier damages. After intrathecal administration of methotrexate CSF is monitored prior to subsequent administration, to help predict toxicity.

Tissue distribution

In the pharmacokinetic concept, a linear relationship between the dose administered, the resulting plasma concentration, the concentration in the biophase and the therapeutic effect is implicit. Even though large concentration differences may be observed regionally this hypothesis may still be valid. However, the distribution-partition coefficient may be influenced by many variables. For example, for children the ratio is often different from that for adults. Comedication as well as endogenous substances may considerably influence the partition ratio of drugs.

Time of sampling

To avoid unnecessary and uncomfortable injection of the patient, sampling is required to be restricted to the utmost minimum. For the outpatients one blood sample is often the most that can be acquired. When drugs are slowly eliminated this single sample may adequately reflect the mean plasma concentration and therefore the amount present in the body. Every drug may require its own proper sampling time after drug administration (Table 12.2). The plasma concentration has to reflect the concentration of the drug in the biophase. Drugs that show a large apparent distribution volume and a rapid absorption rate may show a two or more phasic plasma concentration decay-curve after the absorption maxima, even after long-term treatment. According to the current pharmacokinetic concepts, the biophase may generally be reflected by a second or peripheral compartment. The sampling time has to be chosen so that small changes in initial absorption and distribution kinetics or variations with time after the last intake have little influence on the confidence of the measured concentration or the calculated clearance. From Fig. 12.20 it can be shown that for digoxin, the samples should not be taken before 5 hours after drug intake. Even the moment prior to the next administration can

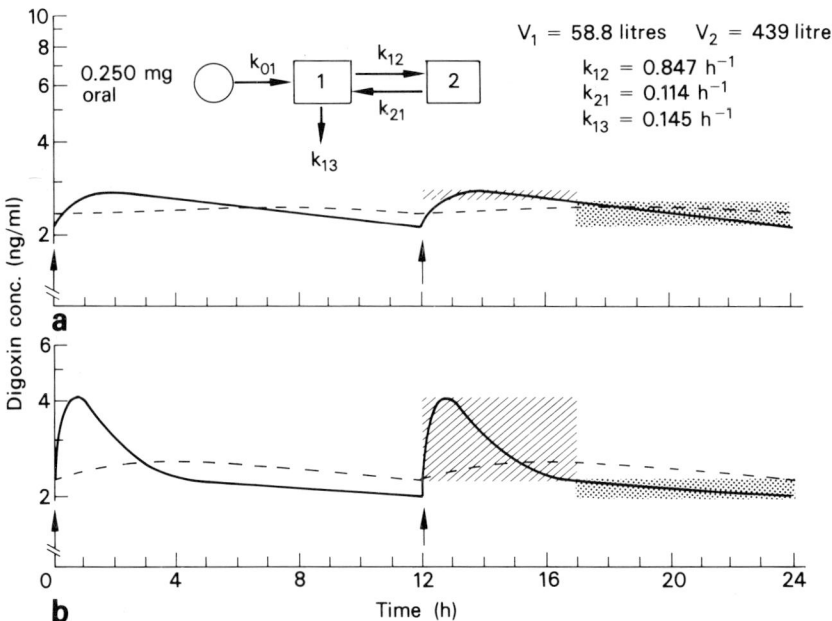

Fig. 12.20 Simulated concentration–time profile of digoxin in compartment 1 (solid line), representing plasma concentration, and in compartment 2 (dotted line) representing the tissues based on parameters obtained from patient material. The reciprocal time constants for absorption (k_{01}) have been varied to mimic (a) a rapidly absorbing formulation (0.25/hour) and (b) a relative slow absorbing formulation (2.0/hour). The patient has taken the drug chronically. Accumulation of the drug is considered maximum. Relatively minor concentration oscillations occur in the tissues even when absorption causes large variations in the initial phase. Therefore, when the drug is given twice daily and the number of samples has to be restricted, sample moments between 5 and 12 hours will best reflect the mean steady state concentration both in plasma as well as in tissue.

still be considered adequate. For drugs that are relatively rapidly eliminated one can improve the confidence values of the concentrations by taking two or more samples during one medication interval. When too large variations in concentration during the medication interval cannot be permitted it can be advantageous to use smaller dosages at more frequent administration periods. The use of 'sustained release' formulations, from the point of view of nursing personnel, may be more economical, but is seldom kinetically justified.

Nutrition

Food intake may have its influence on the absorption rate and the extent of absorption. During chronic medication, rapid absorption is often not desired, to avoid too rapid an onset of possible adverse reactions. When rapid onset of activity is required (e.g. hypnotics), food should be avoided. It has been experienced in nursing centres that when drugs were mixed with meals only an aliquot of the dose (meal) was ingested. Separation of drug intake and meals may reduce the problem.

Pharmaceutical quality

Content and weight uniformity variations may cause variations in plasma concentration of a drug. Drug mixtures are often compounded or reconstituted just prior to administration. The above-mentioned pharmaceutical variables are often considered constant. This in essence is a quality problem that has been extensively documented. It has often been found to contribute to the variance of the mean drug clearance and may be identified in retrospective analyses. Since the confidence limits of content and weight uniformity permit variations of 10–15% it cannot be expected that concentration and clearance data will ever show a smaller range of limits.

Assay quality

The analytical method to determine, specifically, selectively and most accurately, the drug and its metabolites is still the most crucial element in pharmacokinetic research and practice. The current methods of analysis use separation techniques based on solvent extraction, thin-layer chromatography, gas chromatography, high-pressure liquid chromatography and binding to specific proteins or antibodies. They are being continuously improved to increase reproducibility and to decrease the detection limits. An important requirement of the assay is the ability to detect small amounts of substance in the order of 0.5 nanogram to 500 µg in a sample of restricted size: mostly 0.05–2 ml plasma. Reliability and reproducibility of the method is an important factor.

In a similar manner to the established routine in clinical chemistry, standardisation is necessary to compare the results of different laboratories, methods, chemists, times of the day, week or month. The usefulness of such quality control has been proved by the Phenytoin Control Group organised by the department of Clinical Pharmacology of St Bartholomew's Hospital in London, where the variations in the results of over 30 laboratories has been progressively decreased over the last 2 years.

Gas chromatography using flame ionisation detection or electron capture detection for halogenated compounds has become the major routine technique for drug analysis in biological fluids. However, non-reproducible thermolysis of compounds may occur and resolution of mixtures may require derivatisation that introduces problems of synthetic gain.

Radioimmunoassay is a rapidly developing possibility to determine drugs at the submicrogram level. However, limited specificities are still a major disadvantage.

Enzyme multiplied immunoassay techniques (EMIT) have more recently been introduced as a very promising, rapid and confident method for assays of phenytoin, phenobarbital and primidone.

High-pressure liquid chromatography is rapidly gaining a dominating position in biological drug assays with spectrophotometric, spectrofluorophotometric and Coulombmetric detection possibilities in the nanogram and even subnanogram levels.

Chemical stability

Stability of the drug in the sample may become a problem when the drug is degraded before it is analysed in the laboratory (e.g. clonazepam in unstable even when stored in the refrigerator). This argues for adequate provisions during transport and storage, in particular when samples are sent over long distances. Lyophyllisation has been proposed but deep freezing appears to be the most practical way for storage.

Plasma concentration–concentration biophase–effect relationships

In interpreting concentrations of drugs in for example plasma, one always considers a known and fixed relationship between this concentration and the one in the biophase. Assays in saliva and determination of saliva concentration profiles has been proved useful for lithium. For other drugs the conditions remain to be investigated. This biophase is in most cases however still hypothetical. As a result of absorption, elimination and distribution processes, unlike biogenous substances, drug concentrations are subject to continuous regional change. Animal studies have shown that the regional differences in concentration may be dependent on the time after administration. Pharmacokinetic 'behaviour' of the drug in various regions of the body has to be known before the concentration values will be meaningful. Basic sciences have not yet reached the state that non-linear kinetics can easily be applied in clinical conditions. Moreover some drugs exert their effect through a kinetically undefined chain of exogenous and biogenous processes. Deficiency or presence of certain bigenous substances and drugs may alter the plasma concentration–tissue concentration effect relationship. Drugs with large tissue–plasma partition coefficients and/or strong binding to tissue and cell elements may show non-linear binding characteristics in conditions where plasma protein binding appears linear. Unambiguous pharmacological effects that allow quantitation of the influence of a drug on the symptoms of diseased patients are scarce and are subject to criticism because of the large variation in intensity and characteristics of most diseases in patients. Sub- and supratherapeutic (toxic) levels have been associated with similar clinical and electrophysiological symptoms in treatment with antiepileptics as well as cardiacs. Research on patients is needed.

Time required to process the samples

To make use adequately of the concentration and clearance figures in planning treatment of individual patients, the information needs to be available at the time patient and physician meet.

For outpatients, the response may be adapted to the pace of the visits to the clinic. The time lapse can be considered, related to the half-life of the drug. Changes in dosages are only meaningful after 80–90% of the new steady state has been allowed to be established thus after ± 3–4 times $t_{\frac{1}{2}}$. In outpatient clinics, it is advantageous to plan visits and give instructions so that the assay is processed before the new regimen is decided. In acute cases, most assays can be carried out within 1 hour after the sample has been taken. When the identity of the drug(s) is unknown, it may take much more time. Therefore careful clinical judgement and thorough anamnestic interviews should precede the sampling of the patient.

Interpretation of the clearance parameter

Although the clearance can be considered a constant, the condition for which the value applies has to be well defined. Clearance values can be determined under clinical conditions, by using equation 23, from plasma concentration values determined in the laboratory and from therapeutic data supplied by the physician such as dosage regimen: dose D, time interval Δt, body weight and height (enabling the calculation and statistical analysis of body surface). By supplying the data on sex, age, concomitant drugs, nutrition (if abnormal), dosage form and brand, period of previous medication, sampling time, clinical pathology, and condition and clinical chemistry (e.g. renal function, status of patient, i.e. outpatient or inpatient), it will be possible to select, statistically the best homogeneous population enabling the calculation of the most confident clearance value under the defined conditions. The clearance value for a drug can also be derived from C_{ss} versus dose/time per kg body weight from graphs often found in the literature.

From equation 23, it can be seen that the reciprocal of the slope of this linear regression line equals the relative clearance (Fig. 12.5a). The statistics of these regression lines supply the confidence parameter of this clearance value. Absence of linearity of this regression line may also lead to identification of enzyme-capacity-limited elimination (Fig. 12.15). Poor confidence will stimulate the search for variables that may improve the homogeneity of the population.

So far the following variables have been identified for a number of drugs. An attempt has been made to quantify their influence in order to use dosage calculations and dosage correction based on: body weight or surface, age, sex, pathology (e.g. liver and kidney function), absorption characteristics, comedication, influence of physiological concentrations of biogenous substances on tissue distribution and distribution volume among other factors.

Comparison of results from routine plasma concentration determinations with statistically obtained parameters also enables checks to be made on laboratory performance and assay method.

When these qualities are guaranteed by internal standardisation and standard samples it may be possible that deviating clearance values help to identify, diagnose and evaluate:

1.   Clinical condition.
2.   Lack of patient adherence to the prescriber's regimen and total medication profile.
3.   Erratic pharmacokinetics (e.g. non-linear kinetics, multicompartment kinetics, absorption and elimination dysfunctions, first-pass metabolism).
4.   Influence of comedication or nutrition.
5.   Quality of the formulation (limited bioavailability).
6.   Inadequate route of administration.
7.   Instability of the sample.

Before a dosage regimen is corrected, it is advisable to consider and weigh these factors. When changes are made or observed, a new sample taken after more than five times the $t_\frac{1}{2}$ of the drug following the change should be analysed to check its influence on the normal value for these conditions. Next to the identification of the above factors plasma concentrations may support diagnosis of:

8.   Toxic, adequate or subtherapeutic results in particular when clinical symptomatology does not distinguish between states of overdosing or underdosing.

When not identified, these symptoms may lead to increase of the dose or the addition of a related compound that may result in serious problems. When the diagnosis is clinically confirmed it may result in:

1.   Correction of dosage regimen.
2.   Treatment of the disease states.
3.   Enforcement of the intake.
4.   Addition or withdrawal of one or more drugs.
5.   Change to another formulation or route of administration.

Some examples of qualitative variables influencing clearance

Pregnancy

Pregnancy may influence the clearance significantly. In general, during the latter part of pregnancy, the concentration of antiepileptic drugs decreases, requiring an increase of the dose to maintain the therapeutic plasma concen-

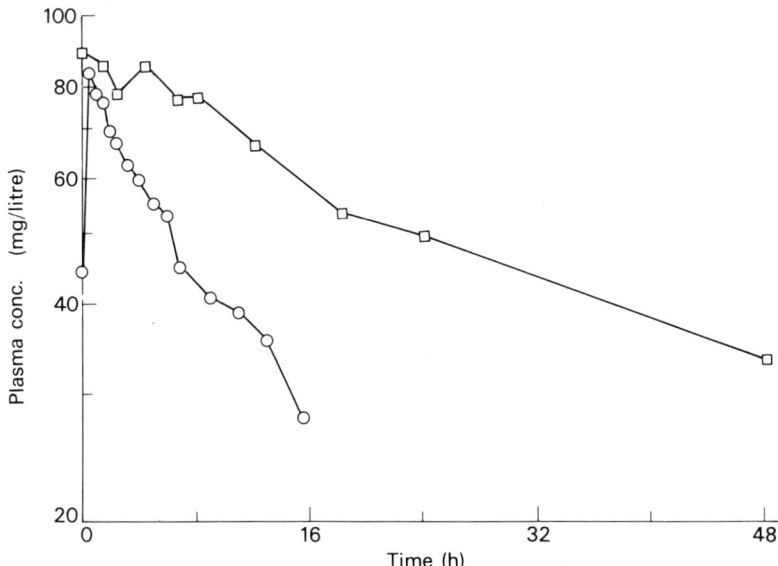

Fig. 12.21   Elimination of 2-propyl pentanoate (Depakine^R) from plasma in a mother (circles) and in the newborn baby (squares) immediately following delivery. The biological half-life of the drug in the child appears much longer (30 hours), compared to the mother (10 hours) (Knop & Edmunds 1976).

tration. This has now been reported for 2-propylpentanoate (Knop and Edmunds 1976), carbamazepine (Christiansen and Dan 1977) and phenytoin (Bardy *et al* 1978). This decrease can partly be explained by the larger distribution of the drug, the increased rate of metabolism also playing a role. After delivery, the clearance capacity and the plasma concentration are restored in a period of about 1 month. A distinct difference in rates of elimination of 2-propylpentanoate (2-pp) can be observed between mother and child directly following delivery (Fig. 12.21). The menstrual cycle also appears to influence the seizure pattern of patients periodically. To our knowledge no information is available about whether this may be reflected by changes in clearance and plasma concentrations during these periods. It is not possible yet to use these phenomena prospectively because of the limited statistical confidence of the presented material.

Alcohol and antiepileptics

The pharmacological interaction of alcohol with antiepileptic drugs is left undiscussed here. Although both adverse affects on seizure frequency as well as increased sedation are possible, there is little known about the qualitative and quantitative influence of alcohol on the kinetics of distribution and metabolism of antiepileptic drugs. In dogs and monkeys an inhibition of the elimination of both ethanol as well as 2-PP has been reported, that could not be confirmed in man (Vree and Van der Kleijn 1977).

Salicylate and 2-propylpentanoate

Concomitant administration of 2-propylpentanoate and acetylsalicylic acid causes an increase in the fraction excreted of the conjugated form of 2-propylpentanoate. The renal excretion of salicylate appears to be decreased by 2-propylpentanoate.

Primidone and phenytoin

When primidone is given to patients it is well known that at least two metabolites, phenylethylmalonic acid (PEMA) and phenobarbitone, are formed. Both compounds have antiepileptic activity. Phenobarbitone, moreover, has a much longer biological half-life than the parent compound. At steady state, the ratio of serum phenobarbitone/primidone concentration is 1.6. When combined with phenytoin this ratio may rise to 2.5–3 at increasing phenytoin concentrations (Reynolds, 1975).

Phenobarbitone, 2-propylpentanoate: phenobarbitone-phenytoin

It has become obvious that 2-propylpentanoate, when added to a concurrent therapy of phenobarbital, gradually causes an increase of phenobarbitone levels. The same phenomenon has been reported for phenytoin (Reynolds, 1975). This increase has been confirmed by other investigators, but the extent may differ between individuals.

Since it has not been decided whether the parent drug, one or more metabolites or the influence on biogenous processes is responsible for the therapeutic effect of 2-propylpentanoate (2-PP), the idea that the influence on the concomitant drug plays a role has to be excluded. In mice not only the plasma level of phenobarbitone is increased when given together with 2-PP but also the concentrations in brain and liver are increased (Fig. 12.22). The tissue–plasma partition coefficients, however, are not affected. In analogous experiments no influence of 2-propylpentanoate on phenytoin concentrations or ratios could be observed (Hulshof 1977).

Phenytoin and various drugs

Phenytoin is very susceptible to the influence of comedication because of its capacity-limited elimination and its high protein binding (Table 12.7). Richens and Houghton (1975) report the influence of sulthiame, pheneturide, diazepam, chlordiazepoxide, carbamazepine, and ethosuximide. Chlordiazepoxide and ethosuximide did not influence the plasma concentration and thus

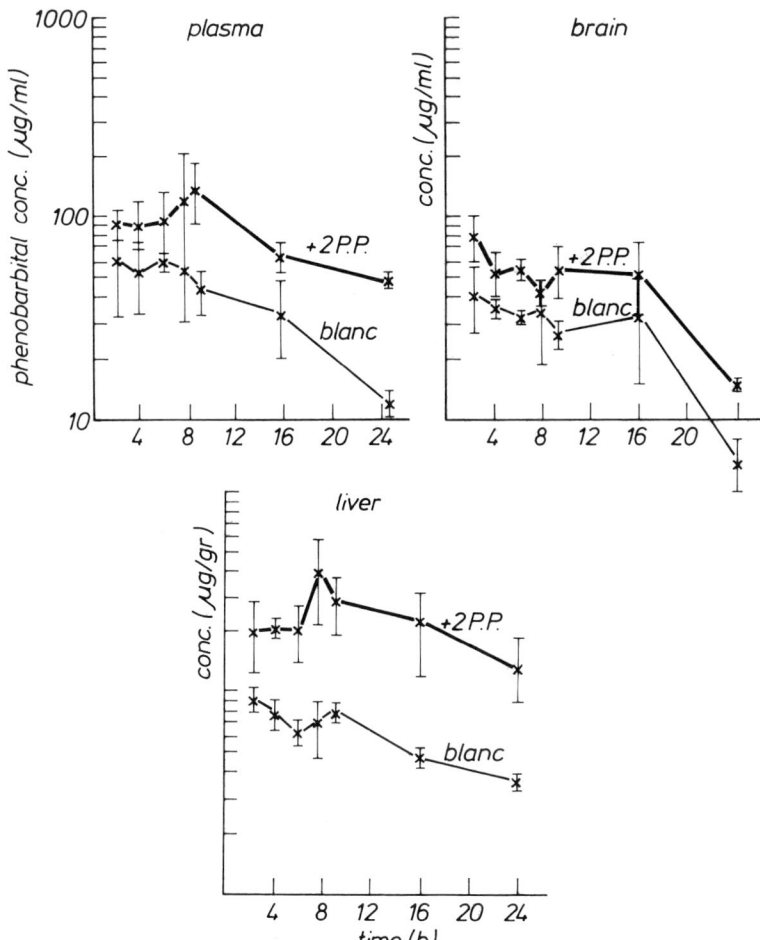

Fig. 12.22 Increase of the concentration–time profile of phenobarbital in rats treated concomitantly with 2-propyl pentanoate (Valproate, Depakine[R]) as compared to rats treated with phenobarbital alone. The brain plasma ratio is not altered.

the clearance in a significant way. Carbamazepine and diazepam increased the clearance, whereas the others caused a decrease (Table 12.5). The observation for carbamazepine is in contrast to data from Guelen *et al* 1975 (Table 12.7).

Drugs demonstrating an increased clearance also showed an increased parahydroxy metabolite:parent drug (p-HPPH:DPH) ratio in urine. The opposite phenomenon was found for those drugs causing a decreased clearance. Many other drugs may interact with the metabolism of phenytoin, causing

Table   12.5 Diphenylhydantoin, comedication correction factor (M). Calculated from data of
Richens & Houghton (1975)

Comedication	M
Sulthiame	0.56
Pheneturide	0.79
Diazepam	1.26
Chlordiazepoxide	1.1 (n.s)
Carbamazepine	1.2
Ethosuximide	0.91 (n.s)

an increase in plasma concentration. Their reported incidences are so low that
they can best be monitored in individual patients by careful clinical and chemical analyses.

Biogenous compounds

Not only do drugs influence the kinetics of distribution and metabolism of
other drugs, but also biogenous substances may change the rate constants,
the distribution volumes and the tissue plasma partition coefficients. This has
been demonstrated in animal experiments. Folic acid, known to be epileptogenic to rats when given in relatively high dosages, can change the partition
of phenytoin between brain and plasma (Guelen and Ten Berge 1979). Phenytoin itself appears to lower folate concentrations in chronically treated patients.
Folate administration to folate-deficient patients, on the other hand, causes
a decrease of phenytoin plasma concentrations (Jensen and Olesen 1970).

Calculation of maintenance dosage regimen

The equation that was derived earlier for the calculation of the individual
dosage regimen, in cases of exponential elimination processes is repeated here:

$$\text{Dose} = Cl^* \times C_{\text{therap}} \times \Delta t \times W \qquad (23)$$

Although more complicated models may sometimes be more justified, simple
one-compartment distribution kinetics can often satisfactorily serve the clinical
purpose.

In epilepsy one tries to maintain about 21 mg of phenobarbitone per kg
body weight and for phenytoin the amount is about 8.4 mg/kg. In cardiology,
0.010–0.15 mg/kg of digoxin is required, depending on severity, to control
myocardial and electrocardial disease conditions. Of these amounts about
14% of phenobarbitone and 60% of phenytoin are eliminated daily and need
to be compensated by dosage at the appropriate frequency. This means that

3 mg/kg of phenobarbitone and 5.2 mg/kg of phenytoin have to be administered every 24 hours. The frequency or the administration interval (Δt interval = 1 frequency) needs to be adapted, so that the oscillations in amount remain within the therapeutic limits (Table 12.1).

Correction of the dose per interval in the case of linear kinetics

Because the plateau concentration is considered proportional to the dose, in cases when the individual clearance differs from the statistical mean and the expected therapeutic concentration or effect has not been reached, the dose can be re-established by:

$$\text{Dose}_2 = \frac{C_2}{C_1} \times \text{Dose}_1 \qquad (45)$$

in which C_2 represents the desired plasma concentration, C_1 the determined value and Dose_1 the original dose assuming the dosage interval will not be changed nor requires change in cases where the biological half-life is short in relation to the interval.

Calculation of the dose during chronic medication in the condition of enzyme-capacity-limited kinetics

Because phenytoin is used chronically, it is necessary to include the concentration-dependent clearance value and thus K_m and V_{max} in equation 23.
    This equation can in these cases be rearranged to:

$$\text{Dose} = \frac{V^*_{max}}{K_m + C} \times \Delta t \times W \times C_{therap} \qquad (46)$$

Because K_m and V^*_{max} differ individually and not enough statistical information is available, this equation can only be used for treatment and subsequent monitoring to start a regimen. Rough mean figures for K_m and V^*_{max} for phenytoin are $K_m = 5$ mg/litre and for $V^*_{max} = 0.264$ mg/kg/h
    Non-linear binding characteristics at the tissue level can occur when linearity exists for plasma protein binding, especially when drugs have a large tissue–plasma partition coefficient. This may complicate the problem and needs intensive investigation.

Correction of the dose per interval in the case of non-linear kinetics

When, in contrast to linear kinetics, the steady state concentration is not proportional to the dose per interval, the new dose (Dose_2) can be found by:

$$\text{Dose}_2 = \frac{(K_m + C_1)}{(K_m + C_2)} \cdot \frac{C_2}{C_1} \cdot \text{Dose}_1 \qquad \text{or} \quad (47)$$

when a third regimen is included by:

$$D_3 = \frac{D_1 . C_2 (C_2 - C_1}{D_1 . C_2 (C_3 - C_1) - D_2 . C_1 (C_3 - C_2)} . \frac{C_3}{C_2} . D_2 \qquad (48)$$

The proposed methods for dosage regimen calculation of phenytoin using non-linear pharmacokinetics should be considered experimental and have to be confirmed as being valuable by further data collection and analysis in controlled clinical conditions. Adjustment of the dosage regimen of drugs known to have non-linear pharmacokinetic properties, like phenytoin, should be done carefully. The clinical experience of the physician will be as important as the pharmacokinetic knowledge without losing sight of the needs of the individual patient. It is obvious that the practice of calculation of dosage with most of the above-mentioned equations goes beyond the daily routine of in- or out-patient clinical treatment.

A number of computer methods which are also feasible for use on programmable electronic hand calculators are available to facilitate dosage calculations (Forrest *et al* 1978).

Calculation of maintenance dosage for combinations of drugs

The influence of drugs on the clearance of other drugs may lead to dose adaptations when the same C_{therap} has to be maintained. Both increase and decrease of the clearance as a result of comedication have been reported. Decrease of statistical confidence of the clearance values is also possible. This may give problems with the interpretation of the therapeutic efficacy.

An attempt has been made to quantitate the influence of well-defined comedications. This would allow calculation of the dose using the following equation with the comedication factor M from Tables 12.6, 12.7 and 12.8.

$$D = Cl^* \times C_{therap} \times M \times \Delta t \times W \qquad (49)$$

Table 12.6   Mean relative clearance (Cl^*) and comedication correction factor (M) for phenobarbitone

Comedication	Cl^* (ml/h/per kg body weight)	M	Cl^* (ml/h per m² body surface)	M
None	5.3	1.00	178.4	1.00
Phenytoin	4.2	0.79	139.9	0.78
Carbamazepine	4.5	0.85	136.3	0.76
Primidone	4.2	0.79	142.8	0.80
Phenytoin + carbamazepine	3.9	0.74	130.6	0.73
Random	4.0	0.75	114.7	0.64

Table 12.7 Mean relative clearance (Cl*) and comedication correction factor (*M*) for phenytoin

Comedication	Cl* (ml/h/per kg body weight)	*M*	Cl* (ml/h per m² body surface)	*M*
None	19.7	1.00	487.2	1.00
Phenobarbitone	18.7	0.95	588.4	1.21
Primidone	22.9	1.16	823.5	1.69
Carbamazepine	17.2	0.87	614.5	1.26
Phenobarbitone + primidone	25.4	1.29	848.9	1.74
Phenobarbitone + carbamazepine	5.8	0.80	411.1	0.84
Phenobarbitone + primidone + carbamazepine	16.2	0.82	487.1	1.00
Random	19.3	0.98	626.6	1.29

Table 12.8 Mean relative clearance (Cl*) and comedication correction factor (*M*) for carbamazepine

Comedication	Cl* (ml/h per kg body weight)	*M*	Cl* (ml/h per m² body surface)	*M*
None	130.8	1.00	4767.2	1.00
Phenobarbitone	145.8	1.12	5792.1	1.22
Phenytoin	190.6	1.46	5375.0	1.13
Primidone	184.6	1.41	5542.0	1.16
Phenobarbitone + phenytoin	207.1	1.58	6099.9	1.28
Random	194.5	1.49	6117.7	1.28

Change of clearance during chronic treatment

Many psychotropic drugs are known to increase the amount of drug-metabolising enzyme, cytochrome P450. Increased enzyme activity also affects the drug which is responsible for enzyme stimulation (autoinduction) while concomitant drugs are also metabolised faster (heteroinduction). Phenobarbitone has been extensively studied for this phenomenon in different laboratory animal species and in humans. In patients this effect can occasionally be demonstrated (Table 12.6), but has never been very impressive. Autoinduction of phenobarbitone, if it can be observed, is only of minor importance. The autoinduction of carbamazepine is much more impressive. When measured after a single dose the biological half-life of carbamazepine appears to be 35–40 hours, whereas after 2–3 weeks this value may change to 20 hours.

A pharmacokinetic model able to describe the time course of change in elimination rate constant is expressed by:

$$k_{el}^t = k_{el}^x - (k_{el}^x - k_{el}^0)e^{-k_1 \cdot t} \qquad (50)$$

in which k_{el}^t is the reciprocal time constant for elimination at any time following the onset of carbamazepine treatment, k_{el}^x the same constant after establishment of a new steady state, k_{el}^0 the original value before starting treatment and k_1 the reciprocal time constant for induction (Pitlick *et al* 1976).

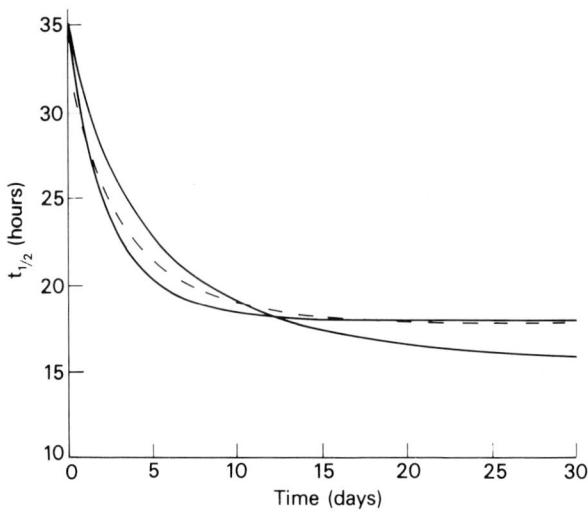

Fig. 12.23   Decrease of the biological half-life of carbamazepine (Tegretol^R) in the course of chronic treatment. The reciprocal time constant for induction k_1 has been varied similarly as can be observed in patients. Solid line, $t_{\frac{1}{2}} = 6.35$ days; broken line, $t_{\frac{1}{2}} = 3.58$ days; dotted line, $t_{\frac{1}{2}} = 2.43$ days.

The rate constant is supposed to increase exponentially ($t_{\frac{1}{2}}$ decreases exponentially). This constant is thought to be associated with the degradation rate constant(s) of the induced enzyme(s). The biological half-life for induction may vary from 2 to 7 days (Fig. 12.23). When given in combination with other drugs like phenobarbitone and phenytoin, $t_{\frac{1}{2}}$ values of 6–15 hours have been reported (Morselli 1975). This auto- and heteroinduction will require individual adaptations of the dosage regimen during this period.

Calculation of maintenance dose for children

Children generally require a relatively larger maintenance dose per kg body weight or m^2 body surface caused by a relatively larger clearance of drugs,

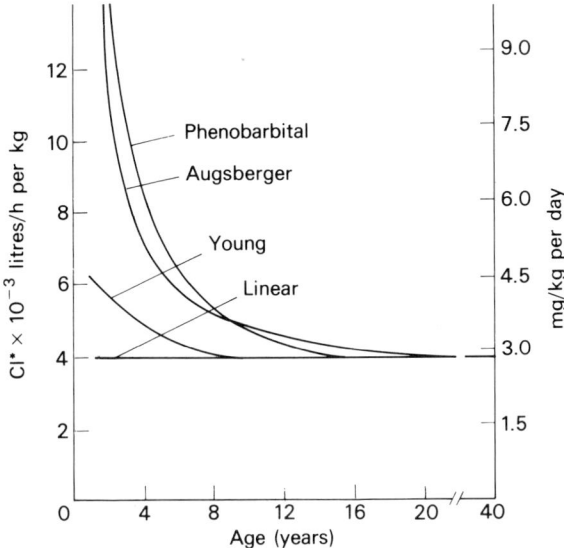

Fig. 12.24   Relationship between relative clearance (Cl*), age and required daily dose to reach a plasma concentration of 30 mg/litre of phenobarbital. The relationship will differ statistically for patients treated with combinations of drugs. The equations of Young ($[n/n+12] \times 100\%$ of adult dose, where n is age) and of Augsberger ($n \times 4 + 20\%$ of adult dose) have been translated in terms of relative clearance.

the net result of a larger relative apparent distribution volume and a larger reciprocal time constant for elimination (k_{el}) (smaller $t_{\frac{1}{2}}$). The correction factor to the mean adult dosage for antiepileptic drugs generally does not obey the classical, growth statistics based on Young's rule (age/(age + 12) × 100 = percentage of the adult dose). It appears that the Augsberger rule (4 × age + 20 = percentage adult dose) generally serves the aims better (Fig. 12.24). When medication with more than one drug is considered, the dosage regimen should be corrected to the specifications of the individual combination. The equation suitable for the calculation of paediatric dosages reads:

$$\text{Child Dose} = \text{Cl}^* \times A \times C_{\text{therap}} \times \Delta t \times W \qquad (51)$$

in which A is the correction factor of the relative clearance for the given age of the patient (Table 12.9), or

$$\text{Child Dose} = P \times \text{Adult Dose}/100 \qquad (52)$$

in which P is the percentage of the dose of an adult (Table 12.9). The mean Adult Dose will generally be found in regular textbooks. For a number of drugs it has been ascertained that the clearance in the elderly can significantly differ from the mean value in adults in an impredictable manner. Therefore clearance surveillance is indicated for this group of patients.

Table 12.9   Percentage P of the adult dose for children and correction factor A for age of the relative clearance

Age	Denekamp	Young	Augsberger	Guelen et al (phenobarbital)	
	P	P	P	P	A
0 mth	11				
3	16				
6	19				
9	22.5				
12	24.5	7.7	24		
18	27.5				
2 yr.	30	14.3	28	28.6	3.50
3	34	20	32	37	2.70
4	38	25	36	46.5	2.15
5	42	29.5	40	54.8	1.82
6	44.5	33.3	44.1	62.5	1.60
7	48.5	36.8	48	69.0	1.45
8	52	40	52	76.9	1.30
9	55	45	55.8	80	1.25
10	60	50	60	85.1	1.18
11	64	55	63.8	93.0	1.08
12	69	60	67.8	95.2	1.05
13	75	65	72.2	97.6	1.02
14	81	70	76	98.6	1.01
15	84	75	80	98.8	1.01
16	90	80	84	99.4	1.006
17	95	85	88	100	1
18	100	90	92	100	1
19	100	100	100	100	1
20	100	100	100	100	1

Calculation of starting dose

Due to the possible initial multicompartment kinetics after a rapid bolus injection, V^* may be smaller than V_{ss} after infusion. It may be possible to meet the therapeutic aim and the effective concentration in plasma by using the equation:

$$\text{Dose} = C_{\text{therap}} \times V^* \times W \qquad (53)$$

or

$$\text{Dose} = 1.44 \times t_{\frac{1}{2}} \times Cl^* \times C_{\text{therap}} \times W \qquad (54)$$

This dose is likely to produce initial side-effects for many drugs. When the clinical condition permits a more gentle start to the therapy it is preferred to start with the maintenance dose and to wait for evaluation of the therapeutic effect until the time required to reach the steady state concentration has passed. An initial higher starting dosage regimen for a limited time period followed by continuation on an adapted maintenance regimen is often preferred in sudden crises.

Time required to reach the steady state concentration

Although the administration of a rapid intravenous bolus injection of diazepam or clonazepam may be indicated in acute critical conditions like status epilepticus, it is impossible to reach equilibrium plateau concentrations throughout the body before a period of at least 4–5 times the $t_{\frac{1}{2}}$ has elapsed and the drug has been given as a sequential intermittent treatment or intravenous linear infusion (Table 12.2). The same holds true when a change in the dosage regimen has been made or when a change in clinical condition or treatment has been instituted.

Time interval of drug administration (Δt)

To meet the conditions of continuous infusion, thus minimising fluctuations in plasma concentrations and effect, the dosage interval should be maintained as constant as possible. Although this creates many domestic problems it should be realised that the preferred schedules for drug administration in hospitals can be given as in Table 12.10. The interval should be adapted to the specification of minimum fluctuations (e.g. 20–10%). This may require a different interval for each drug depending on its $t_{\frac{1}{2}}$. It has been realised that in community practice, due to the problems of migration, complexity of working schedules etc., it is difficult to cope with such a regimen. The habit of prescribing too many drugs to be taken too frequently may lead to problems of patient compliance. Unit dose distribution systems and motivation and instruction have been experienced as improvements. Sustained release preparations and drugs with prolonged half-lives are worth developing as long as the total bioavailability of the drug will not be reduced.

Table 12.10   Preferred schedules for drug administration in hospitals

Dosage frequency	Dosage interval (Δt)	Administration times
4 d.d	Every 6 hours	6.00
		12.00
		18.00
		0.00
3 d.d.	Every 8 hours	6.00
		14.00
		22.00
2 d.d.	Every 12 hours	6.00
		18.00
1 d.d.	Every 24 hours	18.00

Use of the plasma concentrations and relative clearance values as references in clinical practice

A preferred procedure for the accompaniment of patients when starting and during treatment can be scheduled as follows:

1. **a.** Definition of the nature and
   b. the degree of the disease (diagnosis).
2. **a.** Choice of the drug.
   b. Dosage form.
   c. Route of administration.
3. **a.** Definition of therapeutic aim.
   b. Definition of C_{therap}.
   c. Tolerance of the risks.
4. Definition of the tolerated oscillation of the plasma concentration during successive administrations.
5. Determination of dosage interval (Δt) and dosage frequency from the plasma concentration amplitude and biological half-life of the drug (equation 10).
6. Calculation of initial dose (or regimen) and/or maintenance regimen according to equations 53 and/or 23.
7. Determination of time after which steady state plasma concentration can be considered to be achieved $(5 \times t_{\frac{1}{2}})$.
8. Clinical evaluation of the patient after achievement of steady state and assay of plasma sample(s).
9. Calculation of the relative clearance (Cl^*).
10. Comparison of the calculated Cl^* value with the mean figure available from statistical sources as function of the individual variables from the medical record (Table 12.2).
11. Several possibilities have been experienced:

1.1. The therapeutic effect meets the clinical prerequisites in **3a** (above).
1.2. The determined plasma concentration meets C_{therap} as chosen in **3b** (above).
1.3. The relative clearance (Cl^*) can be calculated with equation 23 to confirm the reference value that no errors have been made. It is also useful to check laboratory performance and stability of the sample.
1.4. Conclusion: the patient is doing well and the drug dosage regimen is well calculated.
1.5. A new plasma sample should only be assayed when a change in one or more conditions is observed.

2.1. The therapeutic effect does not meet the clinical prerequisites in **3a**.
2.2. The determined plasma concentration is unequal to C_{therap} as chosen in **3b**.

2.3. The calculated clearance equals the mean clearance value for the given condition.

2.4. Conclusion: the dosage regimen should be corrected by using equation 24.

2.5. A new plasma sample and new clinical examination should be made when the new steady state has been allowed to establish.

3.1. The therapeutic effect meets the clinical prerequisites **3a**.

3.2. The determined plasma concentration is unequal to C_{therap} as chosen in **3b**.

3.3. The calculated clearance equals the mean clearance value for the given conditions.

3.4. Conclusion: the determined plasma concentration appears to be the C_{therap} for this patient. The value should be documented in relation to the diagnosis and other record information on the progress of the patient.

3.5. A new plasma sample and a new clinical examination should only be made when a change in condition is observed.

4.1. The therapeutic effect does not meet the clinical prerequisites **3a**.

4.2. The determined plasma concentration is unequal to C_{therap} as chosen in **3b**.

4.3. The calculated clearance does not equal the mean clearance value for the given conditions.

4.4. Conclusion: clinical and kinetic.

   a. The variables should carefully be re-examined in order to identify possible deviations of the patients.

   b. The new clearance value should be used to calculate the new appropriate dosage regimen with equation 23.

4.5. A new plasma sample and a new clinical examination should be made when the new steady state has been allowed to establish.

5.1. The therapeutic effect does not meet the clinical prerequisites **3a**.

5.2. The determined plasma concentration is equal to C_{therap} as chosen in **3.b.**

5.3. The calculated clearance equals the mean clearance value for the given conditions.

5.4. Conclusion: the clinical and kinetic conditions should be re-examined. The adequacy of the choice of the drug should be carefully evaluated. When the decision is made to try another substance, a new condition is added and the logics should be started from 1. The drugs should be omitted gradually and be replaced by the newly chosen drug. The time span to replace the drug mutually equals the time to reach 90% of the steady state, that is, equal to the time for elimination.

5.5. A new plasma sample should be determined after the steady state of the new drug has been allowed to establish. This sample may also serve to check whether the deleted drug and/or its metabolites are still present.

6.   Theoretically there are four more combinations possible that will require careful examination of the clinical and kinetic conditions dosage adaptation, or further study on the therapeutic adequacy of the treatment.

Summary

The conditions for which the plasma determinations and the calculated clearance values of drugs in patients can be used in the accompaniment and monitoring of treatment are discussed. It appears that many variables are involved in the control of the clinical effect in patients during therapy. Personal interaction between the department of pharmacy and the assay-requesting physician is necessary to make adequate use of the information obtained from both sides. Because of the position of a drug as initiator of a sequence of many metabolic and physiological processes it is even more necessary than for biogenous substances that the conditions under which the concentrations are measured and interpreted are carefully managed. The use of statistically obtained clearance parameters for drugs as a function of age, disease, sex, comedication and others has been of value in the quality control of the assay, for the retrospective monitoring of patients and for prospective management of dosage regimens. Because the quality of the concentration and clearance data also depends on the organisation of drug distribution, registration and administration to patients, it is prefered to have the clinical pharmacokinetics laboratory associated with the department of pharmaceutical services.

REFERENCES

BARDY A. H., HULESMAA V. K. & TERAMO K. (1978) In *Advances in epileptology: 1977*, eds. H. Meinardi & A. J. Rowan. Swets & Zeitlinger, Amsterdam.

BREIMER D. D. (1974) *Pharmacokinetics of hypnotic drugs*. PhD Thesis, Department of Pharmacology, University of Nijmegen, Netherlands.

CHRISTIANSEN J. & DAM M. (1977) In *Antieplileptic drug monitoring*, p. 128. Pitman, London.

DE ZEEUW R. A., WESTENBERG H. G. M., VAN DER KLEIJN E. and GIMBRÈRE J. . F. (1978) 8th Meeting of the European Poison Control Centres, Utrecht, Netherlands.

FORREST A., RODMAN J. & JELLIFFE R. W. (1978) *Programmable Calculations in Clinical Pharmacokinetics*. Paper presented at Midyear Clinical Meeting of the Californian Society of Hospital Pharmacists, San Francisco, October 13–15.

GARRETT E. R., BRES J., SCHNELLE K & ROLF L. L. (1974) *Journal of Pharmacokinetics and Biopharmaceutics* **2,** 43.

GUELEN P. J. M. & JOHANNESEN S. (1971) In *Antiepileptic drug monitoring*. p. 345. Pitman, London.

GUELEN P. J. M. & TEN BERGE E. (1979) *European Journal of Pharmacology* submitted.

GUELEN P. J. M. & VAN DER KLEIJN E. (1977) In *Antiepileptic drugs monitoring*. p. 335. Pitman, London.

GUELEN P. J. M. & VAN DER KLEIJN E. (1978) In *Rational antiepileptic drug therapy*. Elsevier, Amsterdam.

GUELEN P. J. M., VAN DER KLEIJN E. & WOUDSTRA U. (1975) Pharmacology of antiepileptic drugs. In *Proceedings of the Wodadiboff Symposium*, ed. H. Schneider. Springer Verlag, Berlin.

HULSHOF J. A. M., SCHOBBEN F. & VAN DER KLEIJN E. (1977) *Pharmaceutische Weekblad* **112**, 326.

JENSEN O. N. & OLESEN O. V. (1970) *Archives of Neurology* **22**, 181.

JONKMAN J. H. G. (1977) *Thiazinamium methylsulphate, bioanalysis and pharmacokinetics*. PhD Thesis, University of Groningen.

KNOP H. J. & EDMUNDS L. C. (1976) In *Abstracts Symposia and Communications of the 17th Dutch Federation Meeting, Amsterdam*, p. 253.

LEVY G., TSUCHIYA T. & AMSEL L. P. (1972) *Clinical Pharmacology and Therapeutics* **13**, 258.

LUDDEN F. M., HAWKINS D. W., ALLEN J. P. & HOFFMAN S. F. (1976) *Lancet* i, 307.

METZLER C. M. (1969) *A User's manual for NONLIN*. Technical Report 7292/69/7292/005. Upjohn, Kalamazoo, Mich.

MORSELLI P. L. (1975) In *Advances in Neurology*, Vol. 11, eds. J. Kiffin Penry & D. D. Daly, pp. 279–292. Raven Press, New York.

MORSELLI P. L., RIZZO M. & GARATTINI I. (1971) *Annals of the New York Academy of Science* **179**, 88.

PITLICK W. H., LEVY R. H., TROVPIN A. S. & GREEN J. R. (1976) *Journal of Pharmaceutical Sciences* **65**, 462.

REYNOLDS E. H. (1975) *Clinical pharmacology of antiepileptic drugs*. p. 79. J. Springer, Berlin.

RICHENS A. (1975) *Epilepsia* **16**, 627.

RICHENS A. (1978) The St Bartholomew's Hospital Quality Control Scheme for antiepileptic drugs. In *Advances in epileptology: 1977*, eds. H. Meinardi & A. J. Rowan, p. 239. Swets & Zeitlinger, Amsterdam.

RICHENS A & HOUGHTON G. W. (1975) *Clinical pharmacology of antiepileptic drugs* p. 87. J. Springer, Berlin.

SCHOBBEN F., VAN DER KLEIJN E. & GABREËLS F. J. M. (1975) *European Journal of Clinical Pharmacology* **8**, 97.

VAN GINNEKEN C. A. M., VAN ROSSUM J. M. & FLEUREN H. L. J. M. (1974) *Journal of Pharmacokinetics and Biopharmaceutics* **2**, 395.

VAN DER KLEIJN E., GUELEN P. J. M., BAARS A. M., VREE T. B. & TREMOND E. (1975) *Pharmaceutische Weekblad* **110**, 1222.

VAN DER KLEIJN E., PIJNAPPEL H., VAN WIJK H., GUELEN P. & RIJNTJES N. (1976) In *Methods of analysis of antiepileptic drugs*, p. 161. Excerpta Medica, Amsterdam.

VAN DER KLEIJN E., LUCARDIE S., VAN LAKWIJK-VONDROVICOVA E., BAARS L., TERMOND E., GUELEN P. J. M., MULLER N. F. & VREE T. B. (1977) In *Plasma digitalis concentration and digitalis therapy*, ed. T. Godfreind, p. 119. Editions Arscia, Brussels.

VAN DER KUY A. & VAN DER KLEIJN E. (1972) *Pharmaceutische Weekblad* **107**, 697.

VREE T. B., BAARS A. M. & VAN DER KLEIJN E. (1975) *Pharmaceutische Weekblad* **110**, 1257.

VREE T. B. & VAN DER KLEIJN E. (1976) In *Clinical pharmacy and clinical pharmacology*, p. 67. North-Holland, Amsterdam.

VREE T. B. & VAN DER KLEIJN E. (1977) *Pharmaceutische Weekblad* **112**, 313.

WAGNER J. G. (1973) *Journal of Pharmacokinetics and Biopharmaceutics* **1**, 103, 338.

WAGNER J. G. (1975) *Fundamentals of Clinical Pharmacokinetics*. Drug Intelligence Publications, Hamilton, Ill.

IV
Provision of information

13

Drug information services

M. L. ROGERS & C. W. BARRETT

The pharmacist's role in providing information on drugs and medicines is not new. He has traditionally been the prime information source for doctors, nurses and paramedical staff. When drugs were few in number and generally of relatively low potency the number of inquiries was small and could usually be answered quickly by reference to pharmacopoeias and formularies. In recent years two things have happened which have created a need to alter this traditional pattern. Firstly, the number of drugs and medicines has increased enormously. The newer drugs are generally more potent and selective and the medicines into which they are formulated have become more complex. Secondly the literature relating to drugs has expanded at a staggering rate. The sources of this literature are very diverse, including pharmacy, medicine, pharmacology and biochemistry. It covers a wealth of information on these newer drugs, their actions, clinical uses, unwanted effects, interactions with other drugs, comparative efficacy and so on. All this information has to be evaluated in assuring the safe and effective use of medicines and has placed a heavy burden on the prescriber and the pharmacist to whom he traditionally turns for drug information. A quick reference to pharmacopoeias and formularies is no longer sufficient, in many cases, to provide an adequate answer. There has, therefore, been a trend to create new sections within departments of pharmacy where drug information sources can be properly organised and where full-time staff, properly trained and equipped, can provide answers to drug-related questions making full use of the extensive literature now available.

The first information centre to be set up was that at the University of Kentucky Medical Centre, USA, in 1962 (Burkholder 1963; Parker 1965). Its objectives were to collect information, to evaluate and compare drugs, to provide an education and teaching aid for health care personnel, to assist clinicians in the selection of safe and effective medication and to enable pharmacists and pharmacy students to develop their abilities in providing information on drugs and medicines. In addition it envisaged a future role as headquarters for the Kentucky Poison Control Centre, as a possible centre for reporting adverse drug reactions and as a centre for a statewide drug information service.

In February 1964 a special conference on drug information services arranged by the American Society of Hospital Pharmacists was held at The

University of Kentucky Medical Centre (Stauffer 1963, 1964). This led to a rapid development of hospital-based drug information centres. There were proposals for nationwide coordination of drug information activities, in particular the collection, storage and retrieval of information using electronic data processing.

In the late 1960s and early 70s reports of drug information networks were emerging from America. Early experience had shown that drug information centres were relatively expensive to set up and staff could not, to be financially viable, confine their services to one hospital. Greater efficiency of operation could be achieved by extending the facility to a group of hospitals (Pearson 1974) or even to a state, with the inclusion of health care personnel outside the hospital service. Two systems which have received wide publicity are the single centre model, based at the University of Kentucky Medical Centre providing a statewide service (Amerson & Walton 1971), and the Michigan regional network model (Pearson *et al* 1970, 1972a, 1972b). At this time a number of commercial systems for the retrieval of drug information were becoming available (e.g. the Iowa System and the De Haen System which will be discussed later).

Published accounts of developments in drug information centres in Europe have been fewer than in America, but similar, though slower progress has been made. In 1971 the drug information centre at Leeds General Infirmary was combined with a regional poisons information bureau and a 24-hour service was instituted (*Pharmaceutical Journal* 1971). An account of the first operational year of the drug information centre at The London Hospital (Rogers & Barrett) was published in 1972. The objectives of this centre had many similarities to those at Kentucky and were as follows:

1. To enable pharmacy staff to keep abreast of drug information.
2. To provide facilities for staff training.
3. To support the ward pharmacy service.
4. To provide facilities for answering questions from medical, nursing and other professional staff.

On the European mainland, centres in Verona, Geneva, Nijmegen, Tilbourg, Torino, Nancy, Barcelona, Alicante, Madrid and Valencia were identified in 1975 (Garcia-Iñesta) in a survey of resources; but there must have been many others not included.

With the implementation of the recommendations of the working party on hospital pharmaceutical services (DHSS 1970), the idea of organising drug information services at regional level developed in England. A number of principal pharmacists have now been appointed, charged with developing regional services.

These individuals work together as a subcommittee of the Regional Pharmaceutical Officers Group with the Department of Health as the Drug Information Subcommittee (DISC) to coordinate national policy on drug informa-

tion, organise training of pharmacists in information work and avoid unnecessary duplication of effort.

INFORMATION NEEDS

That there is a need for providing information on drugs and medicines is
obvious to anyone working in hospital pharmacy practice. Information is an
aid to decision making. Among those requiring information are physician,
pharmacist, nurse, researcher, other professionals in health care, committees
and patients. The growth in the role played by science in medicine as reflected
in the amount of published work, the number of journals and the vast range
of drug products on the market, has meant that practitioners of medicine and
pharmacy, in common with other scientific disciplines, have experienced difficulty in keeping up with advances in knowledge. The doctor's response, increasingly, has been to turn to the pharmacist for help. Most problems presented by the doctor are concerned with a particular patient, his disease-state
and therapy. The information requested is usually required within a few hours,
so that treatment may be changed or started and is needed in the form of
data, rather than lists of references or paper reprints. Production of an answer
therefore involves selection, interpretation and evaluation of information. The
type of information requested may include any of the chemical or biological
properties of a compound or a comparison of the suitability of several compounds for a specific case, where, for instance, renal or hepatic disease may
complicate choice. The pharmacist too, may require immediate information
on drugs. This may concern straightforward matters such as dosage or availability but also involve formulation or bioavailability data which may not be
found in the manufacturers' literature. Quality controllers may require an
alternative assay or stability data. Nurses need to know the effects and dangers
of drug therapy so as to be able to assess the appearance of adverse effects—
they also must know enough about preparations to teach patients to use them.
Researchers need to retrieve a particular report, or search the literature. Care
has to be taken to ensure that they are not asking for information that they
should rightly be searching themselves. Committees need information to help
them decide policies, produce hospital formularies and award contracts.
Patients need to know how to take the medicines they are given, what they
will feel if the drug works, likely adverse effects and what to do about them.
Measuring and accurately identifying the nature of the need is, however, not
easy. As a prospective undertaking it is virtually impossible and probably
futile. Retrospectively it requires constant analysis if changing needs are to
be properly met.

The drug information centre at The London Hospital was established with
no attempt to quantify the need beyond the subjective assessment of demand
experienced at the time. It also started operating without any publicity beyond

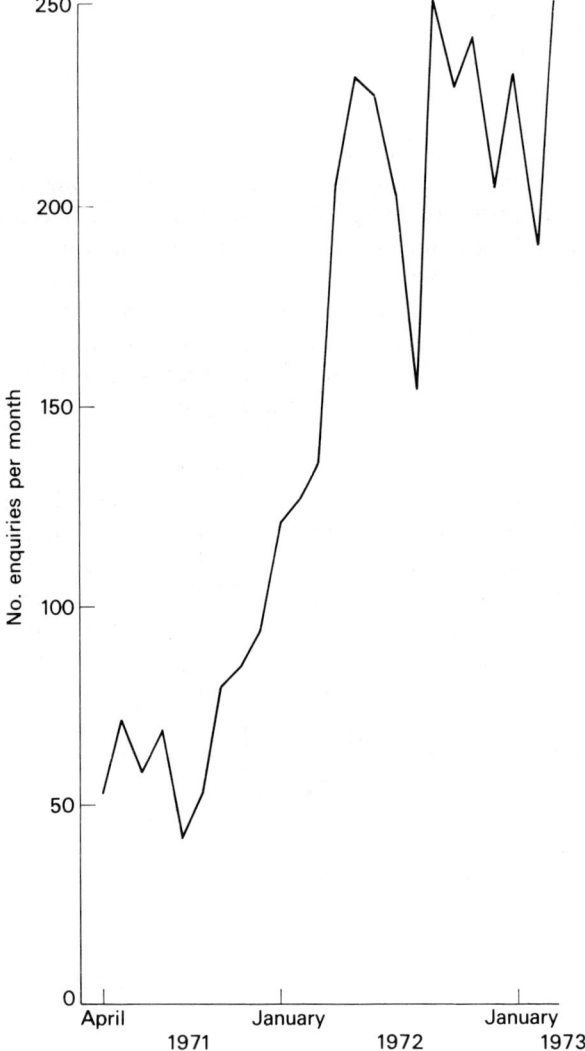

Fig. 13.1   Total number of queries received each month at the London Hospital Drug Information Centre (April 1971 to March 1973).

an announcement in the hospital magazine that fell short of advertising. Instead it was decided to use the 'satisfied customer' as the basic method of making medical staff aware of the services available. Despite this the demands on the centre increased rapidly, as shown in Fig. 13.1

An analysis of answers to questions asked at the London Hospital Centre from June 1975 to May 1976 showed that the users were: doctors 43.7%, nurses 11.0%, pharmacists 38.4% (includes many questions via ward pharmacy ser-

Table 13.1 Who asked for which information?

Category	Pharmacy (%)	Doctors (%)	Nurses (%)	Others (%)	Total (%)
Availability/supply	16.1	14.3	11.4	19.5	13.9
Administration/dosage	14.8	22.3	21.4	7.3	18.2
Adverse effects/toxicity	7.6	14.6	8.6	12.2	10.6
Identification	8.4	6.2	10.0	7.3	7.3
Indication/choice/ contraindication	9.0	11.3	9.0	6.5	13.5
Interactions	3.6	5.3	1.4	6.5	4.1
Pharmacology/ pharmacokinetics	3.5	4.2	4.3	4.1	3.9
Pharmaceutical	24.1	14.5	24.8	22.0	19.0
Other	12.8	7.4	9.0	14.6	9.6

vice), others 6.8%. The type of information they asked for is shown in Table 13.1. The categories are those agreed nationally by the DISC.

Table 13.2 shows that almost half the questions asked required an immediate answer, and that 72% of answers were needed on the same day. It is apparent that the questions are, in a high proportion of cases, concerned with treatment of individual patients. The service has to be able to meet these demands on it.

In designing and setting up a drug information centre it is necessary to establish some priorities in meeting the needs. It is logical that in the first instance it should provide a service for pharmacy staff. Where there is a ward or clinical pharmacy service in operation then the Drug Information Centre provides an essential back-up service. It is probably true to say that a ward pharmacy service does much to identify for drug information staff the type and extent of need for information in the ward. As more information is collected and analysed of the users and non-users of centres and their reasons, it will become easier to identify those areas where unmet needs exist. It will then be possible to prepare and actively disseminate selected information to meet them, as is to some extent being done at present with pharmacy bulletins and related documents.

Table 13.2 Time by which answer was required

Urgency estimate	(%)
Immediate	47.4
Same day	24.7
Next day	7.2
Within a week	14.1
No time limit	6.7

RESOURCES

In order to meet the various demands for information directed at it, a drug information centre should be run by full-time personnel under the direction of a pharmacist. There should be a library of reference and text books (suggestions in the Appendix) used for quick reference answers and also to give background in cases where the information pharmacist is unfamiliar with the nature of a problem. General reference works and specialised textbooks can also be found in the medical library or public reference library. The centre should subscribe to a number of journals thought to be useful for information required in preparation of answers, or as educational material for the staff of the pharmacy department. Some suggestions are made in the Appendix.

If the service needs to cover a topic intensively for a period of time it could be worth surveying the likely journals and applying the Bradford–Zipf Law of Distribution. Briefly, if a collection of papers on the topic is examined and journals marked in order of productivity, three zones can be marked off so that each zone produces one-third of the total papers.

The first, the nuclear (core) zone, contains a small number of highly productive journals, say n_1, the second zone contains a larger number of moderately productive journals, say n_2, and the outer zone a still larger number of journals of low productivity, say n_3. The law of scatter says that $n_1 : n_2 : n_3 = 1 : a : a^2$ where a is a constant.

In the data first analysed, the value of a was about 5.0, so that a typical collection of 248 journals might be divided into eight highly productive 'core' journals, 40 journals of moderate productivity and 200 journals of low productivity, for a particular topic. Brookes (1968) has discussed modifications to the law, but the original simple version stated above is probably adequate for selection of primary journals most useful for a specialised subject.

Choice will also depend on whether there is a medical library in the hospital which can be used by the department, and the journals that it buys. Duplication of subscriptions will normally only be required for a few of the most important journals. The journals which are taken should be retained and bound if possible.

It is possible to use the journals' indexes and commercially available abstract services for retrieval. The main disadvantage of relying on commercially produced indexes is the inevitable time-lag between primary publication of the original report and its appearance in a secondary source such as an abstract. This delay is seldom less than three or four months and is considered to be unacceptable by many information services, not only those in drug information. Another reason for dissatisfaction with commercial indexes to the literature is that they do not index in sufficient depth to allow all the useful information in articles to be found. For these reasons, many information services find it necessary to index journal articles themselves, although it is time consuming. Some people cut up or copy relevant articles and file them. Others prefer to leave the journals intact, and instead file a card carrying the reference to the article. The Regional Drug Information Services Group cooperate in abstracting and indexing journals to produce on a national scale a data base more current than the commercial systems. In either case, the most suitable technique for manual retrieval is probably coordinate indexing (see p. 447 for method). By indexing the articles 'in house' last week's articles are as readily accessible as last year's.

It is useful to maintain a file of manufacturers' literature as a source of product information. This should not include promotional material but may include handbooks on the product or copies of symposia sponsored by the company. The data sheets required by the Medicines Act (1968) are a good rapid reference for approved indications and recommended dosages. Many of them are bound together as a compendium, revised periodically.

Simple card index systems

Card indexes are a useful way of sorting information for retrieval. They are easily added to, form their own index, and can carry an abstract of an article. Simple card index systems on drugs available in this country include the *Index of New Products* (Pharmaceutical Press) and the *Current Abstracts of Pharmacy and Therapeutics* (Guild of Hospital Pharmacists). The first of these is designed to carry basic information on such things as uses, dosage and legal restrictions of new preparations. The information is provided by the manufacturers, and the cards are intended to be useful to pharmacists confronted by a request to supply something they have not encountered. They are much more informative than the *Monthly Index of Medical Specialities* (MIMS) which is used for the same purpose. The second system is an attempt to cover useful articles on drug use or professional topics appearing in a number of well-known medical and pharmaceutical journals. The cards have a title, usually the approved name of a drug, and carry the full title and reference of the article together with an abstract, which is often the author's summary. These cards may be quite useful for tracing reports of a drug for a particular indication. If several card indexes are subscribed to, they are best filed together in one sequence.

Information retrieval systems

Serious searches for information require a wider coverage of journals than that available from *Current Abstracts*. At an intermediate level between the simple and the most comprehensive come several American systems, suitable for use in hospital information centres. These are the Iowa Drug Information Service (often referred to as the Iowa system), the de Haen drug information system: *Drugs in Use*, and *International Pharmaceutical Abstracts* produced by the American Society of Hospital Pharmacists.

The Iowa system covers about 150 English language journals. It has two main indexes, for drug names and disease names. These are cumulatively updated monthly, and the December index issues are retained as part of the permanent index to the system. The indexes are on microfiche (sheet microfilm of the international standard size 105 mm × 145 mm). In addition to the indexes microfiche copies of the complete articles are also supplied. Inclusion of the complete article is a major advantage, firstly because abstracts seldom give the exact information the reader wants to know, secondly because very often in drug information the answer is required quickly. With the Iowa system, if a reference is retrieved, it is available to be read. There is no delay in obtaining articles from outside libraries.

The de Haen *Drugs in Use* system is a microfiche system covering over 400 journals, including a number of foreign language journals. The articles are abstracted on microfiche in the form of a 'structural excerpt'. These are cumulatively updated. The indexes to the system are of drug aims, and diseases, brand names, manufacturer, Chemical Abstract Service (CAS) registry number and therapeutic class. Separately purchased fiche indexes cover drug interactions and adverse effects.

Published comparisons of the Iowa system and de Haen (Tourville & McLeod 1975; Madden & MacDonald 1977) have found that Iowa was more comprehensive and of higher utility. Although de Haen covers more than twice as many journals as Iowa it performed very poorly in comparison. But the Iowa system in turn covered much less of the literature than the large data bases dealt with below, and Madden and MacDonald considered that Iowa should be used in combination with another system or systems. For manual searching they suggested that Iowa plus *Index Medicus* and the *Drug Literature Index* would be most comprehensive.

International Pharmaceutical Abstracts (IPA) is a journal published twice a month, with cumulative indexes every 6 months, covering professional and technical fields of interest to pharmacists. It is also available in microfilm format. It carries abstracts of articles in classified groups such as 'drug interactions', 'pharmaceutical technology', 'information processing and literature' and 'pharmacy practice'. IPA is useful for its cover of subject fields not adequately dealt with in any other system. It includes abstracts from about 1000 journals in pharmacy and medicine.

Unlisted Drugs is an abstracting service which specialises in covering reports of new drugs in the world's literature. It is available as a card index or as a journal with cumulative indexes at 6 months, 1 and 2 years. Substances are included by their research code numbers and by any names devised for them, including brand names. The international cover makes this a useful source for locating those odd names not in *any* of the books.

There are a number of systems, based on computer storage and retrieval, which attempt to be comprehensive. Some of them are available also as printed versions for manual searching.

At one time most of these systems would have been out of reach of hospital-based services, because of the very high subscriptions required. This is now changing rapidly because of the advent of time-sharing networks. In effect anyone can, via experienced operators, search one of these large data bases. Instead of paying a huge annual subscription, one pays just for the time spent searching. In a typical search this may be only a few minutes, at a cost of perhaps £5 to £10. This should be compared with the cost, in qualified personnel's time, of manually searching the same data base.

The technique of searching realtime (or online as it is also called) is usually more fruitful than a manual search, because you can immediately see the results of modifying your search terms (the system is 'interactive'), often, too, one can search and retrieve articles by many more terms in a computer version than in the printed version of the same system because of space constraints in the hard copy. For example, the printed version of *Index Medicus* limits a reference to three entries, but the same reference may be indexed by up to 20 terms in the computer version, and can also be found by asking the computer to look for words in titles and abstracts.

The most useful (because it is widely available) of the large data bases in drug information work is *Index Medicus*. This is a monthly publication of the United States Library of Medicine covering about 2400 journals. It is published as a large paper journal, and also on microfiche, and a cumulative version is also supplied annually. The first computer searchable version of *Index Medicus* was called 'Medlars'. 'Medlars' centres were essentially remote terminals of the *Index Medicus* computer and performed literature searches 'offline'. They could handle complex questions but the response time was slow: search statements and the resulting bibliography went by post. A more recent derivative of *Index Medicus* is 'Medline' (Medlars on line). This is a realtime system: an immediate answer is available on the remote terminals, allowing modification of the search strategy. Medline has largely replaced Medlars as the computer search version of *Index Medicus*.

In England Medline is now searchable as part of Blaise (British Library Automated Information Service). The main difference for the user is that since the computer is in Harlow, Essex, instead of Washington DC, the telephone charges should be lower, and therefore searches should cost less.

Another data base offered by the National Library of Medicine, and also available via Blaise, is Toxline. This is made up of nine subfiles arranged so that they are searched simultaneously. It covers toxicological, analytical and metabolic references to drugs and industrial and agricultural chemicals. The subfiles include Toxbib (toxicity bibliography: the toxicity and adverse reaction reports from *Index Medicus*), CBAC (chemical and biological activities: the pharmacology and toxicity parts of Chemical Abstracts), IPA (adverse effects reports), TMIC (toxic materials information centre) and others cover pesticides and teratogens.

Chemline is an online dictionary which helps by listing the terms needed to search for a substance in the subfiles of Toxline. Toxline goes back to 1971. Earlier data can be searched by Toxback in which the search is entered online but searched offline overnight.

Medical Subject Headings (MeSH) is the thesaurus controlling the vocabulary of the *Index Medicus* systems. It is available separately as a bound annual; the MeSH vocabulary file is also available online via Blaise for use as an adjunct when searching Medline; it will, for example, tell you how a

Table 13.3   Ranking systems in order of number of references found on particular subjects

Smith *et al* (1972)	Ashmole *et al* (1973)
1. Excerpta Medica (Drugdoc)	1. Excerpta Medica (Drugdoc)
2. Medlars	2. Medlars
3. Ringdoc	3. Ringdoc
4. Chemical Abstracts Condensates	4. *Index Medicus*
5. CBAC	5. ASCA
	6. *Biological Abstracts*
	7. *Chemical Abstracts*

concept was indexed before a particular term was added and the date of the change.

There are several comprehensive European computer-based commercial systems available for retrospective searches. Examples are Ringdoc and Excerpta Medica Drugdoc, both primarily intended for industrial users. 'Ringdoc Pharmaceutical Literature Documentation' abstracts 350 well-chosen journals and, by use of microfilm, punched cards or magnetic tape, permits subscribers to search by manual, mechanical or computerised methods. Ringdoc is not available on time-sharing networks at present. The Excerpta Medica system is a computer tape abstract service of the drug literature covering more than 3400 scientific, medical and pharmaceutical journals to provide possibly the most comprehensive reference retrieval system on drugs. Excerpta Medica is now available on time-sharing networks. These abstract publications are listed in the Appendix.

Smith *et al* (1972) and Ashmole *et al* (1973) have compared the various major systems available and both found that the Excerpta Medica system (Drugdoc) scored the highest number of hits and also of 'unique hits' for the pharmaceutical fields they examined (Table 13.3). Madden and MacDonald (1977) found that Drugdoc retrieved about twice as many references as Medlars. But they suggest that the two systems are complementary and best used in combination.

There is a manual version of Excerpta Medica Drugdoc, called the *Drug Literature Index*, which is available in a few libraries.

Chemical Abstracts abstracts 12 000 journals but these are by no means all relevant to pharmaceutical interests. Detailed discussion of sources of information for particular fields of medicine and chemistry is given in books by Morton (1974), Bottle (1971) and Sewell (1975).

Current awareness

One of the greatest problems facing practitioners is keeping up to date with professional and technical developments. Research workers also have a need to know of new work, but their interests are fairly narrow and specific, and this is more easily catered for. There are a number of services which are intended to help by alerting subscribers to relevant papers. Speed of production is important in this activity. Probably the easiest way of providing this alerting function is to copy the contents (title) pages of the journals the service covers. *Current Contents* does this and its speed of production is such that it is often published before the issues of the journals it lists. There are two *Current Contents* of interest to physicians and pharmacists: 'Life Sciences' and 'Clinical Practice'. Unfortunately there is a good deal of overlap in their journal coverage. More useful to practitioners is *Inpharma*. This is a weekly journal of informative abstracts written in house and published very rapidly by ADIS in Australia. Abstracts of articles in major British journals often appear in *Inpharma* within 2 weeks of primary publication. The system covers articles from 1700 journals on drug evaluation and treatment. *Clin-Alert* performs a similar service in the specialised field of adverse reactions and toxicity. Published every 2 weeks, and, like *Inpharma*, sent by airmail, it covers the more important adverse effects mostly within one or two months. Both publications are indexed quarterly, the *Clin-Alert* index being cumulative.

Derwent Publications, who produce Ringdoc described earlier, also publish a series of 42 Profile Booklets (48 issues a year) for current awareness in various aspects of drug research and therapy. Typical titles of the profiles are *Analysis*, *Biopharmaceutics*, *Infection*, *Psychotropics* and *Urology*. Information comes as whole-page abstracts.

An alerting service which takes the idea of profiles further by narrowing the subject field for each is the weekly *Ascatopics*. This service runs about 490 topics and sends subscribers lists of references relevant to the topic they have chosen. A typical topic would be *Drugs in Renal Failure*. The system is a broader version of ASCA (Automatic Subject Citation Alert), which produces an individual alerting service to research workers. This individual current awareness function is called selective dissemination of information (SDI).

Commercial SDI services are nearly always based on computer data bases and computer matching of the user's stated interests with the articles added to the file. It is possible to run manual SDI services, but only for a small number of customers.

INDEXING

The problem with information is that the more one has, the more difficult it is to retrieve specific items. If the service is collecting reprints or producing abstracts then these should be organised so that they can be retrieved when required.

In libraries, books are arranged on shelves in an order which corresponds with a classification scheme. The most common of these schemes are the Universal Decimal Classification (UDC), the Dewey Decimal Classification and the Library of Congress Classification. Anyone who wishes to learn more about these and other classifications is advised to read Foskett (1975) or Maltby (1975). Information pharmacists will need to know a little about these schemes in order to use libraries effectively, but general classifications are not really suitable for application to specialised information services. The disadvantages of general schemes are first that they have too much detail in most subjects which are of no interest to a specialised service, but do not have enough detail in the field of specialisation. They use a rigid citation order which can separate subjects, and except for UDC there is only one order which means that a document will be indexed at only one point in a file. This type of index is called a serial file (or item entry). The needs of specialised information services are for retrieval of documents by any of the concepts describing their contents, either singly or in combination.

Conventional indexing methods are inadequate for the deep indexing required. If the subject description of an article has seven terms, then retrieval must be possible for any one term, any two terms, any three terms in combination and so on up to all seven in any order. Attempts have been made using conventional serial files to provide this facility by permutation of terms; the problem is in the number of entries likely to be required. If we have an article described by three concepts or terms A, B, and C, then there are factorial three (3!) ways of arranging them in a serial file, in strings of coordinated terms (precoordination):

1. ABC
2. ACB
3. BAC
4. BCA
5. CAB
6. CBA

Only by using all permutations in the index can you be sure that if any one concept is looked for it will be found as the entry term, that if any two terms are looked for they will be found in any order, and that all three terms would be found in whatever order they are quoted.

So an article with three concepts requires six index entries in an item entry index. Four terms would require 24 entries, five terms 120 entries, six terms 720 entries, seven terms 5040 entries, eight terms 40 320 entries, nine terms 362 880 entries, ten terms 3 628 800 entries.

Clearly, it is not possible to index to this extent, and yet retrieval of relevant documents is much less certain if the concept required at the time of searching is not one by which the document is indexed.

The solution to this problem was discovered in the later part of the 1940s. In 1945, Vannevar Bush suggested storing by words, and retrieving by combining the words, and, in 1958, Mortimer Taube suggested the expression Uniterm for the standardised words required. This alternative method of indexing does not permutate strings of terms to make multiple entries. Instead, a separate entry is made for each concept or term. Thus if document no. 1234 is described by four terms ABCD, instead of permutating ABCD, to give 24 precoordinated entries in the index, one prepares unit term (Uniterm) entries, one for each concept:

A. 1234
B. 1234
C. 1234
D. 1234

This gives four entries in the index. If it is necessary to search for any one term it can be found. If two or more terms are required combined, they can be found by combining the unit term entries and checking to see if they have the numbers of documents in common. If they do, the document is likely to be relevant. The coordination of terms is only made at the time of searching, and this index is described as coordinate (or postcoordinate). It is also called an inverted file because its organisation is the inverse of a serial file.

This system of coordinate indexing can be applied to many physical forms of index, from file cards to computer data bases. In its simplest form on file cards, it is usual to put the concept, which is either one word (in pure 'postcoordinate indexing') or a compound word or phrase (in the more usual hybrid compromise of 'coordinate indexing'), as a title on the top edge of the card. The rest of the card in divided vertically into ten columns for the digits 0–9. The accession numbers of documents are then written, on relevant cards, in the column with the same number as the last digit of the accession number. This simply makes finding the number easier when looking for it on several cards together (Fig. 13.2).

Providing for searching by combinations (concept coordination) is the most important feature of coordinate indexing, apart from making it physically possible to index in depth to the required extent.

Keyword									
1	2	3	4	5	6	7	8	9	0
	75:42		75:144				74:518		
							75:78		

Bromocriptine									
1	2	3	4	5	6	7	8	9	0
75:291	75:142	74:13				74:587	75:78	74:599	

Acromegaly									
1	2	3	4	5	6	7	8	9	0
		75:23			74:66		75:78		
					75:36				

Fig. 13.2   Coordinated Index Cards.

In fact there are three logical operations which can be performed with coordinate systems, and they are best illustrated by use of Venn diagrams. In Venn diagrams, classes are shown by circles.

Example

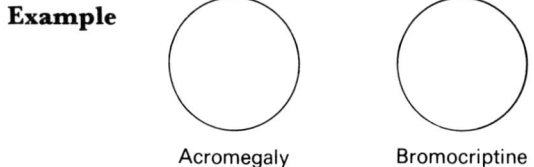

Acromegaly   Bromocriptine

These circles represent the references in a system relevant to the concepts 'acromegaly' and 'bromocriptine' respectively. Strictly, the circles should overlap:

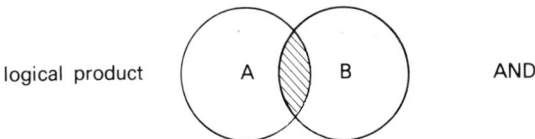

logical product   A   B   AND

The area of overlap represents references which are about both concepts. Thus a search statement (question) 'bromocriptine AND acromegaly?' (logical product) would require a reference to be about both to be retrieved as relevant. However, a search statement 'ampicillin OR cephradine?' indicated by:

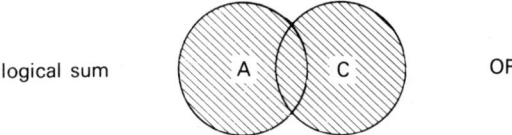

logical sum   A   C   OR

would accept a reference on either subject as being relevant. The shaded areas are of references relevant to the question.

The third type of search possible in coordinate systems is the logical difference:

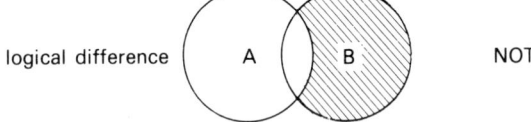

logical difference   A   B   NOT

Here the search statement would be of the form 'All references on bromocriptine but NOT those about acromegaly?'

By choosing broader or narrower terms it is possible to alter the size and overlap of the circles, and look for any combination of terms regardless of what other terms describe the documents. Computer data bases are usually searched by using this method of 'AND' 'OR' 'NOT' logic, because they are organised on the term entry inverted file system.

It is vital to retrieval that the same word or phrase is always used in the system to describe the same concept. If this is not done, synonyms occur and reduce the chance that all relevant references will be found at the time of search.

Most data bases and indexes exercise some degree of word control usually by use of a thesaurus or word list, like Medical Subject Headings (MeSH), the thesaurus of *Index Medicus*. The thesaurus will allow you to look up the term you have thought of and then tell you which synonym is preferred in the system. For example: Crohn's disease (lead-in term): see Enteritis, Regional (preferred term). Word control usually includes drug names, and because many data bases are American, it is hardly surprising that they index drugs by their American names. Remembering this fact can greatly improve retrieval.

Those who would like to know more about the way thesauri are made, are advised to read Gilchrist (1971).

Coordinate indexing (indexing by features) is the basis of a tablet and capsule identification scheme described by Ritchie *et al* (1975) and Allsup *et al* (1977).

ANSWERING QUESTIONS

The drug information centre provides a service to customers. In dealing with inquirers it is important to act in a polite, helpful and confident manner. People tend to ask for what they think the service can provide, rather than what they really want to know. Often the person asking a question will not have thought through the problem sufficiently to ask for specific details. What appears to be a general inquiry may be a specific problem, for which a specific answer would be most helpful.

It is not a good policy to give any but the most straightforward information from memory. The pharmacist is responsible legally for the information given and must take all reasonable precautions.

Interrogating the inquirer

This simply involves making sure one has all the information needed to understand and answer the question. Many inquiries may be inadequately or inappropriately dealt with if the context of the question is not understood. It is not always safe to take the problem stated at face value.

Examples

Q. 'What is the dose of Nystatin tablets?'
A1. (from Data Sheet or MIMS) 'One tablet four times daily (may be doubled).'
A2. 'What is wrong with the patient? ... Candida urinary tract infection ... well, Nystatin is not absorbed from the gut ... may I suggest instead ...'

The second answer is more helpful to the prescriber and to the patient.

Q. Which antidepressive is compatible with methyldopa?'

One could begin here by consulting the drug interaction books ... but is the inquirer aware that methyldopa could be the cause of the depression he is trying to treat? Great tact may be required to check on the knowledge of the inquirer, but this has to be done in such situations to deal adequately with the question.

Begin by asking for details of the patient and the problem. It is helpful to have a printed form as a reminder (Fig. 13.3). Ask the patient's age, sex and diagnosis(es), previous and present treatment. Is the patient in renal or hepatic failure? Is a female patient pregnant or on the pill? What is the patient's body weight? Compare the question and the patient data. Are the present prescriptions reasonable for this patient? Will the drugs interact? Why is the information needed? Knowledge of what the inquirer wishes to do may allow an alternative to be suggested. What does the inquirer really want to know? Modify the original question in the light of discussion and agree the final version with the inquirer. Who is asking the question? This must be recorded so that the answer can be communicated but it helps to bear the user in mind in preparation of the answer so that the level of information supplied is appropriate to the inquirer. (Care should be taken in dealing with personal inquiries from patients about their treatment. After offering reasonable assurance if they have doubts they should be referred back to the prescriber.) When is the answer required by? This will determine the priority of the question. Many people will say 'as soon as possible' and it is necessary then to determine whether the question is really urgent. It may be better to ask 'when is the latest time that the information would be useful to you?' And then aim to answer well within the deadline. Where else has the inquirer tried to find an answer? This can save a lot of time and avoids fruitless repetition.

Answering the question

If the question comes in the form of a letter, do some preliminary work to cover the problem, then phone back the inquirer to check and narrow the field. Simple data can usually be found in reference texts and often in several different sources. Choice depends on previous experience of using the sources for similar problems. It is usually wise to check in an independent text, data found in one source. Even simple numerical data can vary because of misprints, errors in calculation or differences due to different methods of estimation. Where conflicts or different values are found and there is no way of determining which is correct, all values should be quoted and discrepancies pointed out. If many sources quote the same information they could all be copying each other, and they could all be wrong.

Searching the literature

Often a 'look-up' in reference texts is not adequate to answer a question. A literature search for published work will then be required.

In an unfamiliar field it is necessary to be acquainted with the background to the problem before attempting to search, by using reference and textbooks. Look up all unfamiliar words, read a chapter or a review on the general area

N.E. THAMES REGIONAL DRUG INFORMATION SERVICE

Drug Information Centre,
The London Hospital
London, E1 1BB

01–247 5454 Ext. 147
Internal 680

PART A

Card No. [1]   Centre No. [ ]   Inquiry No. [ ][ ][ ][ ]

1 .... 2 ... 3 .... 4 8

Date [ ][ ][ ][ ][ ]   Time [ ][ ][ ]

9 14   15 18

Time answer required by [ ]   1 Immediate   4 Within a week
19   2 Same day   5 No time limit
                               3 Next day

(20–38) Name of caller:
        Address for answer:
        Telephone no:

Patient data (name, age, sex, diagnosis, concurrent therapy, allergies, lab data etc.)

Question

Answer

PART B

Punch Op: Skip to col. 40 after name of caller

Message taken by: [ ][ ][ ][ ][ ][ ][ ]
40 47

PUNCH OP: Skip to column 50

Inquiry:
        1 In person
        2 Via ward pharmacist
(50)   3 Phone
        4 Letter
        5 Telecopier

Caller status:
(51) a) 1 Hospital
          2 Community

      b) 0 Pharmacy
          1 Ward Pharmacist
          2 Consultant
          3 General Practitioner
(52)   4 Senior Registrar
          5 Registrar
          6 Academic staff
          7 House Officer
          8 Nursing
          9 Other

Answer:
        1 Oral
        2 Written
(53)   3 Bibliography
        4 Literature sent

Answer communicated by:
        1 Visit
        2 Phone
(54)   3 Post
        4 Telecopier

Question answered by [ ][ ][ ][ ][ ][ ][ ][ ]
55 62

Date answered [ ][ ][ ][ ][ ][ ]
63 68

Time answered [ ][ ][ ][ ]
69 72

If answer delayed,
give reasons why.   73
1. DIC staff absent   4. Inquirer not available
2. Postal delays of information   5. Other
3. Third party response delays

PART C

Punch Op: Skip to next card

Card no [2]
1

Punch Op: Dup. col. 2–8 from previous card

Drug codes [ ][ ][ ][ ][ ][ ][ ][ ][ ][ ][ ][ ]
9 20

[ ][ ][ ][ ][ ][ ][ ][ ][ ][ ][ ][ ][ ][ ][ ][ ][ ][ ]
21 38

Disease codes [ ][ ][ ][ ][ ][ ][ ][ ][ ]
39 47

[ ][ ][ ][ ][ ][ ][ ][ ][ ][ ][ ][ ]
48 59

Classification of Inquiry
  1) Caller contacted after answer to check
     usefulness of information
(60) a) 1 Initiated or altered therapy because of answer
         2 Information sufficient but not used in therapy
         3 Information insufficient

  2) Origin of inquiry
         1 London Hospital   5 St. Bartholomews
(61)   2 Tower Hamlets   6 Royal Free
         3 Newham   7 UCH
         4 Hackney   8 Other

     62 [ ] AHA no. 1 to 6
             (if out of region put 7)

  3) Type of information – up to 7 items may be circled
(63–78)
     01 Administration/dosage   06 Interactions
     02 Adverse effects/toxicity   07 Pharmaceutical
     03 Availability/supply   08 Pharmacology/pharmacokinetics
     04 Identification   09 Other
     05 Indications/choice of drug/
        contraindications

Punch Op: Skip to col. 79
  5) Medical staff specialty
     01 Anaes. & ITU   15 Paediatrics
     02 Cardiac   16 Pathology
(79) 03 Clin Pharm.   17 Plastic surgery
     04 Dental   18 Psychiatry
     05 Dermatology   19 Radiodiagnostic
     06 ENT   20 Radiotherapy
     07 Endocrinol.   21 Rheumatology
     08 Medicine   22 Thoracic surg.
     09 Nephrology & dialysis 23 Urology
     10 Neurology   24 VD
     11 Neurosurg.   25 Surgery
     12 Obstetric & gynae. 26 Haematology
     13 Orthopaedic & emergency 27 Others
     14 Ophthalmic

Fig. 13.3 Example of a form for recording the nature of inquiries for drug information.

of the problem. Deciding how extensive the search needs to be comes next. This will be determined by how soon the information is needed, to begin treatment for example; it will also depend on the resources available locally or through other organisations. Choose a system likely to be productive for the subject, from those available. How does the system index this kind of subject? What are the preferred terms for the concepts: drug names, disease names, pharmaceutical operations and so on? Many data bases change the way they index particular concepts as the importance of the subject alters. It is good practice to keep a record of the terms searched in each system, and also of the years, volume numbers and sections searched. If this record is kept then it is possible to alter the search terms at any stage in the search, and know which parts must be rechecked with the new terms, even after interruptions to deal with other problems. The decision over which years to search for references will be easier if it is known when a drug was first marketed. For example clinical investigations will have been published around this time, most adverse reaction reports will be more recent. It is usual to work backwards in time, starting from the most recent part of the data base to be searched. Note the references retrieved by use of the preferred terms. If the search is unproductive try alternative headings, different approaches.

Martyn (1967) found that by using the subject indexes of secondary sources, searchers would be able to find, by use of considerable ingenuity, only half to three-quarters of the references available to that publication in the literature. Abstracts journals are therefore not as comprehensive as might be expected.

Scan the references retrieved for relevance to the problem. The authors may cite other papers on aspects of their work; these should be followed up. If more recent work than that retrieved is required, try using the Science Citation Index. This indexes references and lists later papers which cite them. It can thus bring the searcher forward in time. Where the citation index is not available, try to identify the core journals in which most of the references found were published and check the recent issues back to the date of the latest reference retrieved.

Information should be obtained and quoted from the paper in which the original work was reported (the primary source) rather than from an abstract (secondary source) for the sake of accuracy. If the original is unobtainable (for example because of the time limits for the answer) so that a secondary source has to be quoted, this should be made clear to the inquirer in the answer.

Searching the literature is discussed by de Haen (1969) and Sewell (1975). Sewell in particular is useful for further reading on this subject.

When searching for information in secondary sources is not productive, another approach is required. There are many specialist organisations such as research associations, specialist libraries and information bureaux, government departments, professional and trade associations, self-help societies and manufacturers who can help.

Professionals in different health disciplines can be very helpful in contributing opinions or data. It is sensible to keep a record of experts in different fields, and where they can be contacted.

Evaluation of the literature

When the literature search has been completed a further stage is required. The users need data rather than a bibliography in most cases, and an information service is distinguished from a good library by its evaluation of the literature to produce an answer. The medical literature is prone to letters, editorials and other comments about published original work. Although this material is opinion rather than evidence, it is usually included in the secondary sources, and a proportion of any references retrieved will not be reports of original work. These opinions should not of course be included as giving weight to evidence, although they can be useful occasionally.

Original work which is sent to a journal for publication may be scrutinised by referees in some cases. Many journals, however, regard the contributors as being responsible for the design of their studies, applicability of the tests used and the validity of the conclusions. In some cases, any paper submitted may be accepted. Contributors have often had very little training in research methods. In sorting out the work which has been scientifically approached, and whose conclusions are justified, the information pharmacist will need to use all his experience and training. It is important to try to remain sceptical during the evaluation.

Schor and Karten (1966) found that of a sample of 149 original articles from ten highly regarded journals, at least 72% showed a lack of acceptable statistical planning and evaluation. Conclusions were drawn without adequate justification. Of 146 descriptive case reports more than 20% were considered not acceptable. Lionel and Herxheimer (1970) examined 141 reports of clinical trials in four British non-specialist journals and found only 51% satisfactory. Gore *et al* (1977) found that fifteen of the 77 original reports in their sample from the *British Medical Journal* had no statistical anlysis. Of the remaining 62, 32 (52%) included at least one error. In five cases (8%) a claim was made in the summary (abstract) which was not supported by the data presented. This is another good reason for referring to the original document rather than relying on abstracts. Bulpitt (1975) in an article on design of clinical trials stated: 'An inadequately designed experiment usually raises many doubts and it is no wonder that a biological problem often has to be attacked again and again by different observers.' Bulpitt's discussion on designing trials can be used to test how adequately a particular trial was performed. Lionel and Herxheimer (1970) included a checklist of criteria for assessing the acceptability of trials in their report, and Huskisson (1973) has also published a similar checklist. Colton (1974) in his useful book on statistics in medicine devotes a chapter to critical reading of the medical literature, and another to fallacies in numerical reasoning.

The aim in a clinical trial should be that the two groups under simultaneous investigation are as alike as possible except that one group receive the new treatment whereas the other group receive the control treatment. This is in keeping with the scientific method of experiment, where all parameters are controlled except the one being measured.

The nature of clinical trials is very diverse, but the following brief checklist, taken mainly from Colton (1974), may help to remind the evaluator of requirements:

1. What are the objectives of the study? Are they specific or unclear, single or multiple?
2. What is the population to which the authors intend to refer their findings?
3. The design of the trial should be such that the main objective can be met. Are dosage, duration of treatment and so on clearly stated?
4. Was the study an experiment, planned observations or an analysis of records?
5. How was the sample selected? Are there possible sources of selection which would make the sample atypical or unrepresentative? If so, what provision was made to deal with this bias? For example, was there a control group? Were the groups comparable in all respects (size, age, severity of disease and so on)? Was the study double-blind throughout? Did it allow for carry-over effects or first drug preferences? Diagnosis must be established beyond doubt.
6. There should be clear definitions of the terms used including diagnostic criteria, measurements made, criteria of outcome and criteria for withdrawing patients from the trial.
7. The method of measurement should be consistent for all subjects and relevant to the objectives of the study.
8. Are there possible biases in measurement and if so what provisions were made to deal with them?
9. Are the observations reliable and reproducible? Are they presented clearly, objectively and in sufficient detail for the reader to judge them for himself? Are the findings internally consistent, e.g. do the numbers add up in the tables, can the different tables be reconciled?
10. Are the data worthy of statistical analysis? Are the methods appropriate to the source and nature of the data and is the analysis correctly performed and interpreted? Is there sufficient analysis to determine whether 'significant differences' may be due to lack of comparability of the groups?
11. Which conclusions are justified by the findings and which are not?
12. Are the conclusions relevant to the original questions posed by the investigators?

Where the result of a literature search is a collection of conflicting reports it will be found helpful to tabulate the documents and the claims they make, the kind of study used, dosages used etc. Differences in the methods which produced differing results can then clearly be seen.

ACTIVE PROVISION OF INFORMATION

Dealing with inquiries is an important part of the work of the information services. It should usually be the first service offered, because it deals with an existing recognised need. The answering of questions is regarded as a passive activity because it depends on outsiders (the users) initiating the process. More active roles for the information service can also be identified which include:

1. Generally keeping one's users up to date with important developments by disseminating news (current awareness).

2. Identifying deficiencies in the user's professional knowledge as shown by, for example, inappropriate prescribing, and attempting to correct these by articles in bulletins or by producing a formulary of permitted and forbidden products (the articles can form a series which accumulate to become a formulary).

3. Anticipating a demand for routine information about products by supplying it as books, charts or card indexes to be referred to at the point of use, thus saving oneself much repetitive routine question answering.

Current awareness was described in the section on resources above, in relation to commercially produced services. An alerting service tailored to the local pharmacy department or medical firms can be provided by the information centre by scanning relevant journals. The important point is that the product must be current, which means weekly publication or faster if necessary.

Meetings are another useful way of informing people of developments. There are a number of organisations which can provide films and slide-tapes and there is even an information service (Medical Audiovisual Aids Information Service, Mavis) which has details of what is available. Journal club meetings can also be useful.

The cheapest and easiest way of disseminating news is by use of a notice board, and this can be effective if in the right place. Bulletins can also be effective means of communicating with users. They must be attractive and distinctive at first sight. This helps to ensure that they will be read. Even more important, they should be well written, make sensible suggestions and reach clear conclusions.

Articles will be more acceptable to a group of users if it can be seen that representatives of the group were involved in production of the articles, either as authors or members of an editorial board. For example, at the London Hospital the bulletin is edited by pharmacists, but the pharmacy and therapeutics committee forms an editorial board, and the authors of articles are often clinical specialists in the subject of the article.

Guidance on writing will be found by reading and referring to standard works such as *The Complete Plain Words* (Gowers 1973), *Usage and Abusage* (Partridge 1973) and *Modern English Usage* (Fowler 1968). Technical writing is dealt with by Godfrey and Parr (1967) and O'Brien (1974) amongst many others. The main point is to maintain a simple style; use short words rather than long words; keep sentences as brief as possible; use the active rather than the passive form; try not to use similes, metaphors, clichés, foreign phrases or jargon.

If a formulary is to be produced, it should have the support of a group who can enforce its recommendations, for example a Pharmacy and Therapeutic Committee.

A chart may be the most appropriate way of presenting some kinds of information (e.g. the colour coding of insulins). Charts should be as simple and clear as possible; it is usually a mistake to try to be comprehensive in covering a subject by chart.

Point-of-use information suitable for reference on wards or in clinics has been produced as card indexes of data sheet type in a number of hospitals (Edwards & Baker 1962; Greth *et al* 1965; Prisco & Plein 1969; Trice *et al* 1972). Specialised data sets have also been produced on intravenous additives.

Whichever method of supplying point-of-use information is chosen, it is important to make sure that it is updated regularly, and that the revised versions reach all the users who have the older version.

The correcting and updating of information is made easier if the data are held in one place. This is the way computer data bases operate, with the information stored centrally in the computer and referred to via remote terminals at the points of use. Such systems are not common in the health service, but some interesting systems have been developed. At the London Hospital a drug interaction information system is available on ward terminals; in Exeter data sheet type information is provided, and at Queen Elizabeth Hospital in Birmingham prescribing information is available on ward terminals as part of a computer-prescribing system. Outside the health service, a similar information system has been proposed by Padfield *et al* (1976) which would be searchable for textwords.

In the United States, developments occurred earlier in the application of computers to pharmacy practice. Emmanuel and Dauphinais (1968) published results of a survey showing that at that time 62 drug information centres in the USA were using computers for some purpose; many more were planning such use. Knight and Conrad (1975) reviewed the published literature on computer use in pharmacy and found computers being used in drug information for formulary preparation, retrieval of microfilm, drug interactions, usage review, prescribing and individual dosing regimens based on pharmacokinetics.

MONITORING DRUG USAGE

Many hospitals have a pharmacy and therapeutics committee which is concerned with the provision of pharmacy services and safe and effective use of medicines in the hospital. The committee usually has among its members clinicians, pharmacists, nurses and administrators. The existence of a drug information centre, a clinical or ward service and such a committee provide an excellent basis on which to undertake collaborative schemes for monitoring drug usage in hospitals. At regional level monitoring could be by a multidisciplinary committee using data from prescriptions and covering the community too. Many articles, coming mainly from USA and Canada, have been written describing such schemes (Rosenberg *et al* 1969; Burkholder 1967; Parks 1970; Hutchinson 1971). The schemes relate to drug usage and compilation of hospital formularies, adverse drug reactions, drug interactions, and the administration of drugs by addition to intravenous infusion fluids, etc. and are usually carried out in collaboration with medical and nursing staff. The drug information centre may collect, coordinate and prepare the data from which the appropriate committee can make decisions and recommendations. There is as yet little published work from this country of the direct use of information centres in this way but undoubtedly much unpublished work has been carried out. In the field of adverse drug reaction monitoring pharmacists have contributed greatly to the work of the Boston Collaborative Drug Surveillance Program (Jick *et al* 1970), the Aberdeen and Dundee Group (Coull *et al* 1970a, 1970b) and the West Midlands Group (Beeley & Baker 1977). A potential drug usage monitoring role for the Prescription Pricing Authority is suggested in a report on that organisation (DHSS 1977); the scheme would collect data from dispensed NHS prescriptions.

FUTURE TRENDS

At present the specialty of drug information is in a period of dynamic functional and organisational development. Manpower requirements have now been measured (Rogers 1978) and indicate that drug information centres will probably have a supporting role to clinical pharmacists. The clinical pharmacist would be the local link with the users. The information centre would provide back-up for perhaps a Noel Hall Area or even a Region. There is no doubt that full-time cover is required for this supporting role, and this may lead to 24-hour services becoming more widespread.

Links with other professional groups have always been important for drug information services. The links have in the past been informal but the trend is towards a multidisciplinary approach to at least some of the services functions. Clinicians and other specialists have acted as consultants for therapeutic problems and have contributed to, or helped to edit, bulletins and other material for dissemination. In future, multidisciplinary committees may identify needs of user groups in hospitals and the community and decide on the best coordinated approach to meet the needs. Jointly operated services are also a possibility.

The active role of disseminating information to professional groups is increasing in importance. At present the main route for this dissemination is by bulletin articles. There is little information on what proportion of various user groups read, remember and act on this material. The individuals who do not read it are probably the ones who need to most of all, in the view of the information service. The industrial approach to such isolated users is to send representatives to visit them; could this be a future role for information services?

Providing information directly to patients has not been a major activity for drug information centres. Questions from patients about their treatment must be dealt with very carefully. Often the correct approach is to refer them back to their prescriber if they have doubts. But patients do need to be better informed about the medicines they take; this could improve compliance and bring about a sensible attitude towards drug taking, self prescribing, and an increased awareness of the hazards and limitations of drug treatment. Drug information services can contribute by producing 'literature' as package inserts or articles for their own periodical publications or commercial magazines.

These are some of the possibilities currently facing drug information pharmacists. The next few years are going to be important and very interesting ones for the development of this specialty.

APPENDIX

Suggestions to form the core library of a drug information centre

Reference and textbooks

Some of these books are alternatives. Personal preference and budget will affect choice.

Pharmacopoieas and formularies

British National Formulary. BMA and Pharmaceutical Press, London.
British Pharmaceutical Codex. Pharmaceutical Press, London.
British Pharmacopoiea. HMSO, London.
European Pharmacopoiea. Maisonneuve SA Sainte Ruffine, France (Pharm. Press, London).

General reference books and indexes

AMA Drug Evaluations. Publishing Sciences Group, Acton, Mass.

Biopharmaceutics and Relevant Pharmacokinetics, J. G. Wagner. Drug Intelligence Publications, Hamilton.

British Chemicals and their Manufacturers. Chemical Industry Association, London.

Chemist and Druggist Directory (Annual). Benn Bros., London.

Clinical Experience Abstracts. FDA, Washington DC.

Current Abstracts of Pharmacy and Therapeutics. Guild of Hospital Pharmacists, London.

Data Sheet Compendium (Annual). Association British Pharmaceutical Industry (ABPI), London.

Index of New Products. Pharmaceutical Press, London.

Martindale, The Extra Pharmacopoeia, ed. A. Wade. Pharmaceutical Press, London.

Merck Index, The, ed. P. D. Stecher. Merck & Co., Rahway, NJ.

MIMS Monthly Index of Medical Specialities. Haymarket, London.

Pharmaceutical Handbook. Pharmaceutical Press, London.

Physical Pharmacy, A. W. Martin, J. Swarbrick & A. Cammarata. Lea & Febiger, Philadelphia.

Remington's Pharmaceutical Sciences, eds, A. Osol, J. E. Hoover *et al.* Mack. Easton, PA.

Scientific Tables, K. Diem & C. Lentner. Geigy, Basle.

Textbook of Organic, Medicinal and Pharmaceutical Chemistry, C. O. Wilson, O. Gisvold & R. F. Doerge. Lippincott, PA.

Unlisted Drugs. Unlisted Drugs, Chatham, NJ.

Where to Buy: Chemicals and Chemical Plant. Where to Buy Ltd, London.

Pharmacology and therapeutics

Antibiotic and Chemotherapy, L. P. Garrod, H. P. Lambert & F. O'Grady. Churchill Livingstone, Edinburgh.

Clinical Pharmacology, K. L. Melmon & H. F. Morrelli. Macmillan, New York.

Drug Interactions, P. D. Hansten. Lea & Febiger, Philadelphia.

Drug Treatment, ed. G. S. Avery. ADIS, Sydney.

Evaluation of Drug Interactions. American Pharmaceutical Association, Washington DC. (Pharm. Press, London).

Harrison's Principles of Internal Medicine, eds. G. W. Thorn, R. D. Adams, E. Braunwald, K. J. Isselbacher & R. G. Petersdorf. McGraw-Hill, New York.

Merck Manual, The. Merck & Co., Rahway, NJ.

Metabolic Basis of Inherited Disease, The, J. B. Stanbury, J. B. Wyngaarden & D. S. Fredrickson. McGraw-Hill, New York.

Paediatric Prescriber, P. Catzel. Blackwell Scientific Publications, Oxford.

Paediatric Vademecum, B. Wood. Lloyd-Luke, London.

Pediatric Dosage Handbook, H. C. Shirkey. American Pharmaceutical Association, Washington DC.

Pharmacological Basis of Therapeutics, The, L. S. Goodman & A. Gilman. Macmillan, New York.

Prices Textbook of the Practice of Medicine, R. Bodley Scott. Oxford University Press, London.

Principles of Drug Action, A. Goldstein, L. Aronow & S. M. Kalman. Wiley, New York.

Textbook of Medical Treatment, S. Alstead, A. G. MacGregor & R. H. Girdwood. Churchill Livingstone, Edinburgh.

Dictionaries and nomenclature

American Drug Index, C. O. Wilson & T. E. Jones (Annual). Lippincott, Philadelphia.

Approved Names. HMSO, London.

Dorland's Illustrated Medical Dictionary, Saunders, Philadelphia.

or

Butterworth's Medical Dictionary. Butterworth, London.

Index Nominum. Swiss Pharm. Soc.

International Non Proprietary Names for Pharmaceutical Substances. World Health Organisation, Geneva.

Oxford English Dictionary, Concise, Pocket or Shorter. Oxford University Press, London.

or

Chambers's Twentieth Century Dictionary. Chambers, London.

Pharmacological and Chemical Synonyms, E. E. J. Marler. Excerpta Medica, Amsterdam.

Adverse effects, toxicology and identification

Chemist and Druggist Tablet and Capsule Identification Guide (available in Chemist and Druggist Directory). Benn Bros., London.

Clinical Toxicology of Commercial Products, R. E. Gosselin, H. C. Hodge, R. P. Smith & M. N. Gleason. Williams & Wilkins, Baltimore.

Dangerous Properties of Industrial Materials, N. Irving Sax. Van Nostrand Rheinhold, New York.

Imprex; Index of Imprints used on Tablets and Capsules, W. A. L. Collier. Ferrier, Edinburgh.

Isolation and Identification of Drugs, vols. I and II, E. G. C. Clarke. Pharmaceutical Press, London.

Poisoning by Drugs and Chemicals, P. Cooper. Alchemist Publications, London.

Register of Adverse Reactions, Committee on Safety of Medicines. HMSO, London.

Side Effects of Drugs, vols. 1–8 and Annuals. Excerpta Medica, Amsterdam.
Textbook of Adverse Reactions, ed. D. M. Davis. Oxford Medical Publications, Oxford.
Treatment of Common Acute Poisonings, H. Matthew & A. A. H. Lawson. Churchill Livingstone, Edinburgh.

Forensic information

Medicines and Poisons Guide 1978, C. E. Hay. Pharmaceutical Press, London.
Pharmacy Law and Ethics, Dale & Applebe. Pharmaceutical Press, London.

Statistics and clinical trial design

Clinical Trials, F. N. Johnson & S. Johnson. Blackwell Scientific Publications, Oxford.
Medical Research, J. M. England. Churchill Livingstone, Edinburgh.
Principles of Medical Statistics, Sir A. Bradford Hill. The Lancet, London.
Statistics at Square One, T. D. V. Swinscow. British Medical Journal, London.
Statistics in Medicine, T. Colton. Little, Brown, Boston, Mass.

Journals

Adverse Drug Reaction Bulletin. Adverse Drug Reaction Research Unit, Shotley Bridge Hospital, Durham.
American Journal of Hospital Pharmacy. American Society of Hospital Pharmacists, Washington DC.
British Journal of Clinical Pharmacology. Macmillan, London.
British Medical Journal. British Medical Association, London.
Bulletin of the Parental Drug Association. Parental Drug Association, Philadelphia.
Clinical Pharmacology and Therapeutics. C. V. Mosby, St. Louis.
Drug Intelligence and Clinical Pharmacy. Drug Intelligence and Clinical Pharmacy, Hamilton, Ill.
Drug and Therapeutics Bulletin. Consumers Association, London.
Drugs. ADIS, Sydney.
Journal of the American Medical Association. American Medical Association, Chicago.
Journal of Clinical Pharmacy. Blackwell Scientific Publications, Oxford.
Journal of Pharmaceutical Sciences. American Pharmaceutical Association, Washington DC.
New England Journal of Medicine. Massachusetts Medical Society, Boston, Mass.
Pharmaceutical Journal. Pharmaceutical Press, London.
Practitioner. The Practitioner, London.
Prescribers Journal. The Prescribers Journal, London.
The Lancet. Lancet, London.

Bibliography for abstracts

Clin-Alert. Science Editors, Louisville, Kentucky.
Current Abstracts of Pharmacy and Therapeutics. Guild of Hospital Pharmacists, London.
Current Contents. Institute for Scientific Information, Philadelphia.
Drugdoc and Drug Literature Index. Excerpta Medica, Amsterdam.
Drugs in Use. Paul de Haen, Info. Systems, a division of Micromedex Inc., Inglewood, Colorado.
Index Medicus. National Library of Medicine, Washington DC.
Inpharma. ADIS, Sydney.
International Pharmaceutical Abstracts. American Society of Hospital Pharmacists, Washington DC.
Iowa Drug Information Service. Westlawn, University of Iowa.
Ringdoc. Derwent, London.
Toxicity Bibliography. National Library of Medicine, Washington DC.
Unlisted Drugs. Unlisted Drugs, Chatham, NJ.

REFERENCES

ALLSUP V., PARKER J. & WALKER J. (1977) *Pharmaceutical Journal* **219,** 529.
AMERSON A. B. & WALTON C. A. (1971) *American Journal of Hospital Pharmacy* **28,** 267.
ASHMOLE R. F., SMITH D. E. & STERN B. T. (1973) *Journal of the American Society for Information Science* **24,** 29.
BEELEY L. & BAKER S. (1977) Making best use of adverse reaction reports in the West Midlands. In *Symposium on Drug Monitoring in General Practice*. 24 June 1977. Oxford Drug Monitoring Conference. pp. J1–J6.
BOTTLE R. T. (1971) *The Use of Chemical Literature*. Butterworths, London.
BROOKES B. C. (1968) *Journal of Documentation* **24,** 247.
BULPITT C. J. (1975) *British Journal of Hospital Medicine* **13,** 611.
BURKHOLDER D. (1963) *American Journal of Hospital Pharmacy* **20,** 506.
BURKHOLDER D. F. (1967) *Drug Intelligence* **1,** 87.
COLTON F. (1974) *Statistics in Medicine*. Little Brown, Boston, Mass.
COULL D. C., CROOKS J., DAVIDSON J. F., GALLON S. C. & WEIR R. D. (1970a) *European Journal of Clinical Pharmacology* **3,** 46.
COULL D. C., CROOKS J., DINGWALL-FORDYCE I., SCOTT A. M. & WEIR R. D. (1970b) *European Journal of Clinical Pharmacology* **3,** 51.
DE HAEN P. (1969) *Drug Information Bulletin* **3,** 140.
DEPARTMENT OF HEALTH AND SOCIAL SECURITY (1970) *Report of the Working Party on the Hospital Pharmaceutical Service*. The Noel Hall Report. HMSO, London.
DEPARTMENT OF HEALTH AND SOCIAL SECURITY (1977) *Report of the Inquiry into the Prescription Pricing Authority*. Chairman R. I. Tricker. HMSO, London.
EDWARDS L. G. & BARKER K. N. (1962) *American Journal of Nursing* **62,** 68.
EMMANUEL D. C. & DAUPHINAIS R. J. (1968) *Drug Intelligence* **2,** 118.
FOSKETT D. J. (1975) Classification. In *Handbook of Special Librarianship and Information Work*, ed. W. E. Batten. ASLIB, London.
FOWLER H. W. (1968) *Modern English Usage*. Revised Sir E. Gowers. Oxford University Press, Oxford.

Garcia-Iñesta A. (1975) *Fourth Workshop on Hospital Pharmacy Practice and Education*, pp. 34–46. 22–24 October, Alicante.

Gilchrist A. (1971) *The Thesaurus in Retrieval*. ASLIB, London.

Godfrey J. W. & Parr G. (1967) *The Technical Writer*. Chapman & Hall, London.

Gore S. M., Jones I. G. & Rytter E. C. (1977) *British Medical Journal* 1, 85.

Gowers Sir E. (1973) *The Complete Plain Words*. Revised Sir B. Fraser. Pelican Books & HMSO, London.

Greth P. A., Tester W. W. & Black H. J. (1965) *American Journal of Hospital Pharmacy* 22, 558.

Huskisson E. C. (1973) *Journal of Hospital Pharmacy* 31, 143.

Hutchinson R. F. (1970) *Drug Intelligence and Clinical Pharmacy* 4, 322.

Hutchinson R. & Burkholder D. F. (1971) *Drug Intelligence and Clinical Pharmacy* 5, 181.

Jick H., Miettiner O. S., Shapiro S., Lewis G. P., Siskind V. & Sloane D. (1970) *Journal of the American Medical Association* 213, 1455.

Knight J. R. & Conrad W. F. (1975) *American Journal of Hospital Pharmacy* 32, 165.

Lionel N. D. W. & Herxheimer A. H. (1970) *British Medical Journal* 3, 637.

Madden M. & MacDonald A. (1977) *Drug Information Journal* 11, 47.

Maltby A. (1965) *Sayer's Manual of Classification for Librarians*. Deutsch, London.

Martyn J. (1967) *Journal of Documentation* 23, 45.

Medical Audio-Visual Aids Information Service (MAVIS), Centre for Medical Education, Ninewells Hospital and Medical School, Dundee DD1 9SY

Morton L. T. (1974) *Use of Medical Literature*. Butterworths, London.

O'Brien T. (1974) *ASLIB Proceedings* 26, 405.

Padfield J. M., Moss S. H., Norton D. A. & Gill M. S. (1976) *Pharmaceutical Journal* 216, 212.

Parker P. F. (1965) *American Journal of Hospital Pharmacy* 22, 42.

Parks J. S. (1970) *Canadian Journal of Hospital Pharmacy* July–August, 141.

Partridge E. (1973) *Usage and Abusage*. Penguin Books and Hamish Hamilton, London.

Pearson R. E. (1974) *American Journal of Hospital Pharmacy* 31, 399.

Pearson R. E., Salter F. J., Bohl J. C., Thudium V. F. & Phillips G. L. (1970) *American Journal of Hospital Pharmacy* 27, 911.

Pearson R. E., Schalgemeier W., Bendall M. & Mehta P. (1972a) *American Journal of Hospital Pharmacy* 29, 229.

Pearson R. E., Thudium V. F. & Phillips G. L. (1972b) *American Journal of Hospital Pharmacy* 29, 312.

Pearson R. E., Thudium V. F. & Phillips G. L. (1971) *American Journal of Hospital Pharmacy* 28, 513.

Pharmaceutical Journal (1971) 207, 561.

Prisco H. M. & Plein E. M. (1969) *American Journal of Hospital Pharmacy* 26, 160.

Ritchie J., Brodlie P. & Harden R. M. (1975) *Lancet* i, 552.

Rogers M. L. (1978) *Journal of Clinical Pharmacy* 3, 189.

Rogers M. L. & Barrett C. W. (1972) *Pharmaceutical Journal* 209, 37.

Rosenberg J. M. & Hanan Z. I. (1969) *Hospital Pharmacy* 4, 22.

Schor S. & Karten I. (1966) *Journal of the American Medical Association* 195, 1123.

Sewell W. (1975) *Guide to Drug Information*. Drug Intelligence Publications, Hamilton, Ill.

Smith D. R., Beauchamp R. O. jr, Garber J. L. & Dougherty M. A. (1972) *Journal of Chemical Documentation* 12, 9.

Stauffer I. (1963–4) *Hospital Pharmacist* 16–17, 161.

Tourville J. F. & McLeod D. C. (1975) *American Journal of Hospital Pharmacy* 32, 1153.

Trice A. E., Scholes M. & Barrett C. W. (1972) *Pharmaceutical Journal* 209, 73.

14

Poisons information services

C. HETHERINGTON

Poisons Information Bureaux were established in the United States and Finland in the 1950s and the first such bureau in Great Britain was opened in the Casualty Department of the General Infirmary at Leeds in August 1961. The calls to the bureau result from the need to provide emergency treatment, and for some, more intensive hospital-based therapy following ingestion of materials considered toxic by doctors and nurses working in hospitals and general practice. The Atkins Report (DHSS 1962) recommended that, for Great Britain, 'an information service on poisoning should be set up with central arrangements for coordination'. The outcome of this report was the establishment in 1963 of the National Poisons Information Service based on Guy's Hospital, London. Poisons Information Services are now established in London, Edinburgh, Cardiff, Belfast, Manchester, Leeds, Bristol, Newcastle and Dublin.

THE BUREAU

The Poisons Information Service is required to provide answers to the thousands of inquiries each year, for patients who have ingested substances of which the doctor supervising treatment has little or no information concerning toxicity. The materials ingested, particularly by young children, are extremely varied and include anything which is found in the home, e.g. for domestic cleaning, application to the garden, use as medicines, cosmetics, home decorating and a host of other materials which cause parents to seek medical advice when consumed by children.

As calls to the centres result from accidents and are for advice on acute toxicity and appropriate treatment, the Poisons Information Bureau must have data filed away for immediate reference purposes on thousands of materials that could be the cause of such inquiries. Unlike the Drug Information Centre in a hospital pharmaceutical service, all inquiries arrive by telephone and demand an immediate answer in the form of advice on toxicity of the product and the appropriate treatment to be given to the patient. They must provide continuous service 24 hours a day 7 days a week (Fig. 14.1).

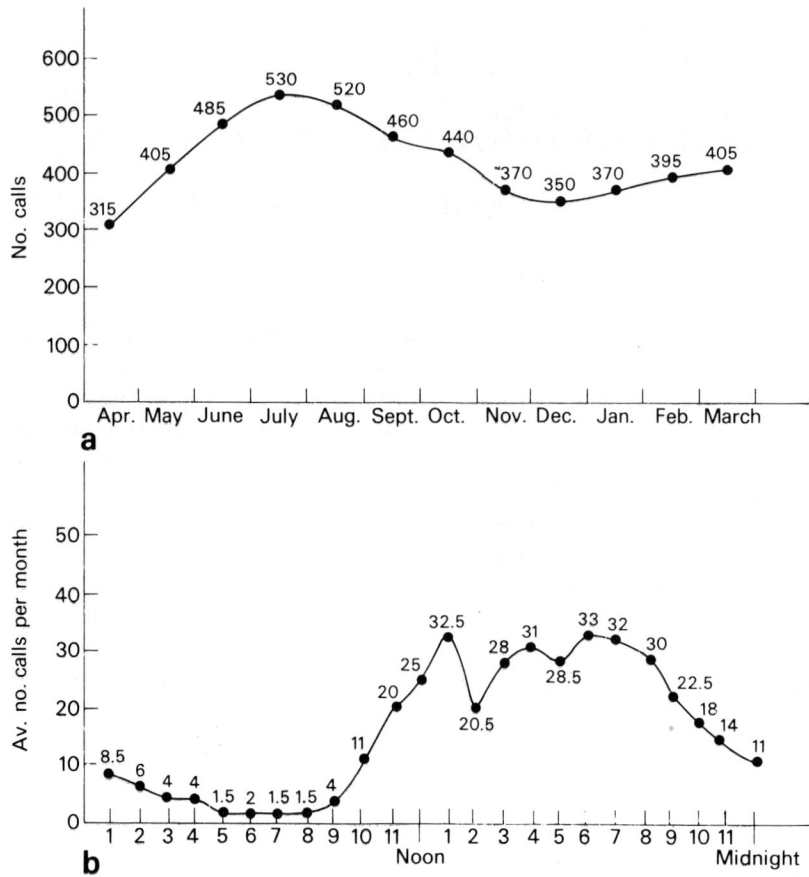

Fig. 14.1 (a) Number of calls per month to the Leeds Poisons Information Bureau during 1973–4. (b) Average number of calls to the Leeds Poisons Information Bureau at different times of the day.

Collecting data

It is possible to divide the data required into broad categories (e.g. chemicals, plants and fungi, pharmaceuticals, agricultural and horticultural products, household items and cosmetics). When collecting information the prime source is the product manufacturer, who can provide formulation data and in the pharmaceutical industry is also often able to offer toxicity data. The majority of manufacturers are very willing to provide details of the constituents of their products when they realise it is required for patient treatment purposes, it is, however, always agreed by the centres that any information provided for the service will be treated in strict confidence. The manufacturer of a household product (e.g. a furniture cream or a washing-up liquid) is usually not in a position to provide toxicity data and often suggests that reference be made to the chemical manufacturer of the constituents to obtain information for the Poisons Information Service. The position is further complicated when manufacturers change the composition of their products without making any announcement, simply considering it part of the general development of an improved preparation. The position in the pharmaceutical industry where the composition of products is declared therefore makes the work of maintaining information files much easier than with the other industries involved.

The data base of a Poison Information Service is made up of entries on thousands of individual products as well as general entries on toxic materials which form the active constituents of many products (e.g. alcohol, turpentine, aspirin and hypochlorite). The index invariably grows larger each year as new products are introduced and the data on old products are retained, since households can keep items for many years before they are involved in an incident requiring help from the Poisons Information Bureau.

Data storage

The method of storing information is fairly standard and is similar to that used in Leeds. Fig. 14.2 shows a typical entry in the files. The National Poisons Information Service uses large Kalamazoo binders (Fig. 14.3a) for storing information sheets which have the advantage that entries cannot be misfiled but the disadvantage that the files are very clumsy to handle. The visible index filing system (Fig. 14.3b) overcomes the latter and when only a limited number of people use the cards it is a reliable and easily handled system of storage.

The data is recorded in a standard format and cross-referenced to active principle cards whenever possible, as this makes the updating of treatment details very much easier and more reliable. For example, should a change in treatment be found superior for salicylate poisoning, using this cross-reference system it is only necessary to update one card, all the other entries for aspirin-containing preparations need not be altered, making the revision much quicker.

Although product formula data is important to the information pharmacist in preparing a poison bureau entry card, of greater importance to the doctor making use of the service are the signs and symptoms of overdosage of the preparation involved. It is necessary therefore to include a detailed statement of the signs of toxicity, relating these where possible to time following ingestion and severity relative to dosage. It is often extremely valuable to know that drowsiness occurs after a certain time or dosage, particularly when there is doubt as to the quantity of material actually consumed, as it helps in assessing the treatment which may be appropriate.

It is necessary during preparation of an entry to study the pharmacokinetic parameters of the agent. These should be included in the entry card for it

LABURNUM		
Family:	Leguminosae
Syn:	Laburnum anagyroides, Cytisus laburnum, Golden rain.
Description (1, 3):	Tree up to 30' high. Green trifoliate leaves on long stalks. Yellow flowers with five petals (May–June). The fruit is a pod about 2–2$^1/_2$ inches long containing up to eight kidney-shaped beans. All parts of the tree are toxic, particularly bark and seeds. The toxic principle is cytisine (an alkaloid similar in action to nicotine).
Habitat:	Commonly cultivated, seldom grows wild.
Minimum lethal dose (4):	Two or three seeds may produce toxic symptoms. Report of a child taking 18 seeds and recovering after treatment.
Toxic effects (2):	Initial stimulation of central nervous system followed by depression and respiratory paralysis. May cause kidney damage.
Symptoms (1, 2, 3):	These may be delayed for several hours and include nausea, persistent vomiting, excess salivation, burning sensation in the mouth, diarrhoea, dilation of the pupils and tachycardia. This may be followed by dizziness, mental confusion, severe abdominal pain, delerium, muscular weakness, convulsions and respiratory paralysis. Kidney damage may develop leading to uraemia.
Pharmacodynamics: (1)	Toxic principle is rapidly absorbed. Excreted by the kidneys and metabolites may be detected in the urine.
Treatment (2, 3):	Prompt treatment is essential. Emetic if no convulsions S.W.O. yes Purgative – give sodium sulphate 30g in 250 ml water (adult dose) Demulcents – milk fluids, activated charcoal. Fluids – oral – in large amounts if urine output satisfactory parenteral – maintain body fluids and electrolytes Oxygen and artificial respiration – if required for severe respiratory depression or stimulant.
Any other treatment:	Full supportive therapy.
Prognosis (3):	Severe and fatal injury may occur after several days due to delayed kidney damage.
References:	(1) British Poisonous Plants, (2) Martindale, (3) Cooper, (4) Lancet 1951 ii 6 ii 57

Fig. 14.2   A method of storing information concerning poisons.

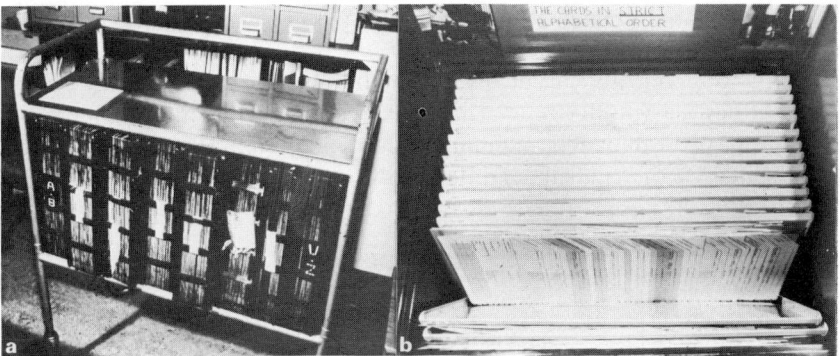

Fig. 14.3 (a) Kalamazoo binders for storing information sheets. (b) Visible index filing system for information storage.

is valuable to know that absorption is in a certain part of the gastrointestinal tract, that excretion is via the kidneys, that toxicity is increased with the concurrent intake of alcohol, that the material is highly protein bound in the blood and that dialysis has been found useless as a means of treatment. All these pieces of information may be used by the pharmacist when answering an inquiry but the most essential information for those who use the service is the emergency treatment for such ingestions and the longer care which should be provided. Treatment information is also recorded in a standard format, thereby allowing the pharmacist answering an inquiry to give specific guidance: e.g. as to whether a stomach wash-out or an emetic is indicated; whether any other drugs are indicated or contraindicated.

Treatment

The information included on treatment is obtained from reference sources (see list at end of chapter) and from suppliers with specialist information (e.g. drug manufacturers from the toxicological investigations of their own laboratories). The pharmacists working in a Poisons Information Bureau need to maintain an up-to-date knowledge of treatment methods by continual scanning of the medical literature for published treatment details and the results of alternative regimes. In some cases precise advice cannot be given because of limited published data being available; it is useful in these cases to follow up inquiries to the service and obtain details of the outcome of treatment of the particular case. It is often possible in such cases to include useful data on the level of toxicity which occurred following particular levels of ingestion. As the minimum lethal dose of many agents is now known, it is valuable to know that patients have recovered after ingestion of certain quantities when treated in a particular way. With the very large number of calls about children (Fig.

14.4) it is essential to know if the effects vary with age and if treatment needs to be modified.

In the complete absence of any information being available on treatment it may be necessary to give general first aid advice and recommend that careful observation of the patient be maintained and general supportive therapy given as indicated by the clinical condition of the case.

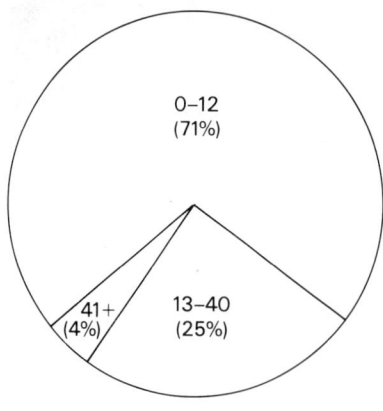

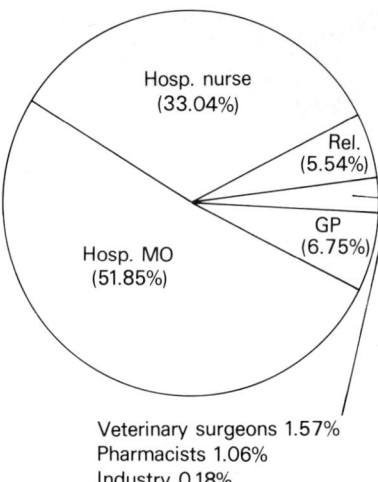

Fig. 14.4   The distribution of calls by age of patient at Leeds Poisons Information Bureau.

Fig. 14.5   The distribution of calls by inquirer at Leeds Poisons Information Bureau.

Answering inquiries

Considerable expertise is required before a pharmacist can handle inquiries to a Poisons Information Bureau. It is essential that they have training and a good understanding of the basic principles of poison treatment. It is advisable to identify the caller before any information is provided as inevitably some calls will come from members of the public (Fig. 14.5). In these cases the help that can be given is mainly reassurance that there is time to get the child to hospital and that the action to take is to drive immediately by car or to dial 999 and ask for an ambulance. In these circumstances it would be very danger-ous and also inappropriate to offer any information on treatment. It is also desirable to determine if the caller is a doctor or someone speaking on his behalf; in some cases it is better to ask for the doctor to take the call, rather than pass information through a third party. The amount of information pro-vided will depend on such factors as, the time since ingestion took place, pre-sence of symptoms, any first aid measures already taken. The extent of detail provided needs to be left to the discretion and skill of the pharmacist answering

POISONS INFORMATION BUREAU					
DATE	TIME 6	TIME 7	TIME 8	AGE 9	
Day 1/2	0.01 1 a.m. 0 1.01 2 a.m. 1	12.01 1.0 p.m. 0 1.01 2.0 p.m. 1		0–3 years 0	
Month 3	2.01 3 a.m. 2 3.01 4 a.m. 3	2.01 3.0 p.m. 2 3.01 4.0 p.m. 3	Male 0	+ 3 yrs/12 yrs 1	
Year 4/5	4.01 5 a.m. 4 5.01 6 a.m. 5	4.01 5.0 p.m. 4 5.01 6.0 p.m. 5	Female 1	+ 12 yrs/21 yrs 2	
	6.01 7 a.m. 6 7.01 8 a.m 7	6.01 7.0 p.m. 6 7.01 8.0 p.m. 7		+ 21 yrs/40 yrs 3	
	8.01 9 a.m. 8 9.01 10 a.m. 9	8.01 9.0 p.m. 8 9.01 10.0 p.m. 9		+ 40 yrs/65 yrs 4	
	10.01 11 a.m. 11 11.01 12 a.m. 12	10.01 11.0 p.m. 11 11.01 12.0 p.m. 12		65 yrs + over 5	

MATERIAL 10		DRUGS 11		HOW TAKEN 12		CALLER 13	
Domestic	0	Salicylates	0	Oral	0	G P	0
Pesticides	1	Barbiturates	1	Topical	1	Hosp. M.O.	1
Agricultural & horticultural	2	Hormones	2	Inhaled	2	Hosp. Nurse	2
		Iron	3	Injected	3	Hosp. Pharm.	3
Cosmetics	3	Tranquillisers	4	Eye	4	Relatives	4
Home remedies	4	Antidepressants	5			Industry	5
Pres. medicines	5	Analgesics	6			Retail Pharmy.	6
Indust. chem.	6	Hypnotics	7			Vets	7
Plant fungi	7	Other	8			Other	8
Other	8						

ANSWER 14		NAME OF MATERIAL	LOCATION OF CALLER
Yes	0		
No	1		

Fig. 14.6 Report sheet for recording the details of an inquiry.

the call. The formula, pharmacokinetic data, either the first aid measures or the long-term treatment all need to be appraised but not necessarily given to the inquirer, for their main concern is to start appropriate treatment; they can always ring back for further information as the resuscitation of the patient proceeds.

As part of the data collection procedures and also to enable calls to be followed up where necessary it is useful to record details of each inquiry on a report sheet as seen in Fig. 14.6. This particular example is designed in such a way that when completed the information can be transferred to punch cards for statistical data analysis. The number of inquiries to Poisons Information Bureau increases each year and this indicates a probable increase in the number of cases seen in hospitals. The decline in recent years of the mortality figures may indicate the success of the service; on the other hand improved care may equally be the reason. However, it is true that casualty officers have been reminded many times by coroners that they should seek information and advice from the Poisons Information Service when treating poisoned patients.

FUTURE DEVELOPMENT

Over the last few years the National Poisons Information Service has developed research laboratories concerned with the investigation of new treatments and the monitoring of blood levels and excretion rates following toxic ingestions (e.g. paracetamol treatment in Edinburgh, paraquat and antidepressant investigations at New Cross, London).

There is a need for considerable improvement in the handling of poisons information and that this could benefit from being more generally associated with the Drug Information Centres developing in the pharmaceutical service of the reorganised National Health Service. The National Poisons Information Service has difficulties in staffing the service with professional staff throughout 24 hours a day—the pharmaceutical services in major centres housing regional specialities such as Drug Information Centres could provide the trained staff necessary for such a service. Development of a Regional Poisons Information Service would demand a corporate effort engaged in the compilation, updating and dissemination of the data, but as this is likely to apply to drug information generally, it would be comparatively straightforward to feed poisons information into the same network. The advantages would be negligible revenue consequences for providing such an improved service and no capital costs, as the Drug Information Centres already exist.

It is likely that microfilming of data will be an important medium for storage of information in the future. It offers the advantage, particularly when held in reel form, of ensuring that no information is mislaid or incorrectly filed. The other great advantage is that it can be readily updated and copied by an economical process. The dissemination of microfilmed data would then offer a particularly attractive system of providing a National Service to regional centres. The Poison Information Bureau may be a specialised section of a Drug Information Centre and can be efficiently provided by the pharmaceutical services. Its characteristics are that it is an impersonal service as all the inquiries arrive by telephone. The response time must be short, as the information is usually required to initiate treatment of a patient with accidental ingestion who has been brought to an Accident and Emergency Department in a hospital.

REFERENCES

DEPARTMENT OF HEALTH AND SOCIAL SECURITY (1962) *Emergency Treatment in Hospital of Cases of Acute Poisoning. Report of the Subcommittee of the Standing Medical Advisory Committee of the Central Health Services Council.* The Atkins Report. HMSO, London.

DREISBACH R. H. (1971) *Handbook of Poisoning: Diagnosis and Treatment.* Lang Medical, Los Altos, USA.

GLEASON M. N., GOSSELIN R. E. & HODGE H. C. (1969) *Clinical Toxicology of Commercial Products.* Williams & Wilkins, Baltimore.

MARTINDALE (1977) *The Extra Pharmacopoeia.* 27th edn. Pharmaceutical Press, London.

MATTHEW H. & LAWSON A. A. H. (1970) *Treatment of Common Acute Poisonings.* Churchill Livingstone, Edinburgh.

15

Drug interactions

I. H. STOCKLEY

The term 'drug interaction' has come to be applied to the change in response to drugs which sometimes occurs when two or more are taken together. It occasionally also occurs when drugs are taken at the same time as particular foods and drinks which contain certain ingredients. If the interference with the action of the drug is sufficiently large then the result will be detrimental to the patient: some drugs completely antagonise the effects of others; alternatively, they may cause exaggerated or even fatal toxic reactions. The expression 'drug interaction' is now usually reserved for reactions which occur between drugs within the body rather than those which can occur in mixtures or intravenous fluids (for which the older, more traditional term 'pharmaceutical incompatibility' is much more appropriate), and by common usage it has come to mean an undesirable interaction rather than one which is deliberately exploited.

Probably the best known interaction of all, the potentially fatal and now notorious 'cheese reaction' with the monoamine oxidase inhibitors which first came into the limelight in the early 1960s, was probably one of the main stimuli for the interest in and recognition of the importance of drug interactions, but the phenomenon is by no means a new one. The increased sensitivity of the myocardium to the effects of the sympathomimetic amines during general anaesthesia was observed in the last century; however, the great majority of clinically important interactions recognised today are associated with drugs introduced during the last two decades. The older medicaments, most of them now largely abandoned, were for the most part relatively ineffective and very much less potent than many of the newer ones, so that interactions between them, if they actually occurred, were relatively unimportant.

The pharmaceutical profession appears to have taken a much greater interest in the problem of interactions than that taken by its medical counterparts. There appear to be two main reasons for this: firstly, the education of the pharmacist is directed towards a comprehensive understanding of drugs, with their detailed pharmacology forming a very large part of graduate and postgraduate training, whereas medical education covers a much wider field of interest with fewer opportunities to study in great depth any particular aspect at undergraduate level. Secondly, as many of the professional pharmaceutical skills are now carried out largely within the laboratories of the drug houses, the pharmacist has turned his attention increasingly towards a widening role as an information scientist with a detailed pharmacological knowledge, one aspect being, inevitably, drug interactions. And so just as the pharmacist has always been responsible for checking drug dosages, so the check on the possibility of drug interactions has become a complementary professional responsibility.

In an ideal world every pharmacist would have detailed information on every interaction at his fingertips (in the same way that pharmacy and nursing students were once expected to memorise drug doses), but it would be an intolerable, if not an impossible, burden on the memory to learn the details of every interaction, and so in practice the pharmacist is obliged to rely on something other than his memory to alert him to the potentially clinically important drug interactions he is likely to encounter. Nevertheless, a general pattern does exist in the growing mass of information on interactions which it is not unreasonable for any pharmacist, even those with the poorest of memories, to recognise and know, and which can form the basis of his practical knowledge of the subject.

A THREE-QUESTION MEMORY CHECK ON INTERACTIONS

If one is faced with the question 'does A interact with B?' there is an extremely simple and easily memorised three-question check which depends on little more than a generally good pharmacological background knowledge of the drugs in question, the answers to which can alert one to the likelihood of an interaction.

Question 1: Do the drugs have similar or opposite effects?

The answer to this question will pick out a large number of the most straightforward and obvious interactions. It is important, however, to bear in mind that a good number of interactions result from drug side-effects, so that in thinking about the drugs one must think of their whole spectrum of pharmacological activity and not just of their main therapeutic use. So, for example, the combined effects of alcohol and drugs used as hypnotics, sedatives and tranquillisers is, clearly, likely to result in enhanced CNS depression, but it should not be overlooked that this will also occur with other drugs whose major effects are not central depression such as the antihistamines, antiemetics analgesics. The potential hazard of these interactions will also depend on the situation of the patient: a small enhancement of the alcohol-induced CNS depression might be of little significance in home surroundings, but of major importance if the patient is driving a car where alertness is at a premium. Another example of this 'additive' type of interaction is found with those drugs with anticholinergic effects, such as the antiparkinsonian agents, together with phenothiazines or tricyclic antidepressants which can, in some circumstances, result in the development of anticholinergic toxicity. One aspect of this toxicity is the development of heat stroke in particularly hot and humid conditions.

The converse of these additive interactions are those with antagonistic effects. An obvious example of this is the interaction between vitamin K and warfarin. The oral anticoagulants are competitive inhibitors of vitamin K (though this is now disputed) and their activity is antagonised by the presence of vitamin K, so that a reversal of adequate anticoagulation can be achieved if the patient is given enough vitamin K. This might easily occur with a multi-vitamin preparation. It also occurs in at least one proprietary remedy for the treatment of chilblains where its presence could very easily be overlooked. So it is most important when asking this first interaction question to look at drugs as a whole, and not be misled by concentrating on one or other of their pharmacological characteristics or usages.

Question 2: Are the drugs titrated to achieve a particular serum level of pharmacological effect?

Drugs included in this category are the oral anticoagulants, the hypoglycaemic agents, the anticonvulsants, antibacterial agents, corticosteroids, lithium etc. These drugs, more than most, depend to a greater or lesser degree for their actions on achieving a nice balance between two extremes; the one being the development toxicity due to overdosage, and the other the inadequate protection of the patient against the disease for which he is being treated because the serum levels are too low. Even a relatively small change in the serum levels may be significant so that particular care should be exercised with these drugs. It is probably true to say that the great majority of the important interactions are found among these groups of drugs because the effects of an interaction are usually relatively easily monitored. So, for example, a patient stabilised on phenytoin to control convulsions began to show the toxic effects of phenytoin overdosage when administered chloramphenicol. The reason being that chloramphenicol is a liver enzyme inhibitor, so that the normal rate of phenytoin metabolism was reduced and, with the same daily dose of phenytoin, the serum levels of the anticonvulsant began to climb until the toxicity began to manifest itself. If an enzyme-inducing antibiotic had been used instead, the likely result would have been partial or total loss of control of the convulsions. In either case there is a clear and obvious result of the interaction, and this is true of most of the interactions in this category where the dosage is fairly critical.

Question 3: Do the drugs affect the same or associated sites of action?

If they do, then the possibility of an interaction may be increased. A considerable number of the newer drugs affect their pharmacological actions at central or peripheral adrenergic neurones (the MAOI, tricyclic antidepressants, alpha- and beta-stimulating sympathomimetic amines, antihypertensive agents, beta blockers, chlorpromazine-like drugs) so that it is hardly surprising that interference sometimes occurs at these sites. The pharmacology of some of these agents is complex, so that there are no hard-and-fast rules about what will and what will not interact, but the fact that their actions are mediated in the same areas should certainly alert one to the possibility of an interaction.

A simple three-question system of this kind will not necessarily pick out every single interaction, but it will certainly select a large number and it depends for its use on nothing but the knowledge and professional skills which the pharmacist already has been trained to possess, and it will enable him to try to answer an interaction question in a structured way.

AIDE-MEMOIRE SYSTEMS

The next best thing to having a comprehensive reference book universally available (a virtually impossible ideal) is one of the simple pocket-sized aide-memoire systems. These have the advantage of being small, cheap (most of them are given away by drug companies) and they will fit into a 'white coat' pocket easily and unobtrusively. Their major disadvantage is the amount and depth of knowledge which they carry, but they can act as a useful memory support when nothing more comprehensive is available.

1. *Drug Interactions and Normal Values Tables* by A. K. McIver, FPS, of the North Lonsdale Hospital, published by permission of Nicholas Laboratories as a free service to the medical and pharmaceutical professions in the form of an alphabetical table printed on card and measuring $8'' \times 5''$. It was first published in a different form in 1965 (and more recently in the *Pharmaceutical Handbook* published by the Pharmaceutical Press) and now requires some updating, but the brief information it contains is accurate and reliable.

2. *Drug Interaction Alert* designed by Dr. Ivan Stockley of Nottingham University. This is a small pocket-sized slide rule or pocket folder carrying outline basic information about the majority of the interactions now known. Seventy-three drugs or groups of drugs are listed, the importance being graded by means of colours and coded by symbols. It is published and distributed as a free service to members of the medical and pharmaceutical profession by Boehringer Ingelheim. There is also a complementary large-scale wall chart containing the same information and intended for display in dispensaries and wards. French, German and Spanish language versions have also been produced.

3. *Drug Interaction Guide* produced and published by Abbott Laboratories. This contains an alphabetical chart of interactions with some references.

4.   *Medisc.* This is a plastic pocket-sized disc which carries basic information on drug interactions and was developed by Dr Brian Whiting and his associates in the University of Glasgow and the Scottish Home and Health Department. It may be purchased from Excerpta Medica Services.

Aide-memoire systems of this type are very valuable indeed, provided that their obvious limitations are recognised. They are only intended as a 'first stage' alerting system which acts as a reminder or directs the attention to an interaction, so that more detailed information can be sought elsewhere. Provided systems like these are not abused, they have a very useful role indeed to play, but it is clear that they require the support of more detailed reference texts.

COMPREHENSIVE REFERENCE TEXTS

The back-up to the simple systems so far described is a small library of reference books. There are now a number of books on the market about drug interactions, but their quality and reliability is very variable and, in my opinion, only a few are of real practical value. The reason is that many authors have not been sufficiently discriminating in their use of data. Isolated case reports, experimental animal data, human data and manufacturers' cautionary statements have been lumped together with well-documented clinical observations, with little or no distinction being made between them, so that without looking up the original papers there is absolutely no way of knowing whether the interaction described or listed should be regarded seriously or not. Some of the worst books even quote each other as 'authorities', which is an unfortunate example of 'the blind leading the blind'. For my money, I would buy the following:

1.   *Evaluations of Drug Interactions* (1976) 2nd edn, published by the American Pharmaceutical Association, and distributed by the Pharmaceutical Press in the UK. This is an accumulating series of authoritative monographs produced by teams of pharmacists, pharmacologists and physicians. The information is of a very high standard and reliable.

2.   *Drug Interactions*, P. D. Hansten (1979) 4th edn, published by Lea and Febiger. This book is in the form of a three-column table and covers a much wider range than the first publication described, but each interaction is treated more superficially. This is an excellent publication and of proven reliability.

3.   *Drug Interactions and their Mechanisms*, I. H. Stockley, first published 1974, republished with supplement 1978 by the Pharmaceutical Press. This is a very inexpensive, soft-bound facsimile of a series of articles which first appeared in the *Pharmaceutical Journal* and contains almost the same range of interactions as those found in Hansten's book, but with a much greater emphasis on the possible pharmacological mechanisms involved.

In a review which appeared in the *American Journal of Hospital Pharmacy* in December 1976, the author who had reviewed the three publications listed above and four other books came to the following conclusions: 'it can be concluded that the content of *Evaluations of Drug Interactions*, Hansten and Stockley, is more comprehensive than the others. Thus, these three would appear to be superior regarding both content and documentation.... Considering both the objective criteria and my impressions of format and indexing, *Evaluations of Drug Interactions* and Hansten were reviewed favourably on all points. Stockley must be considered nearly as complete, and certainly as authoritative....'

It is interesting to note that these three publications are all relatively inexpensive compared with most of the other books on the subject, and it is possible to buy all three for less than the cost of some of the most expensive (and unreliable) books.

UPDATING INFORMATION

Reports of interactions or of studies on known interactions appear virtually every week in the journals of the world, and the difficulty is to keep abreast of the advancing tide of information. Very few hospitals, apart from those associated with a University Medical School or Pharmacy School, have the library facilities which would enable the pharmacist to keep in touch with the latest developments, and in any case few pharmacists (even those in Drug Information Departments) have the time or opportunity to concentrate on this one area of knowledge. For this reason abstracting services and systems are invaluable. But for those who need some guidance on the journals to concentrate on, the following list contains those journals which are worth scanning on a regular basis:

Index Medicus (monthly). Relatively recently this abstracting journal has included a subheading on drug interactions.

Clin-Alert (irregular, about twice a month). This abstracts adverse reactions and interactions exclusively and is invaluable.

Pharmaceutical Journal (weekly). In its 'Drugs in use' section reference is often made to interactions described in other journals. In addition, the 'Prescription products' section is worth looking at, but it must be appreciated that statements about interactions in this section are based on the highly cautionary statements made by drug manufacturers and (though it does not say so) may well be based on animal and not human data. Fuller information from the drug houses very often shows that what appears as a full-blown warning is based on the most slender evidence and reflects the concern of the manufacturer not to get involved in medicolegal problems rather than the seriousness of the so-called interaction indicated. This also applies to their data sheets.

Many interactions are also described in the following journals and since many pharmacists read some of these regularly, it is worthwhile keeping an eye open for interaction reports, particularly in the correspondence section of the journal: *British Journal of Clinical Pharmacology, Australian Journal of Pharmacy, European Journal of Clinical Pharmacology, Journal of Clinical Pharmacology and Therapeutics* (in fact, virtually any journal of clinical pharmacology), *British Medical Journal, The Lancet, Journal of the American Medical Association, New England Journal of Medicine, Clinical Pharmacy and Drug Intelligence,* and the *Journal of the American Pharmaceutical Association*.

All these journals provide details on interactions sometimes, and a regular browse through will in addition provide an excellent and continuing education on current drug usage.

A WARNING

The importance of any 'in vogue' subject is easily exaggerated and this is certainly true of interactions. Fortunately, the whole subject is now beginning to settle down, but the last few years have seen a strong and ill-balanced overreaction to the hazards of using drugs together. Safe and adequate therapy must recognise the possibility of the occurrence of drug interactions, but to pay a disproportionate amount of attention to this aspect of the adverse reactions field is to get the whole topic out of proportion and out of perspective. Diet, dosage, age, sex, disease, genetic background and many other factors may very easily be of greater importance than the interference by one drug with the actions of another. The literature on drug interactions is still suffering from the results of an overreaction and it is, therefore, most important to be discriminating in the use of books, charts and reports if one is not to lose what *is* important amongst the mass of unreliable data. It may sound an almost absurd truism but 'the only interactions which are of clinical importance are those which are of clinical importance'. Extrapolated animal data, isolated case reports, and manufacturers' data sheets, useful as they can be, have been the source of a flood of so-called interactions, and this kind of 'wolf crying' degrades and obscures the useful and valuable information on which safe prescribing depends. The mythology which has pervaded the field of drug interactions is only now being dispelled, so that it is important for the pharmacist to view many of the statements about interactions with reservations, if not with scepticism, until the quality of the clinical data which lies behind them is known.

Index